PEPTIDES
101

PEPTIDES 101

Regenerative Applications in Modern Medicine

by
Mike KS Chan,
Thomas Skutella,
Jonathan R.T. Lakey,
Olha Nishkumai
&
Dmytro Klokol

EUROPEAN™ WELLNESS ACADEMY
Biological Regenerative Medicine

PEPTIDES 101: Regenerative Applications in Modern Medicine

EUROPEAN WELLNESS ACADEMY

Library of Congress Control Number: 2025951550

ISBN (hardcover): 9781662971921
eISBN: 9781662971938

DOI: https://doi.org/10.69669/vj2793

gatekeeper press™

Tampa, Florida

Contents

List of Abbreviations

MO	Mito Organelles
SS-31	Tetrapeptide, also known as elamipretide
PEG	Polyethylene glycol
GPCR	G-protein coupled receptors
RTK	Receptor tyrosine kinases
AMP	Adenosine monophosphate
cAMP	Cyclic AMP
IP_3	Inositol triphosphate
PI3K	Phosphatidylinositol 3-kinases
AKT	Protein kinase B
MAPK	Mitogen-activated protein kinase
ERK	Extracellular signal-regulated kinase
FAK	Focal adhesion kinase
DNA	Deoxyribonucleic acid
RNA	Ribonucleic acid
UV	Ultraviolet
ROS	Reactive oxygen species

mtDNA	Mitochondrial DNA
NHEJ	Non-homologous end joining
MMEJ	Microhomology-Mediated End Joining
MOTS-c	Mitochondrial open reading frame of the 12s ribosomal RNA type-c
AMPK	Adenosine monophosphate-activated protein kinase
SIRT1	Silent Information Regulator 1
PGC-1α	Peroxisome proliferator-activated receptor-gamma coactivator-1alpha
NF- κB	Nuclear factor-kappa B
IL-10	Interleukin 10
TGF-β	Transforming growth factor-beta
IL-1	Interleukin 1
TLR	Toll-like receptor
Th1	T helper type 1 cells
Th17	T helper 17 cells
Th2	T helper type 2
VEGF	Vascular Endothelial Growth Factor
VEGFR	Vascular Endothelial Growth Factor Receptor
NO	Nitric Oxide
EPC	Endothelial progenitor cell
ECM	Extracellular matrix
RCT	Randomized controlled trials
TIMP	Tissue inhibitors of metalloproteinases
SMAD	Suppressor of Mothers Against Decapentaplegic homolog
NOP	Nanomized organ-specific peptides
NP	Nanomized peptides

MALDI-TOF	Matrix Assisted Laser Desorption Ionization-time of Flight
LC-MS/MS	Liquid Chromatography-Tandem Mass Spectrometry
MTP	Mitochondria-targeted peptides
ETC	Electron transport chain
MDP	Mitochondrial-derived peptides
SASP	Senescence-associated secretory phenotype
P53	Tumor protein 53
ULK1	Uncoordinated-51-like kinases
NAD	Nicotinamide adenine dinucleotide
NMN	Nicotinamide mononucleotide
NR	Nicotinamide riboside
ATP	Adenosine triphosphate
FOXO3a	Forkhead box class O 3a
FOXO4-DRI	Forkhead box O transcription factor 4-D-Retro-Inverso peptide
Bcl-2	B-cell leukemia/lymphoma 2
TFAM	Mitochondrial transcription factor A
SHLP	Small humanin-like peptides
PRP	Platelet-rich plasma
PEDF	Pigment epithelium-derived factor
MSC	Mesenchymal stem cell
TEC	Thymic epithelial cell
NRF1	Nuclear respiratory factors
HO-1	Heme oxigenase-1
SOD	Superoxide dismutase
CIP1	Cyclin-Dependent Kinase- Interacting Protein 1
LPPSIMKE	Liver, pancreas, placenta, kidney, intestines, retina

H_2O_2	Hydrogen peroxide-induced oxidative stress
CRISPR/Cas9	**C**lustered **R**egularly **I**nterspaced **S**hort **P**alindromic **R**epeats (Cas 9 -associated protein
FDA	Food and Drug Administration
EMA	European Medicines Agency
ADME	Absorption, distribution, metabolism, and excretion
GMP	Good Manufacturing Practice
ACTH	Adrenocorticotropic hormone
MSH	Melanocyte stimulating hormone
GH	Growth Hormone
GHRH	Growth hormone-releasing hormone
GHS	Growth hormone secretagogues
GHS-R	Growth hormone secretagogue Receptor
PTH	Parathyroid Hormone
IGF	Insulin-like growth factors
HPLC	High-performance liquid chromatography
SPPS	Solid-phase peptide synthesis
sORF	small open reading frames
rRNA	Ribosomal ribonucleic acid
IGFBP3	Insulin-like Growth Factor-Binding Protein 3
MS	Mass spectrometry
CTA	Cell transformation Assay
QC	Quality Control
qNMR	Quantitative nuclear magnetic resonance
NMR	Nuclear Magnetic Resonance
QA	Quality Assurance

JC-1	chemical compound/fluorescent dye used in mitochondrial membrane potential studies
TMRE	Tetramethylrhodamine ethyl ester
MOMP	Mitochondrial Outer Membrane Permeabilization
MIMP	Mitochondrial Inner Membrane Permeabilization
OMM	Osteopathic Manipulative Medicine
Apaf-1	Apoptotic peptidase activating factor 1
Smac	second mitochondria-derived activator of caspases
cGAS-STING	cyclic GMP-AMP synthase stimulator of interferon genes
XIAP	X-linked inhibitor of apoptosis
IFN- β	Interferon-beta
AIF	Arterial input function
Ca2+	Calcium ion
Ki67	protein marker for cell proliferation
PCNA	Proliferating Cell Nuclear Antigen
MHC	Major Histocompatibility
T-cell	Type of white blood cells lymphocytes
ADA	Adenosine Deaminase
PK	Pharmacokinetic
Vd	Volume of distribution
kDa	Kilodaltons
PBMC	Peripheral blood mononuclear cell
ACE	Angiotensin-Converting Enzyme
β-blockers	Beta blockers
NADPH	Nicotinamide adenine dinucleotide phosphate
TNF-α	Tumor Necrosis Factor-alpha

IL-6	Interleukin 6
IL-1β	Interleukin-1 beta
NRF2	Nuclear Factor erythroid 2-related factor 2
AHR/STAT3	Aryl Hydrocarbon Receptor/Signal Transducer and Activator of Transcription 3
MAPK/NF- κB	Mitogen-activated protein kinase/Nuclear factor kappa-light-chain-enhancer of activated B cells
I/R	Ischemia-reperfusion
CVD	cardiovascular disease
PLGA	Polymeric nanoparticles
MTS	Mitochondrial targeting sequences
MI	Myocardial infarction
KLF2	Kruppel-like factor 2
eNOS	Endothelial nitric oxide synthase
VCAM-1	Vascular Cell Adhesion Molecule-1
ApoE	Apolipoprotein E
HNGF6A	Humanin analogue
H9c2	subclonal line of the original clonal cell line derived from embryonic BD1X rat heart tissue
Nrf2/ARE	Nuclear factor erythroid 2-related factor 2/Antioxidant Response Element
NF-κB	Nuclear Factor-kappa B
MDA	Malondialdehyde
HUVEC	Human umbilical vein endothelial cells
Gly14	Humanin-analogue
p16	Senescence marker
p21	Senescence marker

p53	Senescence marker
GMP	Good manufacturing practice
PET	Positron Emission Tomography
MR	Magnetic resonance
GLP-1	Glucagon-Like Peptide-1
GIP	Glucose-dependent Insulinotropic Polypeptide
PYY	Peptide tyrosine tyrosine
miRNA	MicroRNA
SFRP5	Secreted Frizzled Related Protein 5
IFN-c	Interferon-gamma
MCP1	Monocyte Chemoattractant Protein-1
CXCL5	C-X-C motif chemokine ligand 5
C-X-C	cysteine-X-cysteine (family of proteins)
FFA	Free fatty acids
SCFA	Short-chain fatty acids
FAHFA	Fatty acid esters of hydroxy fatty acids
DHOME	12,13-dihydroxy-(9Z)-octadecenoic acid
BCAA	Branched-chain amino acids
JNK	c-Jun N-terminal kinase
IKK β	Inhibitor of nuclear factor kappa-B kinase subunit beta
JAK/STAT	Janus kinase/signal transducer and activator of transcription signaling pathway
ERK1/2	Extracellular signal-regulated kinase 1/2
AKT	Protein Kinase B
OSP	Organ-specific peptides
HMG-CoA	3-hydroxy-3-methylglutaryl-coenzyme A

mTOR	Mammalian target of rapamycin
FGF23	Fibroblast Growth Factor 23
KL1	Klotho domain 1
GLP-1/GIP	Glucagon-like peptide-1/Glucose-dependent insulinotropic polypeptide
PPARα	Peroxisome proliferator-activated receptor alpha
ACE	Angiotensin-Converting Enzyme
DDP-4	Dipeptidyl Peptidase-4
NAFLD	Non-alcoholic Fatty Liver Disease
NASH	Nonalcoholic steatohepatitis
VO_2	Maximal oxygen consumption
HOMA-IR	Homeostatic Model Assessment for Insulin Resistance
BP	Blood pressure
BMI	Body Mass Index
GLUT4	Glucose Transporter Type 4
HED	Human equivalent dose
NOD	Non-obese Diabetic
EPO	Erythropoietin
CCL5	C-C motif chemokine ligand 5
DLT	Dose-limiting toxicity
OGTT	Oral glucose tolerance test
ECG	Electrocardiogram
Hs-CRP	High-Sensitivity C-Reactive Protein
ELISA	Enzyme-Linked Immunosorber Assay
MRI	Magnetic Resonance Imaging
DXA	Dual-energy X-ray absorptiometry

OHdG	8-hydroxy-2'-deoxyguasonine
LDL	Low-Density Lipoprotein
HOMA	Homeostasis Model Assessment
HMG-CoA	3-hydroxy-3-methyglutaryl-coenzyme A
T2DM	Type 2 Diabetes Mellitus
HDL	High-Density Lipoprotein
ATP/ADP	Adenosine Triphosphate/Adenosine Diphosphate
DSMB	Data and Safety Monitoring Board
RP	Retinitis Pigmentosa
DAMP	Damage-associated molecular patterns
NLRP3	NLR family pyrin domain containing 3
RGC	Retinal ganglion cells
RPE	Retinal pigment epithelium
α-MSH	Alpha-melanocyte-stimulating hormone
KPV	Tripeptide (Lysine, Proline, and Valine)
NAP	Neuroprotective peptide
NAPVSIPQ	Neuroprotective protein NAP
ADNP	Activity-Dependent Neuroprotective Protein
AASI	Autologous Specific Immunotherapy
IRBP	Interphotoreceptor Retinoid-Binding Protein
ILM	Internal Limiting Membrane
TDP-43	Transactive response DNA binding protein 43kDA
ALS	Amyotrophic Lateral Sclerosis
NMDA	N-methyl-D-aspartate
AD	Alzheimer's Disease
PD	Parkinson's Disease

HD	Huntington's Disease
UPS	Uniquitin-proteosome system
RNS	Reactive Nitrogen System
APP	Amyloid-beta precursor protein
BBB	Blood-Brain-Barrier
CNTF	Ciliary neurotrophic factor
BDNF	Brain-derived neurotrophic factor
NGF	Nerve growth factor
Pc21	peptide mimetide of CNTF
Aβ	Amyloid beta
GSK-3β	Glycogen synthase kinase-3 beta
BSP1	Black soybean-derived peptide
BACE1	Beta-site Amyloid Precursor Protein Cleaving Enzyme 1
aSynPEP-DB	database of biogenic peptides for inhibiting α-synuclein aggregation
LL-37	Human cathelicidin antimicrobial peptide
TSPO	Translocator Protein
SOD1	Superoxide Dismutase Type 1
VIP	Vasoactive Intestinal Peptide
NSC	Neural Stem Cell
CPP	Cell-penetrating peptides
MnSOD	Mitochondrial superoxide dismutase
ASD	autism spectrum disorder
MCI	Mild Cognitive Impairment
CoQ10	Coenzyme Q10
mPTP	Mitochondrial Permeability Transition Pore

IBD	Inflammatory bowel disease
CD	Crohn's Disease
UC	Ulcerative Colitis
LPS	Lipopolysaccharide
IgA	Immunoglobin A
NOD2	nucleotide-binding oligomerization domain-containing protein 2
DC	Dendritic cell
PSA	Polysaccharide A
Tregs	Regulatory T cells
REG3y	Regenerating islet-derived protein 3 gamma
MYD88	Myeloid differentiation primary-response protein 88
TEER	Transepithelial Electrical Resistance
ZO-1	Zonula occludens 1
AT-1001	Larazotide acetate
H-SNI	Hydrostatin-SNI (a snake-venom-derived peptide)
GLP-2	Glucagon-Like Peptide-2
MPO	Myeloperoxidase
MBCP	derived from buffalo milk
AMP-18	Gastrokine-1
Ac2-26	Annexin A1 mimic
NIPEP-IBD	synthetic peptide targeting integrin β1
SJMHE1	Helminth-derived peptide
DSS	Dextran Sulfate Sodium
Keap1-Nrf2	Kelch-like ECH-associated protein 1/Nuclear factor (erythroid-derived 2)-like 2
HMD	Heavy Metal Detoxification

DAI Disease activity index

OA Osteoarthritis

RAGE Receptor for Advanced Glycation Endproducts

NLR Neutrophil to Lymphocyte ration

NSAID Non-steroidal anti-inflammatory drugs

MMP Matrix metalloproteinases

ADAMTS metallonoproteinases with thrombospondin motifs

SPF Specific-pathogen-free

HGH Human Growth Hormone

BPC-157 synthetic peptide (Body Protective Compound 157)

PEDF 29-mer Pigment epithelial-derived factor-derived short peptide

GHRP-6 Growth Hormone-Releasing Peptide-6

CJC-1295 synthetic peptide analog of GHRH (growth hormone-releasing hormone)

HA Hyaluronic acid

CTX-II C-terminal telopeptide of Type II collagen

COMP Cartilage Oligometric Matrix Protein

WOMAC Western Ontario and McMaster Universities Arthritis Index

KOOS Knee Injury and Osteoarthritis Outcome Score

TCR T-cell receptor

CD4+ Cluster of Differentiation 4 positive

CD8+ Cytotoxic T cells

NK Natural Killer

IFN-y Interferon-gamma

FOXN1 Forkhead box protein N1

OS Overall survival

HO-1	Heme oxygenase-1
PINK1	PTEN-induced kinase 1
PTEN	Phosphatase and TENsin homolog
DTH	Delayed-type hypersensitivity
CRP	C-reactive protein
CBC	Complete Blood Count
GAG	Glycosaminoglycan
DEJ	Dermal-epidermal junction
GAIS	Global Aesthetic Improvement Scale
SPMCE	Skin-placenta-mesenchyme-collagen-elastin
SPM	Skin-placenta-mesenchyme
GHK-Cu	copper peptides
GEA	Global Eyelash Assessment
CJD	Creutzfeldt-Jakob Disease
JAK2	Janus kinase 2
STAT	Signal transducers and activators of transcription
IRS1, IRS2	Insulin receptor substrates
SOCS	suppressor of cytokine signaling
SHP1, SHP2	protein tyrosine phosphatases
HIV	Human Immunodeficiency Virus
AIDS	acquired immunodeficiency syndrome
rhGH	recombinant human GH
AGHD	Adult populations with GH deficiency
SDS	Standard Deviation Score
DAC	Drug Affinity Complex
BW	Body Weight

TB-500 Thymosin Beta-4

IU International units

WADA World Anti-Doping Agency

TUE Therapeutic Use Exemption

IGF-1 LR3 Insulin-Like Growth Factor 1 Long Arg3

About the Authors

Mike KS Chan, Researcher, Author, and Educator, Founder and Chairman of the European Wellness Biomedical Group; Senior Technical Consultant at EWBG; Head of Scientific committee of preventive, regenerative and anti-aging medicine and Asian Chairman (ESAAM); Adjunct Professor of Lincoln University College (Malaysia); Associate Professor of AASCP, USA (American Academy of Stem Cell Physicians), Chairman for A4M, USA (American Academy of Anti-Aging Medicine) for Thailand/Asia, Japan's Regenerative Medical Association MMJ (Multi-Dimensional Holistic Medical Team Japan) and co-Founder of FCTI Precursor Stem Cells (Europe), Author of over 70 books and over 150 publications, has experience of 45 over years in Stem cells Research in Germany, Switzerland, European Union, Soviets, China, Mexico, USA, Japan, Middle East since early 80's, presenter for over 10000 presentations and scientific lectures globally at most major conferences of the World on anti-aging and precision medicine. He is also a pioneer in Regenerative Medicine and Cellular Therapies in a big way in the 80's into Asia Pacific, the Middle East and Australia.

Thomas Skutella, MD, PostDoc (Max Planck Institute for Psychiatry, Munich, Germany), Full Professor at Heidelberg University, former group leader in the Neuroscience Research Center (Charite Berlin, Germany), director of the Center for Regenerative Medicine (Tübingen, Germany), Head of the department of Neuroanatomy in the Institute for Anatomy and Cell Biology (Heidelberg, Germany),

Group for Regeneration and Reprogramming, Medical Faculty, Institute for Anatomy and Cell Biology, Heidelberg University (Germany).

Jonathan R.T. Lakey, B.Sc., M.Sc., Ph.D. (University of Alberta at Edmonton, Canada), Professor Emeritus, Department of Surgery, University of California Irvine (CA, USA); Department of Biomedical Engineering, University of California Irvine (CA, USA), Director of Research at the Clinical Islet Program in the Department of Surgery at the University of California, Irvine (CA, USA), Outstanding Leadership in Alberta Science Award from the Alberta Science and Technology Leadership Foundation, the Outstanding Achievement Award from the Canadian Diabetes Association, and Royal College of Physicians and Surgeons.

Olha Nishkumai, MD, PhD, Professor, Doctor of Medical Sciences, Board Certified Specialist Cardiologist, Rheumatologist, and Internal Medicine specialist; Full Professor at the Department of Internal Medicine No. 2 at Bogomolets National Medical University (UA); Medical Consultant at the European Wellness Biomedical Group.

Dmytro Klokol, MD, Specialist in General Surgery (Board Certified, MoH UA), PhD (Emergency and Reconstructive Surgery), GCP (Malaysia, USA), PostDoc (Regenerative Medicine, NL, EU); Certified expert in Interventional procedures in Regenerative Medicine and chronic pain management (Spain, EU); Certified Educator at International Accreditation Organization (IAO, USA); HRDCorp certified educator and trainer (Malaysia); International Board for Anti-aging and Regenerative Medicine (IBARM, USA) certifying academic board member.

Peptides 101: Regenerative Applications in Modern Medicine provides a foundational overview of peptide biology and their expanding therapeutic roles in regenerative and functional medicine. The book reviews peptide structure, synthesis, and signaling pathways, with emphasis on their applications in tissue repair, immune modulation, neuroprotection, and metabolic regulation. Integrating current research with clinical perspectives, it highlights safety profiles, evidence-based protocols, and emerging trends in peptide therapeutics. Designed for clinicians, biomedical researchers, and students, this text bridges basic science and translational medicine to illuminate the regenerative potential of peptide-based interventions.

Instead of Prologue: The Molecules of Return

Between the cracking of our joints, the dimming of our sight, and the slow unraveling of memory in our later decades, there lies a question that has haunted humanity since we first became conscious of time: *is aging truly inevitable*? Or have we, somewhere along the evolutionary path, simply forgotten how to maintain ourselves?

Across the millennia, we accepted aging as a Natural Law, like gravity or the cycle of the Moon. But perhaps aging is not a law at all, perhaps it is more like rust on metal or plaque on a tooth: not inevitable, just unaddressed. This book explores a growing body of evidence suggesting that aging, far from being an unavoidable fate, is instead a molecular cascade, a set of signals, malfunctions, and cellular miscommunications that might be modulated, slowed, or even reversed. And at the heart of this emerging paradigm lies a class of ancient and intelligent molecules: peptides.

As Robert Anton Wilson mentioned in his historic address to the Libertarian Party's Presidential Nominating Convention in 1987, the short chains of amino acids, the *peptides* are the forgotten language of biology, the signals of the body and "if you do not have enough of them, your life is pretty miserable". They are not new inventions, nor futuristic nanotechnologies. They are older than language itself, predating not just human civilization but multicellular life. They are the messengers of the body's internal world—always subtle, elegant, and precise.

To truly appreciate the promise of peptides in regenerative medicine and longevity, one must understand how they differ from the tools of modern pharmaceutical medicine. Whereas drugs are often designed to dominate biology, blocking enzymes, hijacking receptors, or silencing symptoms, the peptides speak in the native dialect of the cell. They do not force, they suggest. They do not invade, they harmonize. If pharmaceuticals are generals shouting commands, peptides are diplomats restoring order.

This contrast between synthetic pharmacology and biological harmony is more than a scientific detail, it is a true philosophical divergence. For over a century, we have pursued medicine as war. We've declared war on cancer, on bacteria, on cholesterol, on aging itself. But war, even when won, leaves behind debris. The side effects of many drugs are not collateral, they are intrinsic to their mechanism. Peptides, in contrast, offer a medicine of partnership. They are not chemicals to overpower, but signals to guide.

The story of peptides begins in the late 19th century, when Emil Fischer, a meticulous German chemist, first began to decode the structures of amino acids and peptides. His work revealed the fundamental architecture of life: that molecules had shape, and that shape mattered. Without Fischer's insight, we would not understand how a tiny shift in the order of amino acids could transform a harmless peptide into a therapeutic agent or a toxin. He opened the door to the molecular era.

But it was in 1921 that the world first witnessed the profound power of peptides in clinical medicine. In a small Toronto lab, Frederick Banting and Charles Best isolated insulin from the pancreas of a dog. That singular peptide, just 51 amino acids long, saved a diabetic boy from certain death. For the first time, a naturally occurring peptide had been extracted, purified, and injected to restore life. Insulin was not just a treatment; it was a revelation. It showed us that disease could be corrected, not suppressed.

Decades later, another figure—Günter Blobel (the German-American Nobel Prize Winner 1999 in Physiology or Medicine from The Rockefeller University in New York), a cell biologist of uncommon precision unlocked a mystery that puzzled generations: how does a cell know where to send its proteins? His discovery of "signal peptides", tiny sequences that direct proteins to the correct cellular address, was like discovering postal codes inside the body. Just like a zip code, GPS or the IP address. Without them, enzymes end up in the wrong compartments, like packages lost in a vast warehouse. Blobel's (not to confuse with Bobel Gunter) insight was not just a biological breakthrough, it revealed something profound: location is not incidental; it is essential. Healing, to be effective, must be targeted. And peptides know how to target.

This idea, the notion of organ specificity runs like a golden thread through the tapestry of peptide medicine. Some peptides speak only to the brain. Others resonate with the heart. There are peptides that awaken the immune system from its age-induced slumber, and others that coax failing cartilage to rebuild. This is not a one-size-fits-all approach. It is not mass production; it is bespoke restoration. The body is not a battlefield, but a symphony. And peptides are its conductors.

To understand the full promise of these molecules, we must turn our gaze inward to the mitochondria.

For decades, mitochondria were described as the powerhouses of the cell, as though they were little more than energetic furnaces. But they are much more. Mitochondria are the oldest tenants in our cells, descendants of ancient bacteria who, over a billion years ago, formed a pact with early eukaryotic life. In exchange for shelter, they offered energy. This endosymbiotic marriage built every animal, plant, and human that has ever lived. But like all old relationships, it can fray. The lifespan of the entire *cell* depends on the healthspan of mitochondria.

When mitochondria begin to fail through age, stress, toxins, or inflammation, the consequences are catastrophic. The cell begins to misfire. Energy production declines. Oxidative stress increases. Organs shrink. The immune system becomes confused. And the diseases we label as "age-related" begin to appear: Alzheimer's, Parkinson's, diabetes, cancer. These are not separate ailments. They are different expressions of a common failures—the breakdowns in mitochondrial function and cellular communication. The healthspan tightly connected to the lifespan and they both rely on the *cellspan*.

Here too, peptides offer a unique intervention not to mask symptoms, but to repair function. Consider humanin, a small mitochondrial-derived peptide discovered at UCLA by researchers studying neurodegeneration. Humanin appears to protect neurons from the toxic effects of amyloid proteins. It reduces inflammation and increases cellular resilience. In animal models, it prolongs life. Then there is MOs, other mitochondrial peptide that improve insulin sensitivity, muscle function, and even physical endurance. In a sense, these peptides are the mitochondria's own voice forgotten messages, rediscovered.

Another remarkable molecule, SS-31 (also known as *elamipretide*), was developed by scientists Peter W. Szeto and Calvin Lee. It targets the inner mitochondrial membrane, binding to cardiolipin and restoring membrane integrity. In failing hearts, it improves energy production. In aging muscles, it restores strength. In injured neurons, it offers hope. These are not speculative miracles; they are active agents in trials, small beacons lighting a vast terrain of regenerative medicine.

The beauty of this approach lies in its simplicity. Rather than designing new drugs to suppress symptoms, we are rediscovering ancient molecules that remind the body how to heal itself. It echoes the healing philosophies of ancient traditions, from Ayurveda to Chinese medicine where illness was not an invader, but an imbalance. Their goal was not to kill the disease, but to restore harmony. The same principle now returns, not through herbs and chants, but through precision peptides and genomic analysis.

Peptides also evoke the ancient medical maxim of Philippus Aureolus Theophrastus Bombastus von Hohenheim later rephrased by Samuel Hahnemann into *similia similibus curantur*—"like treats like". If the thymus fades with age, we might restore immune vigor with thymic peptides. If cartilage breaks down, perhaps chondrocyte-supporting peptides can rebuild it. As I often said in thousands of lectures all over the World: "*A to A, B to B, and C to C*". This is not mere poetic symmetry; it is a logic embedded in the biology itself. A joint does not want a generic anti-inflammatory; it wants a message that speaks cartilage. A brain in decline does not want sedation; it wants the whisper of neurogenesis. A heart crying of ischemia does not want generic cells, it wants to sing like young after being regenerated by the heart stem cells! The precision is the key as we continue to be more and more specific and specialized: "*A1 to A1, B2 to B2, N12 to N12 . . .*" and so on until the complete wellness through cure and regeneration is achieved!

Yet, even this profound vision comes with caution. We must not leap into peptide medicine as though it were a panacea. The ethics of intervention remain. The Hippocratic principle *Primum non nocere*—do no harm, still applies. But peptides, by virtue of their specificity, their short half-lives, their natural presence in the body, offer a safer and subtler path. They are not zero-sum weapons. They are whispers, not shouts.

As I write this in this book as well as in over 70 other books, the global medical establishment remains largely anchored to the pharmaceutical model. The reason is not scientific inertia, but economic gravity. Peptides are difficult to patent. Their production is complex. Their storage, delicate. They do not yield billion-dollar monopolies. But truth has a way of outlasting commerce. And the truth is that biology wants to heal, it simply forgets how.

Throughout this book, as well as throughout the other 70 over books and over 150 articles that I have written, we will explore how peptides are discovered, how they are synthesized or extracted, how they are delivered and metabolized. We will look at case studies, some miraculous, others sobering. We will meet the scientists, the skeptics, the patients, and the pioneers. We will navigate the fine line between hope and hype. And we will challenge the deeply embedded belief that aging is unchangeable.

Medicine, at its most profound, is not a crusade to stretch the clock's hands endlessly forward. It is the gentler, deeper art of returning significance to the moments we already hold. To walk with steadiness, to summon a memory without struggle, to love without the haze of exhaustion, to shape something new with our own hands—these are not extravagances. They are the birthrights of being human, the quiet miracles that give our days their texture and worth.

In this unfolding era, peptides stand as subtle emissaries between what is ancient in us and what is still possible. They are reminders that within our biology lies a long, unbroken story, the one that began in the earliest tides and continues to write itself in every cell. And in their delicate signaling, they hint at a future in which growing older need not mean growing smaller, a future where age is not synonymous with surrender but becomes instead a continuation of strength, clarity, and presence.

The philosopher Seneca once observed that although we are powerless to stretch the length of our days, we remain free to deepen the life within them. What he could not have foreseen is a world in which this ancient wisdom meets the frontiers of modern science. A world where molecular messengers, born in the primordial seas billions of years ago, now whisper possibilities that blur the line between vitality and longevity. These tiny architects of life, once content simply to shape the earliest cells, may one day grant us not only more life in our years, but perhaps even more years for that life to unfold.

And so, let us begin. Not with promises, but with possibility. Not with fear, but with curiosity. The path of peptide medicine is not just about molecules. It is about memory, the body remembering itself, the cell remembering how to heal, and humanity remembering that science, at its best, is not control—it is communion.

Let the body speak. Let us listen.

Prof. Dato Sri Dr. Mike KS Chan
Author & Researcher

CHAPTER 1

The Molecular Renaissance: Peptides as Pioneers in Regenerative Medicine

From Molecular Fragments to Therapeutic Frontiers

For several decades I have been observing how regenerative medicine has progressed from a vision to a rapidly evolving field, with therapeutic strategies now extending beyond stem cells, gene editing, and biomaterials into a previously under-explored frontier: bioactive peptides. These short amino acid sequences, once considered mere degradation products of proteins, are now recognized as powerful biological messengers with the capacity to orchestrate complex regenerative cascades across tissues and organ systems. Their potential is particularly amplified in their nanomized, organ-specific, and even xenogeneic forms—the topics that this book explores in detail.

The era of molecular precision in medicine has cast new light on peptides, whose small size belies their profound biological impact. From modulating inflammation to directing stem cell behavior, peptides are emerging as molecular "switches" capable of turning on the body's intrinsic healing pathways. Their appeal lies in their dual identity: they are small enough to penetrate barriers and avoid the immunogenicity often associated with larger biologics, yet complex enough to engage specific receptors and signaling networks with high fidelity [1][2][3].

As regenerative medicine seeks more refined tools for organ repair, tissue engineering, and metabolic regulation, peptides, especially those derived from mitochondrial sequences and organ-specific extracellular matrices present a unique opportunity. This chapter introduces the foundational principles, biochemical properties, clinical promise, and future trajectory of peptide-based therapeutics in regenerative medicine.

Peptides: The Forgotten Molecules Reborn

Historically, peptides have occupied a modest role in therapeutic development, largely overshadowed by either small molecules (with their oral bioavailability and rapid pharmacokinetics) or large biologics (such as monoclonal antibodies). However, the inherent advantages of peptides are becoming more apparent as technologies for their synthesis, modification, and delivery advance [4].

Peptides are composed of 2 to 50 amino acids linked by peptide bonds. Their intermediate size allows for high target selectivity with a relatively low risk of off-target toxicity. Unlike small molecules, peptides can mimic endogenous ligands more precisely, enabling them to bind to receptors, enzymes, and ion channels with higher affinity and specificity [5][6]. Their degradability, once a limitation, is now seen as a benefit in certain settings, allowing for transient but potent biological modulation without long-term accumulation or systemic burden.

Furthermore, peptides can be customized at nearly every level: amino acid sequence, secondary structure, chemical modifications (e.g., PEGylation, lipidation), and conjugation with delivery vehicles or targeting moieties [7]. This modularity makes them particularly adaptable for precision and personalized medicine, where therapeutic effects must be tailored not just to a disease, but to a tissue, a cell type, or even a signaling microdomain.

Recent discoveries in mitochondrial peptides, stem cell-derived secretomes, and nanomized xenogeneic extracts are propelling peptides into the spotlight. Their regenerative capabilities, once speculative are now supported by preclinical studies and early-stage clinical investigations that demonstrate measurable improvements in tissue repair, inflammation resolution, and metabolic reprogramming [5].

Mechanisms of Action: Beyond Signaling

Sometimes as enzymes, at times as hormones or transcription factors, peptides exert their regenerative effects through several overlapping mechanisms, many of which are cell type- and tissue-specific [8][9]. The following pathways are commonly modulated by therapeutic peptides:

Receptor-Mediated Signaling

One of the most fundamental mechanisms by which peptides exert biological effects is through receptor-mediated signaling, particularly via G-protein coupled receptors (GPCRs), receptor tyrosine kinases (RTKs), and various cytokine receptors. These receptors serve as molecular "antennae" on the cell surface, translating extracellular peptide signals into a cascade of intracellular events [10].

For example, peptide ligands like bombesin, somatostatin, and neuropeptide Y bind specific GPCRs, activating second messengers such as cyclic AMP (cAMP), inositol triphosphate (IP_3), and calcium ions. This leads to changes in gene transcription, cytoskeletal reorganization, and metabolic reprogramming. In regenerative contexts, this signaling cascade can promote Cell survival by activating anti-apoptotic pathways (e.g., PI3K/AKT), Proliferation via MAPK/ERK signaling, Cell migration through actin remodeling and focal adhesion kinase (FAK) activation, differentiation of stem or progenitor cells into tissue-specific lineages. In therapeutic formulations, synthetic or naturally derived peptides may mimic endogenous growth factors or hormones, providing targeted modulation without the off-target effects of full-length proteins or small molecules [11][12].

Epigenetic Regulation

Emerging evidence suggests that certain peptides, particularly those derived from mitochondrial transcriptional regulators, chromatin modifiers, or nuclear-targeted proteins can modulate gene expression not only through direct receptor interaction but also through epigenetic mechanisms. These include histone acetylation and methylation, regulated indirectly via peptide-induced signaling cascades; DNA methylation patterns, altered by influencing the availability of methyl donors (e.g., via folate or SAM pathways); non-coding RNA regulation, especially microRNAs that control gene silencing at the post-transcriptional level [13].

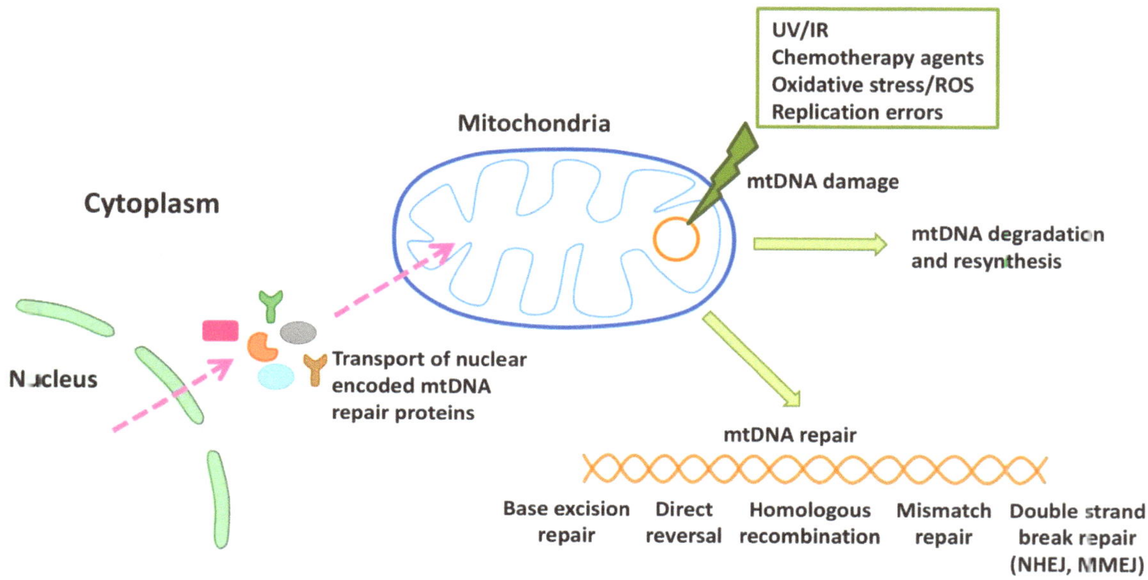

Fig 1.1. *Mitochondrial Genetic and Epigenetic Regulations (source: Wagnber et al., 2022).*

A compelling example is the mitochondrial-derived peptide MOTS-c, which modulates gene expression through activation of AMP-activated protein kinase (AMPK) and downstream epigenetic modifiers like SIRT1 and PGC-1α, key regulators of chromatin state and mitochondrial biogenesis [14][15]. These effects contribute not only to metabolic improvements but also to enhanced cellular plasticity, which is crucial in tissue repair and regeneration.

Immune Modulation

The immunomodulatory role of peptides is central to their utility in regenerative medicine, especially in managing the chronic low-grade inflammation that underlies many age-related and degenerative conditions. Peptides can regulate immune responses by suppressing pro-inflammatory transcription factors like NF-κB, a master regulator of cytokine production, adhesion molecule expression, and leukocyte recruitment; promoting anti-inflammatory cytokines, such as IL-10, TGF-β, or IL-1 receptor antagonist, which support tissue repair and limit fibrosis; and mModulating innate immune receptors, including Toll-like receptors (TLRs), thereby altering dendritic cell maturation and macrophage polarization [16][17].

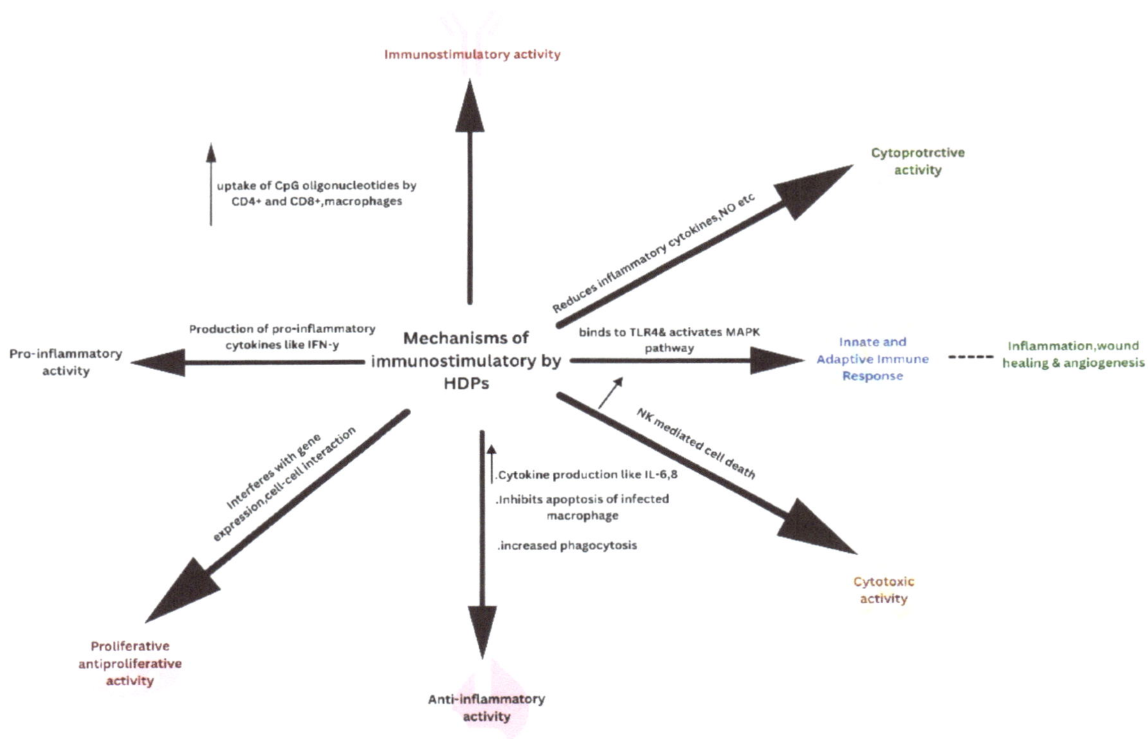

Fig 1.2. *Immunomodulatory mechanisms of the host defense peptides (source: Chatterjee D. and Sivashanmugam K. (2024) Immunomodulatory peptides: new therapeutic horizons for emerging and re-emerging infectious diseases. Front. Microbiol. 15:1505571. doi: 10.3389/fmicb.2024.1505571).*

Some peptides derived from placental extracts or immune cell secretomes have been shown to shift the immune milieu from a pro-inflammatory Th1/Th17 dominance toward a reparative Th2/Treg profile [17]. This immunological “reset” not only facilitates regeneration but also prevents autoimmune responses in inflamed or degenerating tissues.

Angiogenesis and Tissue Perfusion

Tissue regeneration is inextricably linked to vascular support, and many therapeutic peptides act as angiogenic agents, enhancing neovascularization and microcirculation in ischemic or injured tissues. These peptides either mimic endogenous pro-angiogenic factors or enhance their expression. Mechanisms include activation of VEGF/VEGFR signaling, promoting endothelial proliferation and tube formation; stimulation of nitric oxide (NO) synthase, increasing vasodilation and perfusion; and recruitment of endothelial progenitor cells (EPCs) to sites of injury [18].

For instance, Thymosin β4-derived peptides and VEGF-mimetic peptides have shown efficacy in myocardial ischemia, peripheral artery disease, and wound healing models. In clinical applications, angiogenic peptides have been incorporated into hydrogels, scaffolds, and nano-carriers to achieve sustained and localized release, improving perfusion and oxygen delivery to regenerating tissues [19].

Matrix Remodeling and Anti-Fibrotic Action

The extracellular matrix (ECM) is not merely a structural scaffold; it is a dynamic environment that regulates cell behavior, mechanical properties, and biochemical signaling. In regenerative medicine, matrix-binding peptides play a pivotal role in maintaining ECM homeostasis and preventing pathological fibrosis.

These peptides modulate Matrix metalloproteinases (MMPs), enzymes responsible for ECM turnover. Some peptides can upregulate MMP-2 or MMP-9 to clear scar tissue, while others inhibit excessive MMP activity to prevent tissue degradation; tissue inhibitors of metalloproteinases (TIMPs), balancing matrix breakdown and deposition; TGF-β signaling, a central pathway in fibrogenesis; and anti-fibrotic peptides may inhibit TGF-β receptor activation or downstream SMAD signaling.

As shown in preclinical models of lung fibrosis, hepatic cirrhosis, and dermal scarring, these peptides improve tissue elasticity, reduce collagen over-deposition, and facilitate functional tissue architecture restoration [20][21][22]. Their integration into biomaterials and injectable gels further enhances their clinical relevance, allowing for minimally invasive therapeutic delivery, extracellular matrix turnover and fibrosis prevention [22].

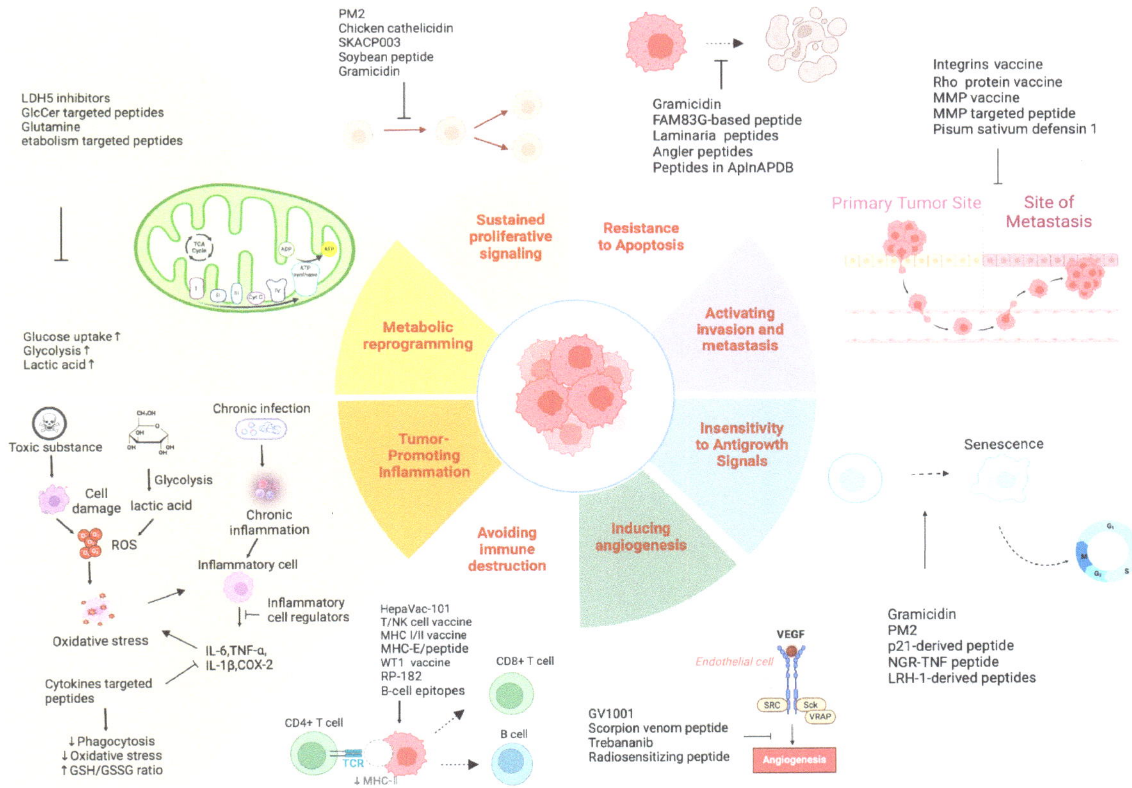

Fig 1.3. *Some oil the mechanisms of action of peptides: including combating sustained proliferative signaling, resistance to apoptosis, metabolic reprogramming, activating invasion and metastasis, tumorpromoting inflammation, insensitivity to antigrowth signals, avoiding immune destruction, and inducing angiogenesis (source: Chen X et al., Reviews on Cancer, 2024).*

These mechanisms are not mutually exclusive. Indeed, the polyvalent action of certain peptides, particularly those derived from stem cells or mitochondria, may explain their observed efficacy in complex, multifactorial conditions such as chronic inflammation, neurodegeneration, and metabolic syndromes.

Nanomization: A Paradigm Shift in Peptide Stability and Bioavailability

A major barrier to peptide therapeutics has historically been their instability in biological environments. Most peptides are rapidly degraded by proteases, possess poor membrane permeability, and are quickly cleared by renal filtration. To overcome this, researchers have turned to nanomization—a process of reducing peptides into nanoscale assemblies or incorporating them into nanoscale carriers to enhance their bioavailability, protection, and tissue targeting.

In the context of regenerative medicine, nanomized peptides can be delivered via self-assembling nanofibers, polymeric nanoparticles, liposomes, or hydrogel matrices. These platforms not only protect peptides from enzymatic degradation but also enable controlled release, allowing for sustained therapeutic effects with fewer administrations.

For example, ultrafiltered nanomized organ-specific peptides (NOPs) derived from porcine heart, brain, liver, and other tissues have demonstrated remarkable bioactivity in preclinical studies, showing regenerative effects when administered via sublingual or parenteral routes [23]. Mass spectrometry analyses confirm that these nanomized fractions contain a reproducible set of low-molecular-weight peptides (<10 kDa), often preserved under cold-chain or lyophilized conditions for extended stability [24].

Figure below illustrates the schematic of nanomization and its benefits for peptide stability, delivery, and receptor engagement.

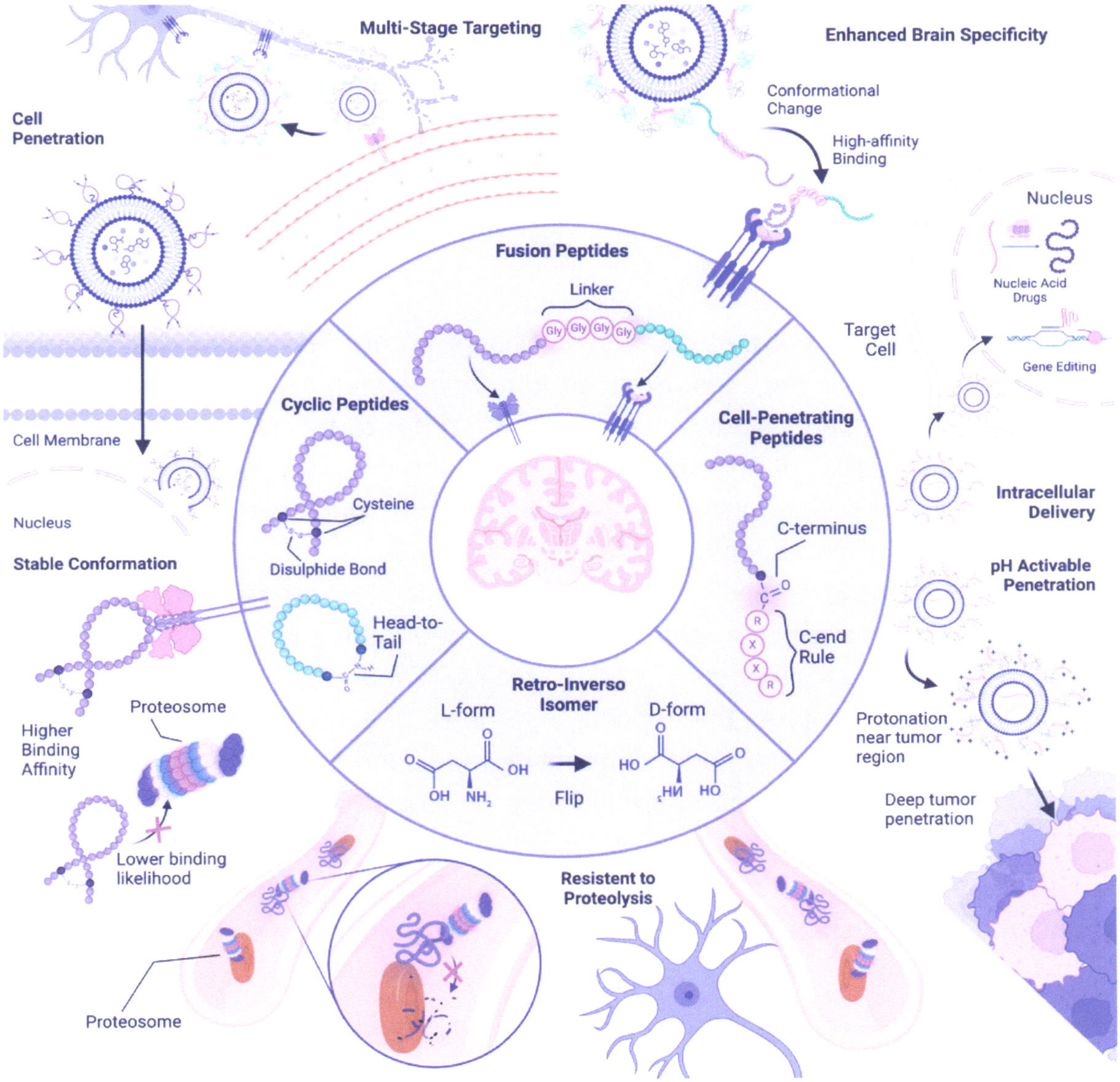

Fig 1.4. *Nanomization of therapeutic peptides improves biological stability, membrane permeability, and targeted delivery in regenerative applications. Overview schematic depicting different types of NPs carrying diverse therapeutic cargos that are functionalized with peptides (source: Tang, S., Han, E.L. & Mitchell, M.J. Peptide-functionalized nanoparticles for brain-targeted therapeutics. Drug Deliv. and Transl. Res. (2025).)*

Moreover, nanomization facilitates non-invasive delivery routes. Unlike larger proteins that must be injected, nanomized peptides can be absorbed via mucosal membranes, transdermal patches, or microneedle arrays thus greatly expanding their practical use in clinical settings.

Xenogeneic and Organo-Specific Peptides: Rewriting the Source Code

Perhaps the most novel and disruptive concept in this field is the use of xenogeneic organ-specific peptides. Sourced from non-human tissues, these peptides are extracted, purified, and reduced to nanomized size for therapeutic use. The central hypothesis is that tissues contain organ-specific peptide signatures that can reprogram or support the corresponding human organ system without requiring full organ transplantation or cell grafts.

Some of the comprehensive studies demonstrated that organ-specific peptides extracted from xenogeneic heart, brain, liver, and kidney retained bioactivity in both in vitro and in vivo models [25]. Using MALDI-TOF and LC-MS/MS mass spectrometry, we have mapped the peptide fingerprints of each extract and monitored their stability over time and under different storage conditions [26]. Remarkably, the profiles remained consistent, supporting the concept that these peptides form a reproducible therapeutic substrate [27].

Table below could summarize the molecular weight distribution, isoelectric point, and thermal stability profiles of several xenogeneic peptide formulations.

Table 1.1. Characterization of Nanomized Organ-Specific Peptides (NOPs) (from: Volchenko et al., 2023).

Tissue Source	Avg. MW (Da)	pI Range	Stability (4OC, 12 mo)	Delivery Route
Heart	3,400	4.5-6.8	>90% intact	Sublingual
Liver	2,900	5.2-7.0	~80% intact	IM

Tissue Source	Avg. MW (Da)	pI Range	Stability (4OC, 12 mo)	Delivery Route
Brain	3,200	4.8-6.0	>88% intact	Intranasal/IV
Kidney	3,100	5.5-7.2	>86% intact	Sublingual

Importantly, these peptides are not simple "extracts" but highly refined molecular subsets, typically <10 kDa, that pass filtration, pathogen testing, and mass spec validation before use. Early-phase safety studies have shown no significant immunogenicity [28].

Mitochondria-Targeted Peptides: A New Axis in Regenerative Therapeutics

Mitochondrial dysfunction is one of the central pillars of aging and a key driver of chronic degenerative diseases. It represents both a consequence of accumulated cellular damage and a propagator of further dysfunction via increased oxidative stress, impaired ATP production, and activation of pro-senescent and pro-inflammatory pathways. In this context, mitochondria-targeted peptides (MTPs) and nano-formulated organellar modulators have emerged as innovative biologics capable of reversing or attenuating these pathogenic cascades.

Studies have shown that mitochondria-targeted peptides can enhance mitochondrial respiration, restore redox balance, and promote mitophagy, the selective removal of damaged mitochondria, hence increasing the *mitochondriaspan* that is tightly related to *cellspan* [29][30]. These peptides often localize specifically to the mitochondrial inner membrane or matrix, interacting with components of the electron transport chain (ETC) or regulatory proteins such as PGC-1α and SIRT1, which are essential for mitochondrial biogenesis and metabolic regulation.

Peptides such as SS-31 (elamipretide), MOTS-c, and other mitochondrial-derived peptides (MDPs) demonstrate the feasibility of using peptide-based interventions to restore mitochondrial homeostasis. Elamipretide, for instance, binds to cardiolipin in the inner mitochondrial membrane, stabilizing the structure of cristae and reducing ROS leakage—a property that has been shown to improve mitochondrial function in models of ischemia-reperfusion injury, heart failure, and neurodegeneration [31].

MOTS-c, encoded by mitochondrial DNA, functions as a signaling peptide that regulates insulin sensitivity and metabolic adaptation. It exerts systemic effects that include activation of AMP-activated protein kinase (AMPK) and inhibition of the folate cycle highlighting its role as a mitokine with endocrine-like properties [32]. Intriguingly, MOTS-c levels decline with age, and replenishing this peptide in preclinical models has led to improvements in metabolic function and physical performance.

These advances have led to a conceptual shift in regenerative medicine: from tissue repair focused on the extracellular environment and stem cells, toward a deeper intracellular and organellar rejuvenation strategy. By restoring mitochondrial integrity, MTPs and organ-specific nano-peptides hold the potential to reinvigorate energy metabolism, suppress inflammation, and delay or even reverse cellular senescence.

Senescence, Inflammation, and the Aging Microenvironment

The therapeutic promise of peptide-based approaches is amplified when viewed through the lens of cellular senescence and chronic inflammation, the two hallmarks of aging that are tightly linked to mitochondrial dysfunction.

Senescent cells are characterized by permanent cell-cycle arrest, resistance to apoptosis, and the acquisition of a senescence-associated secretory phenotype (SASP). The SASP includes a complex mixture of cytokines, chemokines, proteases, and growth factors that perpetuate local inflammation, disrupt tissue architecture, and impair regenerative capacity [33].

Mitochondrial dysfunction is both a cause and consequence of cellular senescence. Increased ROS production damages nuclear and mitochondrial DNA activates the p53 and NF-κB pathways, and reinforces the senescent state. Moreover, impaired mitophagy leads to the accumulation of dysfunctional mitochondria, establishing a self-amplifying loop of bioenergetic decline and inflammatory signaling [34].

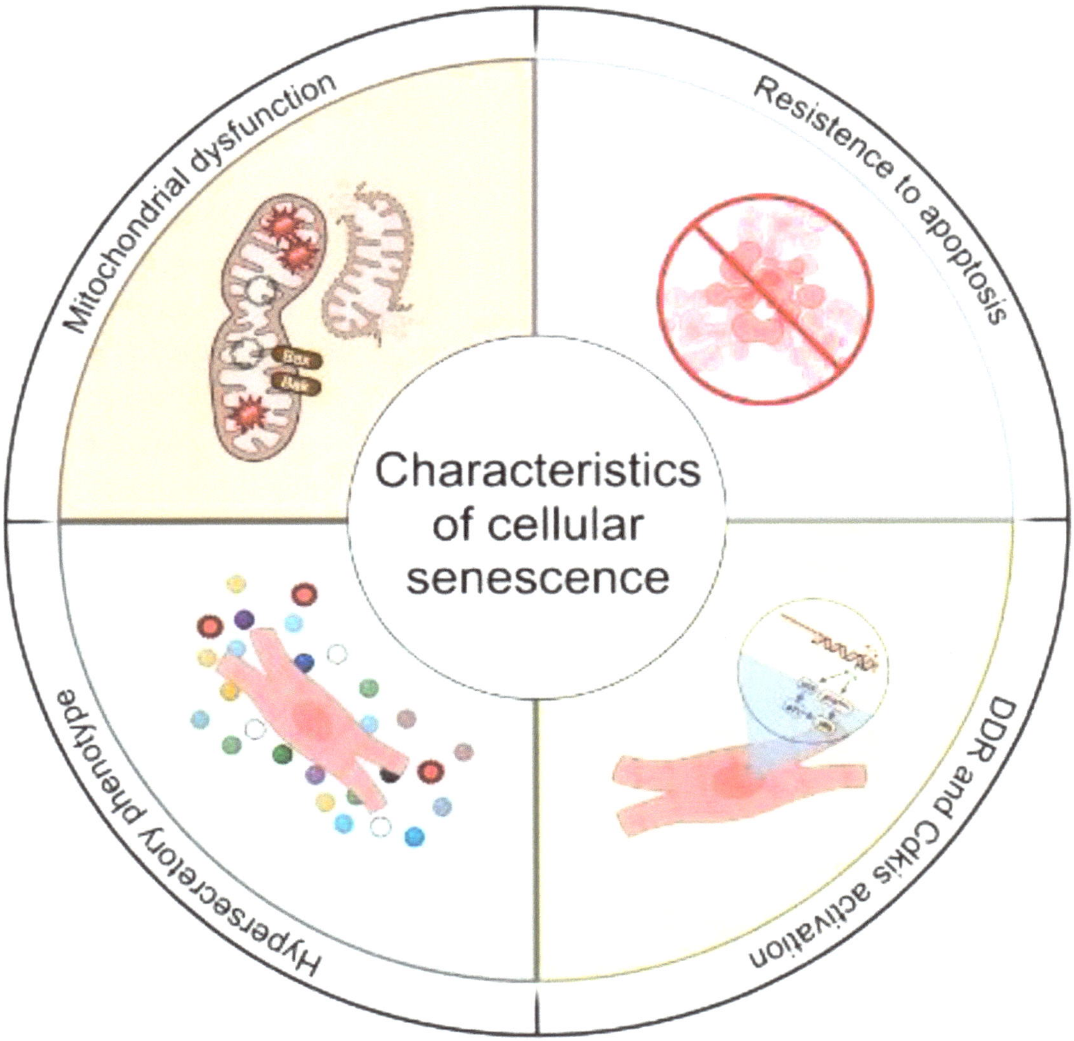

Fig 1.5. *Cellular Senescence, Mitochondrial Dysfunction, and Their Link to Disease*

Cellular senescence and mitochondrial dysfunction are closely intertwined in aging and chronic degenerative diseases. Senescent cells exhibit impaired mitochondrial dynamics, elevated production of reactive oxygen species (ROS), and pro-inflammatory secretory behavior, together collectively forming a toxic feedback loop that accelerates tissue damage and systemic decline. Peptide-based therapeutics offer a unique ability to intervene at multiple nodes in this pathological network, providing both symptomatic relief and root-cause modulation [35].

Enhancing Mitophagy to Alleviate Mitochondrial Burden

One of the earliest and most critical responses to mitochondrial stress is the activation of mitophagy, a selective form of autophagy that targets dysfunctional mitochondria for degradation. With aging or cellular stress, however, mitophagy becomes inefficient, leading to the accumulation of damaged mitochondria, which in turn propagate oxidative stress, inflammation, and metabolic inefficiency [36].

Certain peptides, particularly those derived from mitochondrial regulatory proteins, AMPK activators, or autophagy modulators have demonstrated the ability to reinvigorate mitophagy pathways. This occurs primarily through activation of PINK1/Parkin signaling, a canonical pathway that tags depolarized mitochondria for lysosomal degradation; stimulation of autophagosome formation via upstream regulators like ULK1 and Beclin-1; promotion of mitochondrial fission, enabling segregation of dysfunctional fragments and their clearance [36][37].

For example, mitochondrial-targeted peptides like MOTS-c and humanin analogs have been shown to activate AMPK and induce autophagy-related gene expression [38]. These effects reduce intracellular ROS, minimize DNA damage, and attenuate the pro-inflammatory senescence-associated secretory phenotype (SASP).

By reducing the mitochondrial burden, these peptides not only restore redox homeostasis but also protect nearby cells from the paracrine effects of senescent signaling, thereby containing the spread of cellular aging across tissues.

Restoring NAD$^+$ Levels to Reactivate Sirtuins and Biogenesis

Nicotinamide adenine dinucleotide (NAD$^+$) is a coenzyme central to redox metabolism and mitochondrial function. During aging, NAD$^+$ levels decline significantly, impairing sirtuin activity and compromising mitochondrial quality control. Peptides that modulate NAD$^+$ pathways provide a powerful means to reverse energy deficits and stimulate cellular rejuvenation.

These peptides act through several mechanisms, such as upregulation of NAD$^+$ biosynthesis, either directly or through enhancement of precursors like NMN or nicotinamide riboside (NR); activation of SIRT1 and SIRT3, key NAD⁺-dependent deacetylases involved in mitochondrial biogenesis, DNA repair, and antioxidant defense; and induction of PGC-1α, the master regulator of mitochondrial replication and oxidative phosphorylation [39].

By restoring the NAD⁺ pool, these peptides shift cells away from glycolysis toward oxidative energy metabolism, improving ATP output and cellular resilience. Furthermore, SIRT1 deacetylation of p53, FOXO3a, and NF-κB reduces pro-senescent and inflammatory signaling, aligning the intracellular environment toward regeneration over degeneration.

For instance, certain stem cell-derived or placental peptides have been observed to modulate NAD⁺/SIRT1/PGC-1α pathways in vitro and in animal models, leading to improvements in mitochondrial density, fatty acid oxidation, and insulin sensitivity [40]. These effects are especially promising in metabolic disorders, neurodegenerative diseases, and sarcopenia.

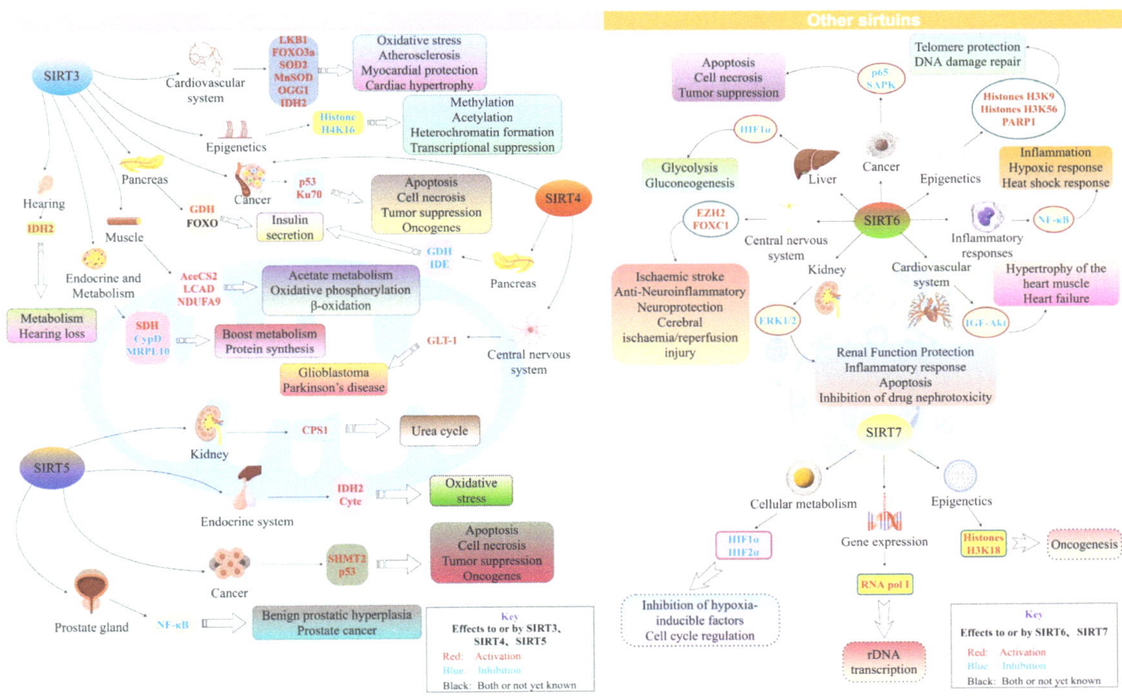

Fig 1.6. *The targets and clinical effects of the SIRTs family (SIRT3-SIRT7) in the tissues and organs of the human body (source: Chen M et al., 2024)*

Acting as Senomorphics and Senolytics: Rewriting the Fate of Senescent Cells

Perhaps the most exciting and rapidly evolving application of therapeutic peptides lies in their potential to function as senotherapeutics—agents that specifically target senescent cells for modification or elimination. These agents fall into two major categories:

- Senomorphics: Peptides that modulate the behavior of senescent cells without killing them. They suppress SASP factors, reduce metabolic stress, and restore partial functionality.
- Senolytics: Peptides that induce apoptosis selectively in senescent cells, thereby clearing dysfunctional cells from tissues and improving the regenerative niche.

Several peptides are under investigation or development for these purposes. FOXO4-DRI, a synthetic peptide, disrupts the FOXO4–p53 interaction, leading to apoptosis of senescent cells while sparing normal ones [41]. Bcl-2 mimetic peptides can sensitize senescent cells to apoptotic cues by inhibiting pro-survival signals that maintain their viability. AMPK-activating peptides can suppress NF-κB-driven SASP secretion, transforming senescent cells from pro-inflammatory to quiescent states [42].

The implications of these interventions are profound. In murine models, senolytic peptides have demonstrated improvements in physical function, lifespan extension, and reversal of age-associated tissue fibrosis. In human skin models, peptide-based senomorphics reduce wrinkles, improve elasticity, and normalize epidermal turnover.

Importantly, unlike many small molecule senolytics, peptide-based senotherapeutics offer higher target specificity, reduced off-target toxicity, and tunable pharmacodynamics due to their modular structure and customizable delivery options.

As our understanding of aging and chronic disease progresses, it is increasingly evident that targeting cellular quality control mechanisms is more effective than merely suppressing symptoms. Peptide therapeutics, by enhancing mitophagy, restoring NAD^+ balance, and eliminating senescent cells, offer a multifaceted approach to this challenge. In combination or sequential regimens, these peptides could form the foundation of preventive aging protocols, preserving mitochondrial integrity and delaying senescence onset; regenerative rehabilitation, facilitating recovery from ischemic injuries, chemotherapy, or surgery; and even chronic disease reversal, especially in conditions driven by metabolic collapse, such as diabetes, Alzheimer's disease, and chronic kidney disease.

Ongoing clinical trials and translational studies continue to evaluate dose optimization, long-term safety, organ specificity, and synergistic effects with existing therapies (e.g., stem cells, NAD^+ boosters, and autophagy inducers).

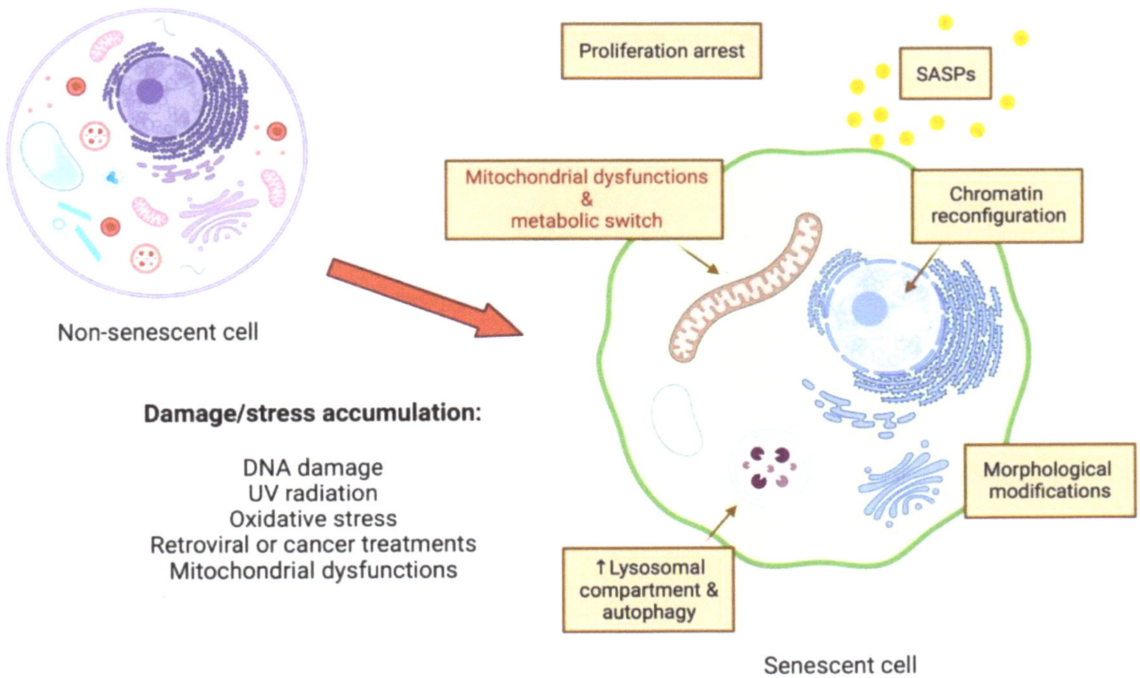

Fig 1.7. *Mechanisms of peptide action on mitochondrial dysfunction and senescence: mitochondrial-targeted peptides improve bioenergetics, reduce ROS, activate mitophagy, and modulate SASP-related cytokine production (source: Protasoni, M., & Serrano, M. (2023). Targeting Mitochondria to Control Ageing and Senescence. Pharmaceutics, 15(2), 352. https://doi.org/10.3390/pharmaceutics15020352)*

From Bench to Bedside: Preclinical and Translational Evidence

Recent studies have begun to validate the safety and efficacy of nano-formulated organ-specific peptides and mitochondrial modulators in both animal models and early human trials.

In aged murine models, administration of nano peptides derived from xenogeneic heart, liver, and brain tissues led to improvements in muscle strength, cognitive performance, and mitochondrial respiration [43][44]. These effects were accompanied by reduced markers of senescence (p16^INK4a, β-galactosidase activity) and increased expression of mitochondrial biogenesis markers (PGC-1α, TFAM).

A recent canine safety study examined chronic administration of organ-specific peptides, confirming the absence of systemic toxicity, allergic responses, or off-target effects [45]. Histological analyses of major organs showed no evidence of inflammation, fibrosis, or structural disruption, supporting the suitability of xenogeneic peptide products for human translational applications.

Importantly, early-phase human trials have demonstrated favorable safety profiles for several mitochondrial-targeted peptides. For example, elamipretide has been studied in heart failure, mitochondrial myopathy, and dry age-related macular degeneration, showing signs of clinical efficacy and acceptable tolerability (Karaa et al., 2018). Peptides derived from stem cell secretomes and placental tissue have also advanced to clinical testing, particularly in contexts such as chronic wounds, neurodegeneration, and immunosenescence.

Table 1.2. Clinical and Preclinical Studies on Mitochondrial and Organ-Specific Peptides

Peptide Type	Model/Disease	Key Outcomes	Reference
SS-31 (Elamipretide)	Mitochondrial Myopathy	↑ ATP, ↓ ROS, ↑ mobility	Campbell et al., 2019
MOTS-c	Metabolic Syndrome	↑ AMPK activation, ↑ insulin sensitivity	Lee et al., 2015

Peptide Type	Model/Disease	Key Outcomes	Reference
Xeno Heart Nano-Peptides	Murine Aging Model	↑ grip strength, ↑ mitochondrial density	Popov et al., 2023
Stem Cell-Derived Peptides	Skin Wound Healing	↑ collagen remodeling, ↑ angiogenesis	Zhang et al., 2020
Xeno Brain Nano-Peptides	Canine Safety Trial	No toxicity, No immunogenicity	Volchenko et al., 2024

Toward a Peptide-Based Regenerative Paradigm

The convergence of advances in peptide chemistry, nanotechnology, and mitochondrial biology has ushered in a new era for regenerative medicine, the one that prioritizes molecular precision, intracellular rejuvenation, and organ-specific modulation. Peptides, once dismissed for their instability and delivery challenges, now represent one of the most promising classes of regenerative biologics.

Their ability to engage cellular signaling pathways, restore mitochondrial function, and counteract senescence makes them uniquely suited for treating the complex, multisystem decline associated with aging and chronic disease. As the field continues to evolve, future directions will include improved peptide design: Using AI and high-throughput screening to optimize sequences for stability, selectivity, and efficacy. Secondly, combination therapies that employ pairing peptides with stem cells, gene therapies, or senolytics to achieve synergistic effects, and personalized peptide regimens, thus tailoring interventions based on individual *omics* data, organ-specific deficits, and regenerative capacity.

Ultimately, peptide-based therapies may form the backbone of 21st-century regenerative medicine, providing safe, scalable, and targeted solutions to some of the most intractable problems in modern healthcare.

Organelle-Specific Peptides: Mitochondria as Master Regulators of Regeneration

As mitochondrial research continues to expand, the therapeutic focus has shifted from simple energy production to recognizing mitochondria as signal-transducing organelles that influence nearly every aspect of cellular health. These include cell cycle regulation, stem cell differentiation, calcium homeostasis, and apoptosis resistance, all of which are crucial in regenerative processes. A seminal review by Chan M., and Lakey et al. (2025) framed mitochondria as not merely "powerhouses" but "central command units" for the coordination of wellness and aging. Mitochondrial peptides, particularly those targeted via nano-delivery are now recognized as multi-functional agents capable of recalibrating dysfunctional cell states across tissues [43].

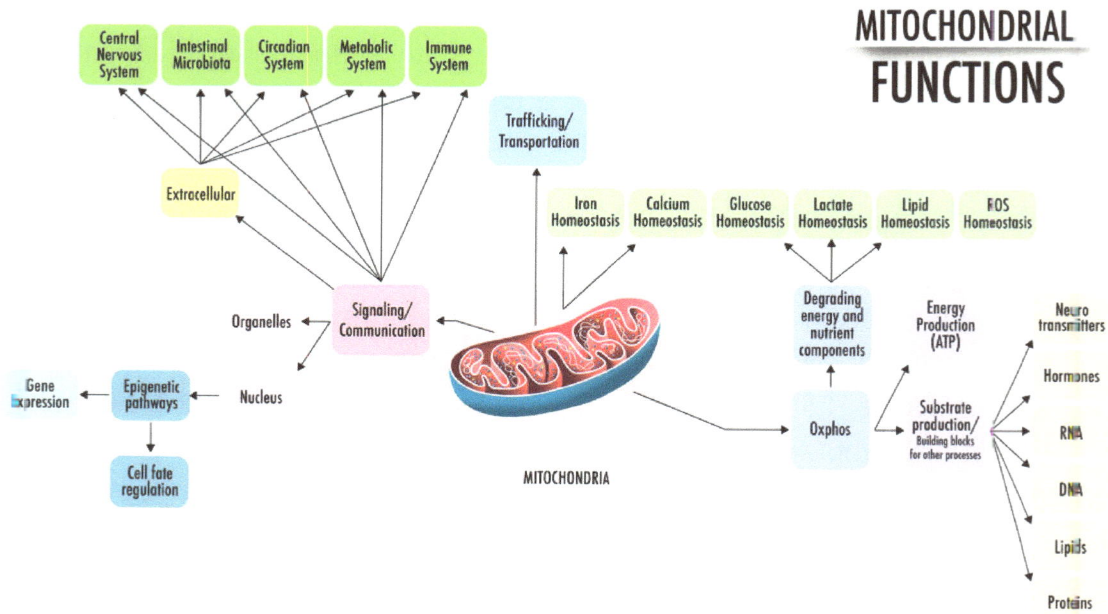

Fig 1.8. *Mitochondrial signaling overview: How organelle-targeted peptides influence cellular health across tissues such as liver, heart, brain, and muscle (source: Casanova A, Wevers A, Navarro-Ledesma S and Pruimboom L (2023) Mitochondria: It is all about energy. Front. Physiol. 14:1114231. doi: 10.3389/fphys.2023.1114231)*

One of my most compelling advancements in peptide-based regenerative medicine is the recognition of tissue-specific mitochondrial architecture and function, and the subsequent development of organ-adapted mitochondrial peptide therapeutics. Unlike the traditional view of mitochondria as uniform energy-producing units across cell types, recent high-resolution structural and proteomic studies have revealed remarkable heterogeneity in mitochondrial morphology, protein composition, cristae structure, and metabolic output depending on the cell's function and tissue origin [43].

For instance, in cardiomyocytes, mitochondria are densely packed and exhibit highly structured cristae, enabling sustained ATP generation to support continuous contractile activity. In neurons, mitochondrial networks are distributed along axons and dendrites to meet localized energy demands and calcium buffering at synapses. Hepatocytes rely on mitochondria for robust metabolic flexibility, supporting gluconeogenesis, β-oxidation, and detoxification. In immune cells, mitochondrial shape and location shift dynamically in response to activation, playing key roles in cytokine production and apoptosis [46].

This tissue-dependent mitochondrial specialization suggests that regenerative interventions targeting mitochondrial health must likewise be customized by organ system. Peptides that restore mitochondrial function in skeletal muscle, for example, may not be equally effective in the brain or liver unless they are tailored to the unique bioenergetic and signaling landscape of those tissues.

This realization has led to the emergence of mitochondrial organelle (MO) therapies—the peptide-based therapeutics designed to match the metabolic and structural signature of mitochondria in specific tissues. These formulations often incorporate:

- Naturally derived mitochondrial peptides, such as those extracted from xenogeneic sources (e.g., porcine, bovine, or placental mitochondria).
- Synthetic mimetics of mitochondrial stress response factors (e.g., MOTS-c, humanin, SHLPs).
- Nano-carriers and vesicles engineered to protect peptides from degradation and enhance delivery to target tissues and intracellular organelles.

Among the most sophisticated advancements in modern regenerative science, SBI and MF-Plus stand at the forefront as exquisitely crafted formulations designed for those who seek more than wellness, for those who instead seek renewal at the cellular level. These exceptional therapies unite rare mitochondrial-derived peptide complexes with elegantly engineered nano-vesicles, creating a finely tuned system that supports cellular vitality, tissue rejuvenation, and the graceful defiance of time itself.

While stem cell therapies, which were introduced by me to Asia in the 1990s remain the pinnacle of regenerative potential, SBI and MF-Plus offer a luxurious, non-cellular alternative for discerning individuals. They deliver a level of refinement, precision, and performance that transcends conventional anti-aging solutions. Together, they embody a new standard of longevity: one where science meets artistry, and rejuvenation becomes not merely possible, but beautifully attainable. When discussing regenerative therapies, I often liken the hierarchy of biological tools to the world of automobiles. Organ-specific progenitor/precursor stem cells, empowered with their remarkable precision and regenerative depth are the Lamborghinis of modern medicine: powerful, elegant, and engineered for extraordinary performance. Organ-targeted peptides, refined to speak the exact molecular dialect of the tissues they serve, are the Mercedes—sophisticated, reliable, and impressively efficient in restoring balance and vitality. By comparison, the broader, more generic peptides and traditional cell extracts function well enough, but they belong to a different class entirely: the dependable Proton Saga of regenerative solutions, still in some cases practical, respectable, and useful, yet far from the exhilaration, precision, and transformative capability offered by the Lamborghini and Mercedes tiers of advanced cellular and peptide therapies.

The key features of *Mito Organelles* peptides:

- **Organelle-Specificity**: MOs from MF-Plus contains mitochondria-targeted peptides that are pre-selected or modified to correspond with mitochondrial phenotypes found in aging heart, brain, liver, and skin tissue.
- **Nano-Encapsulation for Targeted Delivery**: The formulation employs nanoliposomes and organelle-permeable vesicles, which ensure peptide stability, minimize immunogenicity, and facilitate intracellular uptake, especially into dysfunctional mitochondria.

The mechanisms of action of these peptides include stimulation of mitochondrial biogenesis via PGC-1α and NRF1 pathways; suppression of senescence by downregulating p16^INK4a^ and p21^CIP1^ expression and enhancing autophagy; restoration of redox balance by decreasing mitochondrial ROS and enhancing antioxidant defenses (e.g., via Nrf2 activation); and reactivation of stem and progenitor cells through improved mitochondrial function and paracrine signaling enhancement [47].

Among the systemic and local effects that MOs from MF-Plus has been observed to the most prominent are the improvement cellular metabolism in energy-deficient tissues, reversing the early markers of cellular aging and apoptosis, and enhancing the microenvironment in stem cell niches, particularly in bone marrow and neural tissues, promoting the endogenous regenerative capacity [46][48].

Initial preclinical data and early clinical case series suggest that MF-Plus holds promise across a range of applications. For instance, in neurodegeneration—by enhancing mitochondrial function in neurons, reducing oxidative stress, and improving cognitive outcomes. Or in cardiomyopathy—by supporting myocardial bioenergetics, reducing ischemia-reperfusion injury, increasing the heartspan and promoting cardiac repair. In cases of liver disease—by attenuating mitochondrial-driven steatosis and improving detoxification in aging hepatocytes. In dermatological practice - by rejuvenating aged skin through enhanced collagen synthesis, angiogenesis, and fibroblast mitochondrial function.

The dual focus of Mito Organelles is combining systemic rejuvenation with organ-specific regeneration that reflects a broader paradigm shift in regenerative medicine: moving away from single-target interventions and toward bio-synergistic therapies that restore the native complexity of tissue and cellular function.

Clinical Outlook of MO Peptide Therapy

The burgeoning field of peptide-based therapeutics stands at a critical inflection point. On one hand lie rapidly accumulating data showing that mitochondrial-targeted peptide extracts, such as the 300 kDa Mito Organelles (MO) family, can pass standard in vitro safety screens, including the cytotoxicity assays and cell transformation assays, without inciting malignancy. On the other, modern characterization tools, such as mass spectrometric fingerprinting, proteomic stability profiles, organ-specific peptide mapping (e.g., Nano-Organ Peptides, NOPs) are now enabling the precise validation of identity, purity, and potency. Together, these lines of evidence create a foundation of confidence: properly produced, well-defined mitochondrial peptides have shown promising safety and favorable molecular behavior in preclinical settings.

However, as with any emerging therapeutic modality, humility is not simply scholarly decorum—it is an essential guardrail. The complexity of biology ensures that rare or long-term adverse phenomena may lie outside the reach of standard acute assays. Even when *in vitro* and short-duration *in vivo* experiments are reassuring, subtle effects—chronic low-level inflammation, immune sensitization, off-target mitochondrial interactions, epigenetic drift, or unforeseen interactions with co-morbidities require careful attention.

Mito Organelles (MO) as a therapeutic concept act as an exemplar of both promise and the need for rigor. These cellular ultrafiltrates (up to ~300 kDa or more depending on the preparation) are derived from multiple organs, i.e. heart, brain, kidney, thymus, placenta, lungs, connective tissue, and combinations such as LPPSIMKE (liver, pancreas, placenta, kidney, intestines, retina).

Moreover, MO extracts appear to confer beneficial effects under stress. When human cells exposed to mild oxidative stress (e.g. low-dose H_2O_2) were co-treated with MO extracts, viability improved. This suggests not only absence of harm but potential trophic or protective signaling under adversarial conditions.

From a clinical application perspective, the properties of MO extract technology pave the road toward several promising avenues:

By rejuvenating mitochondrial function through improving oxidative phosphorylation, reducing ROS accumulation, enhancing mitophagy, and improving the unfolded protein responses, Mito Organelles may slow hallmarks of aging at cellular level. For example, stem-cell derived MO fractions have been shown in preclinical models to reduce cellular senescence and restore metabolic efficiency in aged stem cell populations.

Because MO extracts are organ-specific, they potentially offer therapeutic support in degenerative conditions. For instance, MO extracts from cardiac tissue could help, in theory, to improve cardiomyocyte mitochondrial health in heart failure; similarly, brain-derived MO might assist neurodegenerative conditions where mitochondrial dysfunction is central.

Since mitochondrial health intersects metabolism, immune signaling, and oxidative damage, MO peptides may serve as adjuncts in metabolic syndromes (e.g., diabetes, fatty liver), inflammatory diseases, or disorders of chronic oxidative stress. Early data indicate MO extracts do not only lack cytotoxicity but improve resilience under oxidative challenges.

Aging skin, wound healing, cosmetic and aesthetic medicine often target mitochondrial decline and extracellular matrix damage. MO extracts, by improving mitochondrial support, reducing oxidative damage, and enhancing cell viability, may improve tissue healing and appearance.

More broadly, MO technology could be integrated into preventive medicine for its ability to support mitochondrial health even before disease onset. This may translate into delayed onset of cardiovascular disease, neurodegeneration, or other age-related pathologies.

These clinical possibilities rest on the twin pillars of molecular fidelity and therapeutic context. It is essential that MO preparations preserve key peptide signatures (m/z peaks, fragmentation profile, relative abundance), stability under storage and handling, and lack of impurities or residual toxic components. Dosing must be optimized, delivery routes considered (systemic vs local), and interactions with existing therapies assessed.

Finally, to move from promise to proven therapy, the field must commit to long-term, well-designed clinical trials, post-market surveillance, and real-world evidence. Rare adverse events, latency of cancer risk, immune modulation over time, and inter-individual variability (based on age, genetics, mitochondrial haplotype, comorbidity) must be monitored. Only through such sustained rigor can peptide therapies, particularly a complex extract technology like Mito Organelles, realize their full potential: enabling not just symptomatic relief, but restoration of function, resilience, and perhaps extension of health span in human beings.

The story of peptide therapeutics is one of balance: confident in what we know through rigorous evidence, yet humble before what we do not. Mito Organelles embodies both the advances and the responsibilities: offering regenerative promise, but demanding careful scientific, clinical, and ethical stewardship if turned into safe, transformative human therapies.

Table 1.3. Summary of Functional Benefits of Mitochondrial Peptide Therapy by Organ System

Organ System	Primary Benefits	Supporting Peptides	Delivery Method
Brain	Promotes Neuro-protection, Increase BDNF, Reduce ROS	MOTS-c, MF-plus	Intranasal, IV
Heart	Increase Cardiolipin stabilization, reduce fibrosis	SS-31, MF-plus	Subcutaneous
Liver	Detox	NOPs, MOTS-c	Oral, Sublingual
Skin	Increases Collagen, Reduces Senes-cence, Promotes Angiogenesis	Placental peptides	Topical, Intradermal

Integration with Other Regenerative Modalities

What distinguishes peptide therapy in the current regenerative landscape is its versatility and compatibility with other advanced approaches. When used concurrently with stem cell therapy peptides can act as "priming agents", enhancing the homing, survival, and differentiation potential of transplanted stem cells [49]. The combination with gene editing peptides may enhance the intracellular uptake or nuclear delivery of gene-editing tools such as CRISPR/Cas9. With exosome therapy together, peptides can be incorporated into or extracted from exosomal preparations to create hybrid biologics that deliver combined effects.

Peptides also provide a more cost-effective and scalable solution compared to autologous cell therapies, especially when produced using recombinant or synthetic techniques. Importantly, many novel peptides show low immunogenicity, allowing for repeated use without the risks associated with immune rejection or cytokine storms.

Regulatory and Safety Considerations

While the scientific rationale for peptide-based therapeutics is increasingly well-established supported by advances in molecular biology, bioinformatics, and regenerative medicine their pathway to clinical adoption is still navigating uncharted regulatory territory. Unlike small molecules, which have a long-established pharmacological and regulatory framework, or large biologics such as monoclonal antibodies, peptides occupy a unique and somewhat ambiguous regulatory gray zone.

Peptides straddle the boundary between biologics and synthetics. They are often derived from endogenous proteins, yet engineered or synthesized to enhance stability, bioavailability, or specificity. This duality poses a challenge for regulatory bodies such as the U.S. Food and Drug Administration (FDA) and the European Medicines Agency (EMA), which are tasked with classifying and evaluating therapies under frameworks originally designed for more conventional drug types. As a result, the regulatory pathway for peptides remains in evolution requiring careful calibration of both preclinical rigor and clinical validation.

To meet the safety and efficacy thresholds expected of modern therapeutics, peptide-based treatments must demonstrate:

- Reproducible pharmacokinetic profiles, including absorption, distribution, metabolism, and excretion (ADME).
- Toxicological safety across short- and long-term exposure windows, in both rodent and non-rodent species.
- Defined mechanisms of action, particularly for multifunctional or organ-specific peptides.
- Manufacturing traceability, with clear documentation of source material, synthesis methods, and quality control checkpoints.

Despite these regulatory hurdles, several intrinsic features of peptides position them favorably for eventual integration into mainstream clinical practice.

- First, peptides generally exhibit predictable and benign metabolic profiles. Most are rapidly broken down by ubiquitous peptidases into naturally occurring amino acids, thereby avoiding the formation of toxic intermediates or long-lived metabolites. This rapid enzymatic degradation reduces the risk of cumulative toxicity—a common concern with small molecule drugs that linger in tissues.
- Second, because of their transient half-lives and efficient clearance, peptides rarely accumulate systemically, even with repeated dosing. This pharmacokinetic property is especially advantageous in chronic or regenerative therapies, where long-term exposure may be necessary to achieve sustained tissue remodeling or immune modulation.
- Third, emerging toxicology data, including findings from controlled animal studies have consistently demonstrated favorable safety margins for many naturally derived peptides. For instance, in vivo studies assessing xenogeneic mitochondrial peptides have reported no evidence of systemic toxicity, genotoxicity, or organ-specific adverse effects, even at doses exceeding therapeutic thresholds. These findings support the hypothesis that peptides, particularly those derived from evolutionarily conserved sequences, are inherently biocompatible and well-tolerated.

As the field matures, there is increasing movement toward Good Manufacturing Practice (GMP)-compliant production pipelines for peptide therapeutics. The shift from experimental preparations to pharmaceutical-grade manufacturing brings with it several key benefits:

- Batch-to-batch consistency, critical for clinical reliability and reproducibility.
- Defined molecular fingerprints, including mass spectrometry validation and sequencing data, allowing for regulatory traceability.
- Sterility and purity standards that align with those for injectable biologics.

This move toward industrial-scale, GMP-certified peptide synthesis is not merely a technical upgrade; it is a necessary precondition for regulatory acceptance. Agencies such as the FDA are unlikely to approve peptide therapies without stringent controls on identity, purity, potency, and stability, all of which require modern manufacturing protocols.

Furthermore, regulatory precedents are gradually being established. Many peptide-based therapies have successfully navigated approval pathways in the U.S. and Europe. Their success provides a roadmap for the next generation of organ-specific, mitochondria-derived, or xenogeneic peptide therapies, even if those molecules are more complex or multifunctional in nature.

Another emerging trend is the development of peptide-drug conjugates, peptide-loaded nanoparticles, and hybrid biologic systems, all of which blur the line between conventional biologics and novel molecular entities. These advances are already prompting regulatory bodies to revise their definitions and adapt their review processes, creating tailored pathways for complex peptide formulations.

Ultimately, the successful clinical translation of peptide therapeutics will depend on sustained collaboration between research scientists, bioengineers, pharmaceutical manufacturers, and regulatory experts. As the biological insights continue to accumulate and as clinical evidence grows to support efficacy in degenerative, metabolic, and immunological diseases, the momentum for regulatory adaptation will become increasingly irresistible.

The story of peptide regulation is not one of rigid barriers, but of gradual integration, a co-evolution between science and policy that reflects the frontier nature of regenerative medicine itself.

Reimagining Regeneration Through Peptides

The science of tissue regeneration is undergoing a profound evolution. Traditionally centered around stem cells, growth factors, and bioengineered scaffolds, the field is now being reshaped by a new class of biologically active agents: short-chain peptides. Once viewed merely as protein fragments or signaling intermediates, peptides are increasingly recognized as master regulators of cellular behavior, capable of orchestrating healing processes across molecular, cellular, and tissue scales.

This chapter has introduced the conceptual and mechanistic foundations of a new therapeutic paradigm, one in which naturally derived, nanomized, and organ-specific peptides function not simply as adjuncts to regenerative strategies but as primary drivers of repair, rejuvenation, and resilience. These peptides are not artificial constructs; they are biologically intelligent molecules refined through evolution and isolated from sources with high regenerative potential, including:

- Xenogeneic tissues (e.g., sheep and rabbit's organs)
- Stem cell secretomes and exosomal fractions
- Placental extracts, rich in trophic and immunomodulatory signals
- Mitochondria-derived peptides and organelle-targeted biomolecules

As this chapter has outlined, these peptides exhibit a remarkable ability to induce both systemic and organ-specific rejuvenation. They have been shown to:

- Modulate core aging processes such as cellular senescence, inflammaging, and mitochondrial dysfunction
- Promote tissue repair by activating progenitor cells, enhancing angiogenesis, and modulating extracellular matrix remodeling
- Exhibit favorable pharmacokinetic and toxicity profiles, supporting safe, repeatable administration
- Be produced with high purity and scalability under GMP conditions, accelerating their translational potential

Rather than acting as blunt instruments, peptides represent precision biological tools able to influence gene expression, intracellular signaling, epigenetic regulation, and intercellular communication in context-specific ways. Their effects are not limited to symptomatic relief but extend to functional restoration at the level of mitochondrial health, stem cell niche integrity, immune homeostasis, and even metabolic recalibration.

This introductory chapter lays the groundwork for a deeper exploration. In the chapters that follow, we will examine the role of these peptides in specific clinical domains. We will talk about Neurodegenerative disorders, where peptide-based interventions offer new hope for preserving neuronal function and reversing glial senescence. Also about the cardiomyopathy and ischemic injury, where mitochondrial-targeted peptides are being leveraged to restore cardiomyocyte bioenergetics; Metabolic syndrome, in which organ-specific peptides improve insulin sensitivity, hepatic function, and adipose tissue remodeling. Even the dermatological and aesthetic regeneration, where peptide complexes stimulate dermal fibroblasts, improve barrier function, and reverse visible signs of aging.

As the field of regenerative medicine advances, a core principle continues to emerge with growing clarity: peptides are not passive byproducts of biology, but active therapeutic signals. They are modular, multifunctional, and programmable, capable of targeting dysfunction at its source, not merely compensating for it, but reversing it.

Their capacity to modulate biology at the level of molecular networks rather than single targets makes them uniquely suited for the complexity of human aging and disease. As we stand at the threshold of this new era, peptides promise to bridge the gap between biological theory and clinical application heralding a future where regeneration is not only possible but precisely controllable.

CHAPTER 2

The History of Peptide Therapy: From Insulin to Organ-Specific Bioactive Formulations

Prologue: A Century of Peptide Vision

Dear Reader, before I take you for a deep dive into the ocean of therapeutic applications of peptides, I feel compelled to tell you about the discovery and history of peptides as bioactive medicinal molecules. So, once upon a time...

When Frederick Banting and Charles Best first discovered that extracts of pancreatic islets could reverse fatal hyperglycemia in dogs, few could have foreseen how that humble breakthrough would evolve into a vast field of molecular medicine. Yet in the decades that followed, insulin initially a crude animal extract became the blueprint for peptide therapeutics, ushering in an era in which short amino-acid chains could mediate life, repair, and renewal.

Over the next hundred years, the science and dreams of peptide therapy would traverse early organ extracts, thymus immunomodulators, Swiss cell therapy pioneers, recombinant analogues, xenogeneic nano-peptides, and mitochondrial signal peptides. This chapter tells that story not merely as a chronology of discovery, but as a narrative of ambition, controversy, and increasing precision.

The Dawn: Insulin and the Peptide Revolution

In the early 1920s, diabetes was a death sentence. Patients succumbed to starvation, ketoacidosis, and multi-organ collapse. The idea of injecting a pancreatic extract to rescue life seemed almost poetic. But in 1921, Banting and Best isolated crude pancreatic extracts; in 1922, they administered the first human injection to a 14-year-old boy, Leonard Thompson, with dramatic effect [50]. That extract contained not a pure peptide, but a blend of proteins, enzymes, and contaminants but the medicine worked.

As techniques improved, purification yielded more refined formulations. By the 1930s and 1940s, porcine and bovine insulin became standard, with cross-species use accepted because of structural similarity. In Germany and Switzerland centers of pharmaceutical chemistry investigators began dissecting insulin's structure, determining its disulfide bonds, and attempting synthetic analogues. The awarding of the Nobel Prize to Banting and Macleod in 1923 cemented insulin's place in medicine and validated peptides as a class of therapy.

Insulin's path illustrates key themes: that a peptide can replace a deficient hormone; that tissue origin, chemical purity, immunogenicity, stability, and delivery are all vital; and that clinical translation requires overcoming biological complexity. Over subsequent decades, insulin analogues with faster or longer action, chemically modified side chains, and insulin pumps emerged. But the seed had been planted: a peptide could be medicine.

Not long after insulin, attention gravitated toward the pituitary gland. By the early 1900s, researchers such as Sir Henry Hallett Dale had observed that extracts of the posterior pituitary (drawn from oxen or other animals) could trigger uterine contractions in cats and other mammals, hence suggesting that the gland secreted a substance powerful enough to initiate labor (Dale, 1906). A few years later, William Blair-Bell in 1909 and others observed that similar extracts controlled postpartum bleeding and promoted milk ejection [51].

These early observations were clinical and phenomenological: pituitary extracts were used, albeit crudely; their utility was clear, but their molecular identity was still uncertain. The leap came in 1928, when a team at Parke-Davis, led by Oliver Kamm, separated two active substances in posterior pituitary extracts: one which caused uterine contractions and milk letdown (which came to be called "oxytocin"), and another which acted as a vasopressor/antidiuretic (vasopressin).

Vincent du Vigneaud's work in the early 1950s took the discovery to fruition. In 1952-53, he determined the amino acid sequences for oxytocin and vasopressin each a nine-amino-acid peptide with a disulfide bridge between two cysteines at positions 1 and 6 [51][52]. In 1953, he also achieved chemical synthesis of oxytocin, making it the first peptide hormone to be synthesized in the lab a testament to both ingenuity and growing capacity in peptide chemistry. For his efforts, he received the Nobel Prize in Chemistry in 1955 [52][53].

But the story of oxytocin and vasopressin was more than a molecular triumph. Over ensuing decades, they became entrenched in obstetrics (use in labor induction, controlling hemorrhage), in water-balance physiology (vasopressin analogs in diabetes insipidus), in social and behavioral science (oxytocin's roles in bonding, stress, emotional regulation) the proof that small peptides could influence not only glands but mind, body, emotion [51].

Around the same era, another peptide came into medical view, the adrenocorticotropic hormone (ACTH), which stimulates the adrenal cortex to secrete cortisol and other glucocorticoids. Early in the 1940s, bovine pituitary extracts were found to contain a factor that could stimulate adrenal activity in Addison's disease. By 1942 ACTH was isolated from the bovine hypophysis [54].

Over the next decade, scientists determined the full 39-amino-acid sequence of ACTH. Work in Germany and elsewhere focused on fragmentation: researchers found that the biologically active portion of ACTH could be reduced to its N-terminal 24 amino acids without losing core adrenal-stimulating activity.

In parallel, the concept of prohormone precursors emerged. POMC (proopiomelanocortin) was recognized as the gene that encodes several peptides (including ACTH, melanocyte stimulating hormone (MSH), endorphins). The discovery that peptides could be produced from larger precursor proteins that are then enzymatically processed expanded the peptide world: suddenly biology had encoded multiplexed peptides in single genes—a mechanism of economy, regulation, and diversity [55].

ACTH entered therapeutic use during the mid-20th century for adrenal insufficiency, but also found wider off-label and experimentally driven applications: in some inflammatory conditions, rheumatism, asthma, eczema. Its potency, however, raised safety issues (glucocorticoid overproduction, side effects), reinforcing that peptide therapies are powerful but require control [56].

As insulin, oxytocin, vasopressin, and ACTH established that peptides could replace missing hormones or trigger potent physiological actions, mid-20th century researchers probed the signals regulating those peptide hormones, especially those emerging from the hypothalamus [57].

Growth hormone (GH) itself had been known pituitary extracts promoting growth in hypophysectomized animals were used in children with growth deficiencies. But its regulation was mysterious. In the 1960s and 1970s, with the development of hypothalamic extracts, scientists isolated growth hormone–releasing hormone (GHRH) and discovered somatostatin, the inhibitory peptide. Alongside, synthetic peptides called growth hormone secretagogues (GHS) were created, including but not limited to small synthetic peptides like GHRP-6, which could stimulate GH release even in modes different from GHRH [58].

Finally, in 1999, researchers discovered ghrelin, an endogenous peptide produced mainly in the stomach, which binds to the growth hormone secretagogue receptor (GHS-R) and stimulates GH release and appetite. The identification of ghrelin completed a regulatory circuit: hypothalamic releasing factor, inhibitory peptides, the pituitary hormone, and peripheral signal peptides that feedback into the system [59].

These discoveries underscored themes that would return repeatedly: cumulative regulation, feedback loops, tissue-specific expression, and the importance of small peptides in inter-organ communication.

Around the mid-20th century, additional peptide hormones were discovered and characterized, further expanding the therapeutic landscape.

- **Parathyroid hormone (PTH)**, although larger in length and complex was isolated and used for disorders of calcium metabolism.

- **Calcitonin**, secreted by thyroid parafollicular cells, was characterized as a peptide hormone that lowers blood calcium, opposing PTH.
- **Insulin-like growth factors (IGFs)** were discovered to mediate some of insulin's metabolic effects and to regulate growth, whose peptides are evolutionarily related to insulin.

These peptides, while differing in size, origin, and function, established that hormone peptides were a broad class: endocrine, paracrine, autocrine; large or small; with receptors and feedback systems; and that they could be therapeutic.

Dear Reader, let me take you to the Germany, circa late 1940s, where in a lab in Göttingen or Munich: a young biochemist pores over chromatography runs of pituitary extracts, trying to isolate an adrenal-stimulating factor. The lab's fridge is cold; the bioassay is delicate; animals survive or die depending on whether the extract is potent enough. Samples degrade; contamination is constant. Yet in those cramped, often under-funded labs, insulin, ACTH, GH fragments are being teased out.

In Switzerland at the same time, chemical firms were trying to synthesize earlier peptides; universities in Basel, Zurich, Geneva had chemists specializing in peptide bond formation, disulfide bond folding, etc. Letters between these labs show fascination mixed with frustration: the yield of synthetic ACTH is low; sequences sometimes ambiguous, cross-reactivity with animal sera complicates measurements; purity is elusive.

Vincent du Vigneaud, writing in his Nobel lecture, recalled midnight hours spent amid flasks and Dean's charge, under weak lamplight, testing oxytocin analogs in uterine strip contractions. Splicing off amino acids, altering disulfide bridges, all to see which changes abolished contraction, which preserved it. His story became legend: the first chemical synthesis of a polypeptide hormone was not just a technical feat, but a proof of principle: that molecules of life could be built.

The early peptide wave taught several lessons that still guide modern peptide therapeutics:

- **Structure matters**: sequence (which amino acids in which order), folding (disulfide bridges, secondary structure), charge, receptor binding, and size all influence activity and stability.

- **Source and species matter**: bovine, porcine, ovine versions differed slightly; immunogenicity could be significant; cross-species differences in sequence sometimes mattered.
- **Purification is hard**: early preparations had mixed peptides, proteins contaminants. Many early side-effects likely came from impurities, variability, or immunologic reactions.
- **Delivery and stability**: many early peptides degraded quickly in vivo: synthetic analogues or modifications (half-life extension, chemical stabilization) were needed; routes of administration (injection vs. oral) were key.
- **Clinical translation is lengthy and often unpredictable**: animal efficacy did not always translate; safety, dosing, organ targeting, feedback regulation, side-effects all needed careful study.

The discovery of insulin acted like a pebble dropped into a still pond with its ripples carried far. Laboratories everywhere sought other hormones, other bioactives. The notion that molecules made of amino acids, extracted from small glands, or from the pituitary, or even synthesized, could be universal mediators of physiology, opened doors to research into growth, stress, immune function, reproduction, metabolism. What followed, in mid-20th century Europe, was a proliferation of physiological exploration: extracting pituitary glands to study growth disorders; hypothalamic extracts to understand pituitary control; adrenal extracts to regulate metabolism; thymus extracts for immune modulation. Each new peptide discovered or synthesized added to the lexicon the oxytocin for labor and bonding; vasopressin for fluid balance; ACTH for stress and adrenal function; GH for growth; somatostatin for inhibition; then newer factors like GHRH, ghrelin, the IGFs.

In reflection, the early decades after insulin were a period of discovery, mistake, revision, and rapidly increasing clarity. The peptidologist pioneers did not know then about nanomization, mitochondrial peptides, or organ-specific xenogeneic fractions but in each discovery, hints of these later ideas were present: that peptides are small enough to pass across membranes, have local and systemic effects, that tissue source matters, that structure defines function.

Organ Extracts and the Swiss/German Tradition of Tissue Therapy

While insulin became the anchor of peptide therapeutics, parallel traditions explored organ extracts, believing that tissues harbor "vital substances" beyond single hormones. In late nineteenth-century Europe, Charles-Édouard Brown-Séquard famously injected himself with testicular extracts, claiming improved vitality. Though scientifically dubious, his experiments sparked interest in organotherapy [60][61].

In German and Swiss clinics, extracts of adrenal, thyroid, pituitary, and gonadal tissues circulated as tonics or therapeutic supplements. These preparations were rarely pure peptides; rather, they were mixtures of proteins, peptides, lipids, and small molecules. Yet they introduced the concept that tissues might contain bioactive "factors" that could influence physiology beyond simple hormone replacement.

By the early 20th century, German pharmaceutical houses were marketing gland extracts in Europe. In Switzerland, where biomedical innovation and spa culture intersected, physicians experimented with fetal tissues, embryo-derived organs, and cell suspensions. The Swiss Riviera, Montreux, Vevey, Lausanne became a microcosm of therapeutic experimentation. In that milieu, one surgeon's audacious vision would leave a controversial yet enduring imprint: Paul Niehans.

Paul Niehans and the Era of Live Cell Therapy

Paul Niehans (1882–1971) remains one of the most dramatic and controversial figures in the history of regenerative therapy. Born in Bern, the son of a physician, Niehans studied both theology and medicine—an early sign of his hybrid intellectual curiosity. After service in World War I with the Red Cross, he settled in Montreux/Vevey and launched clinical experiments that would become "fresh cell therapy" (*Frischzellentherapie*).

One pivotal anecdote stands central in Niehans lore. In the early 1930s, Fritz de Quervain (the eminent Swiss thyroid surgeon) faced a patient who developed tetany following accidental removal of parathyroid glands during thyroid surgery. Conventional medicine had no remedy. Niehans, called upon, injected crushed parathyroid tissue derived from a newborn animal. To the astonishment of clinicians, the tetany subsided almost immediately. That event, much retold, became the symbolic origin of his cell therapy method [62][63].

This dramatic story, whether entirely factual or partly mythologized, cemented Niehans's belief: that animal cell extracts, ideally fresh, could restore function in human tissues. He began injecting suspensions of embryonic or fetal tissue from sheep, lambs, or calves, targeting organs that corresponded to presumed human dysfunction. He broadened his methods: intra-muscular, subcutaneous, organ-specific suspensions, and later lyophilized (freeze-dried) extracts.

In Montreux he founded what would become Clinique La Prairie. His reputation grew rapidly. Word spread that Niehans treated patients included Pope Pius XII, Charlie Chaplin, Winston Churchill, Konrad Adenauer, and other high-profile figures. The Times magazine ran a feature titled "Medicine: The Healing Lamb" describing Niehans's practice of injecting embryonic sheep cell preparations into patients as a rejuvenation therapy [64].

Such celebrity endorsements amplified his reach and reinforced aura. Yet his methods existed in a liminal zone, it was neither quackery utterly nor fully orthodox medicine. Niehans published method manuals, dosage protocols, and anecdotal reports in editions distributed among European clinics and some biohacking circles.

As the demand for "live cell therapy" grew from therapists and medical tourists, practical limitations emerged. Fresh fetal tissue is perishable and requires immediate processing. To distribute treatments beyond local proximity, Niehans and collaborators began producing lyophilized, or freeze-dried, extracts. While less potent in theory than live cells, they were far more transportable and storable.

By the 1950s, Niehans was collaborating with pharmaceutical concerns such as Rhein-Chemie (Germany) to package dried cell extracts. The analogy often used: "fresh milk vs. powdered milk" (Time piece, "Healing Lamb") fresh cell suspensions were more potent but less practical; dried extracts were more manageable but diluted [64].

These dried or stabilized extracts (sometimes labeled "Cellorgan," "CLP Extract," or "Revitalisation formulations") became part of the clinic's offerings. In 1931, the clinic's early work had only used fresh cells; by 1947, preserved cells were injected; by 1949, freeze-dried cells were introduced.

Clinique La Prairie's own narrative emphasizes this progression: in the 1950s, Niehans treated Pope Pius XII; the clinic's international recognition soared; in the

1960s and beyond, extract "Revitalisation" products evolved (https://swissmedexpert.eu/about-clinique-la-prairie).

From the outset, Niehans's work attracted both fascination and critique. Critics in academic medicine questioned the lack of controlled trials, reproducibility, and safety. Concerns about immune reaction, infection risk, xenogeneic pathogen transmission, and inconsistent potency were voiced quietly, harshly, and persistently.

In retrospect, Niehans's legacy is complex: partly a cautionary tale, partly a spark for modern regenerative biology. Some of his ideas, such as organ specificity, extract potency, micro-signals from tissues were able to survive when reframed in molecular and safety-conscious forms.

I consider it a rare privilege in my scientific journey to have worked alongside, and learned directly from, the torchbearers of Paul Niehans' pioneering legacy. Men like Franz Schmid, whose disciplined, almost monastic devotion to cellular extraction protocols echoed the old Swiss school of biological precision, and Dr. Lansberger, who once walked the marble halls of Clinique La Prairie as Niehans' junior colleague. They were not just historians of this field, they were living archives. I remember Dr. Schmid guiding my gloved hands through the careful lyophilization of thymic peptides, explaining, in his clipped Bernese cadence, why temperature curves mattered more than brand names. Dr. Lansberger, ever the philosopher-physician, once shared with me a yellowing notebook of Niehans' sketches—anatomical maps of organ-specific peptide signatures long before mass spectrometry validated them. From these mentors I did not simply learn techniques—I inherited a worldview that one that sees peptides not merely as molecules, but as carriers of the language of regeneration, whispered across decades by those who first dared to decode it. In later part I have passed over that knowledge to over eighty thousands physicians all over the world to whom I have presented more than a thousand lectures worldwide traveling from continent to continent and in-between flight check-ins and airport layovers converting my thoughts into notes that later will be formed into hundreds of books and articles and become a foundation for dozens of patents and discoveries.

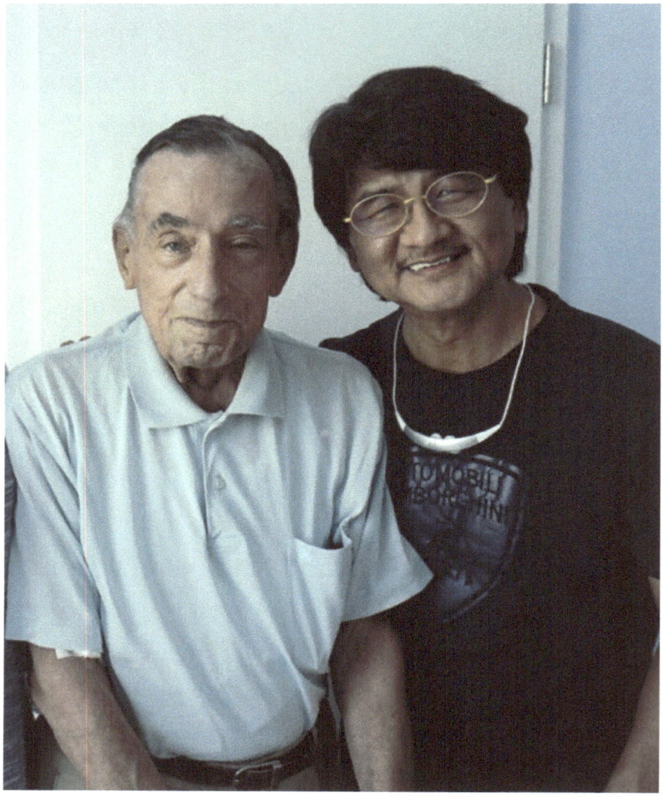

Photo of Prof. Dr. Mike KS Chan and Prof. Albert Landsberger together.

To appreciate the personality and cultural force behind peptide therapies, consider a few archival vignettes such as sheep flocks in Gruyère and dawn harvests. The image is almost cinematic: technicians in the mist of dawn in the Swiss countryside, selecting pregnant sheep, performing rapid fetal retrieval, macerating organs in sterile atmosphere, suspending tissues for injection. This image recurs in memoirs, promotional materials, and clinic lore. While likely dramatized, it reflects Niehans's insistence on freshness, immediacy, and the ritual of regenerative therapy [64]. Clinique La Prairie's heritage mentions that in 1931 the first fresh cells were injected; in 1947 preserved cells; 1949 freeze-dried cells; 1953 Pope Pius XII treated; 1960 CLP research begins; 1966 Niehans retires (dies 1971) (La Prairie history, SwissMedExpert). Niehans's fame soared partly due to high-profile patients and publicity. The 1955 Time article "Medicine: The Healing Lamb" recounted how "persons of value" (Pope, Kings, artists) were flown in to receive injections of fetal sheep cell suspensions. The media framed it as a crossroads of medical boldness and spiritual rejuvenation [64]. In Germany, news of Chancellor Konrad Adenauer's alleged treatment with sheep fetal injections stirred public interest. Authorities eventually banned such practices, citing health risks and unproven benefits (*New Scientist, 25th January 1997, "Germany bans sheep cell injections"*). These stories reflect the interplay of social prestige, medical mystique, therapeutic optimism, and the challenge of separating anecdote from evidence. Naturally, and it goes with our says, the contemporary preparation of xenogeneic cellular material has advanced far beyond anything imaginable in the 1990s. What was once a promising frontier has matured into a discipline defined by meticulous precision, elevated refinement, and uncompromising safety standards. Today's protocols, that are described in many of my previous books, employ sophisticated purification technologies, ultra-selective fractionation methods, and state-of-the-art biosecure processing environments developed and practiced by the Baden labs and FCTI Inc., hence transforming each preparation into a highly curated, scientifically orchestrated product. The result is not merely an improvement, but an evolution: a level of craftsmanship and reliability that positions modern xenogeneic cellular material in an entirely different league from its early predecessors, offering a standard of excellence aligned with the expectations of today's most discerning practitioners and clients.

Thymus Peptides: From Immune Modulation to Regenerative Application

Parallel to organ extracts arose a more molecularly grounded branch of peptide therapy: peptides from the thymus gland, with immune regulatory effects and therapeutic potential.

Immunologists had long noted the role of the thymus in T-cell maturation, central tolerance, and lymphoid organ development. Yet only by mid-20th century did researchers seek "thymus factors" that might modulate immunity therapeutically.

Using calf thymus tissue and mild acid or water extractions, scientists isolated peptide mixtures that promoted immune cell proliferation. One of the early commercial formulations was Thymalin, a mixture of thymus-derived peptides, marketed as an immunocorrector [65].

From Thymalin, scientists used chromatographic fractionation (e.g., reversed phase HPLC) to isolate small, bioactive peptides: most notably L-Glu-L-Trp, later synthesized and marketed as Thymogen. These smaller synthetic dipeptides demonstrated many of the immunomodulatory activities of the parent extract: enhanced T-cell differentiation, improved IL-2 and IFN secretion, neutrophil chemotaxis, phagocytosis, etc.

Another related synthetic peptide, Vilon, was also developed based on thymus extract research [66].

In the late 1970s and early 1980s, researchers isolated Thymosin β-family peptides (β4, β8, β9, etc.) from calf thymus. The PNAS article of 1982 described the isolation of thymosin β8 and β9 peptides, homologous to β4, expanding understanding of how small peptides could have actin-modulating, cell motility, immunoregulatory, or wound-healing effects [67].

Thymosin α1, a 28–amino acid peptide derived from prothymosin α, was the first thymosin fully sequenced and used clinically. It stimulates dendritic cell function, T-cell response, and has been used in viral, oncologic, and immunodeficiency contexts [68].

The 2024 comprehensive Review of Thymic Peptides and Hormones outlines how thymic peptides act through multiple mechanisms: stimulating T-cell maturation, NK cell activity, dendritic cell activation, and even promoting angiogenesis and wound healing [68]. The review notes that despite decades of research, thymic peptide preparations often maintain excellent safety profiles, even with long-term use and continue to be investigated in immunodeficiency, autoimmunity, transplantation, oncology, infection, and regenerative contexts [69].

Clinical use of thymic peptides has included adjuvant therapy in hepatitis B and C, and immune enhancement in cancer patients. While trial sizes are often small and data variable, few serious adverse events have been recorded [70]. Thus, thymus-derived peptides demonstrate a relatively clean history: from crude extracts to defined peptides to clinical deployment, with a clear immune and repair rationale.

My wife Prof. Dr. Michele Wong and I have already explored every key concept related to the thymus and *thymusspan* in depth in one of our previous volumes on Thymus Therapy [71].

Peptide Chemistry, Technology, and the Expansion Era

In the mid-20th century, several enabling technologies converged to accelerate peptide therapy:

- Solid-phase peptide synthesis (SPPS), introduced by Bruce Merrifield in 1963, allowed peptides to be built stepwise on a solid resin, dramatically improving yield, scalability, and complexity [72].
- Advances in purification and analytical chemistry (HPLC, reversed-phase chromatography, mass spectrometry) permitted finer separation, identification, and quantification of peptides.
- Recombinant protein engineering, enabled by molecular biology and gene cloning in the 1980s, removed dependence on animal extracts for hormones and growth factors. Insulin became one of the first recombinant therapeutics, fully human in sequence, expressed in yeast or bacteria.
- Chemical modifications (PEGylation, lipidation, cyclization, D-amino acid substitution) extended half-lives, reduced proteolysis, improved bioavailability, and expanded the practical viability of peptides as drugs.

By the late 20th century, peptide drugs were no longer curiosities but practical pharmaceuticals. According to a review "Therapeutic peptides: historical perspectives . . . , 2018," more than 60 peptide drugs had been approved in the U.S. and other markets; in parallel, over 150 were in active clinical development [73][74].

This expansion confirmed peptides' viability, but also brought sharper recognition of their limitations: low oral bioavailability, short circulation half-life, proteolytic degradation, and cost constraints.

Nonetheless, peptides became standard in endocrinology, oncology (e.g., somatostatin analogues), infectious disease (e.g., peptide antivirals), and more. As the 21st century advanced, researchers began exploring more exotic classes: nanomized peptides, organ extracts re-purposed, mitochondrial peptides, and peptide modulators of senescence.

Mitochondrial Peptides: From Hidden Genomic Messages to Therapeutic Agents

In the 2000s and 2010s, advances in genomics, proteomics, and high-throughput sequencing revealed that mitochondrial DNA (mtDNA) were once thought to encode only canonical respiratory proteins also harbored small open reading frames (sORFs) encoding short peptides. These mitochondria-derived peptides (MDPs) became a frontier in molecular medicine.

In 2001, Hashimoto et al. reported a small peptide, Humanin, encoded within a region overlapping the 16S rRNA, that protected neurons from Alzheimer's-associated amyloid-β toxicity. Humanin binds pro-apoptotic factors like Bax and IGFBP3, inhibits apoptotic cascades, and mitigates oxidative injury [75].

The discovery captured imaginations: mitochondria, beyond energy production, could issue molecular signals, the peptides that influence cell survival, aging, and stress response. Over the next decade, numerous studies would explore humanin's roles in metabolic syndrome, neurodegeneration, cardiovascular disease, and aging.

In 2015, the peptide MOTS-c ("mitochondrial open reading frame of 12S rRNA type-c") was identified. MOTS-c modulates metabolism, thus improving insulin sensitivity, enhancing AMPK signaling, and regulating nutrient stress responses (MOTS-c research, 2021). It has systemic effects; in mice, MOTS-c supplementation improved metabolic parameters and increased resilience to stress.

Around the same time, other small humanin-like peptides (SHLPs) encoded in 16S rRNA regions were discovered, each with distinct expression profiles and physiological roles. The new paradigm: mitochondria execute not only bioenergetics but endocrine and paracrine signaling via peptides.

These discoveries reopened the question: can mitochondria or mitochondrial peptides be used therapeutically? The early success of humanin analogues and MOTS-c in preclinical models suggests yes.

The Rise of Nano-Organic Xenogeneic Peptides

As molecular techniques matured, researchers returned to the dream of tissue-specific extracts but with modern rigor. Xenogeneic tissues (e.g., porcine, bovine, ovine organs) were harvested, processed to isolate low-molecular-weight peptides (often < 10 kDa), filtered, and further nanomized or nanoencapsulated. These nano-organ peptides aim to preserve organ-specific bioactive signature while eliminating impurities and immunogenic elements.

Whereas Niehans's fresh-cell approach operated by bulk suspensions, modern methods use mass spectrometry fingerprinting, peptide fractionation, sterilization, nanoparticle carriers, and preclinical safety testing. In effect, the field has returned to the organ-derived concept but stripped of bulk cells and guided by molecular analytics. Therefore, the concept that peptidespan influences lifespan through its effects on cellspan is becoming progressively substantiated by emerging scientific data. Though the literature is still nascent, some published studies demonstrate organ extract peptide stability (via MS analyses), safety in animal models, and early functional signs (e.g., improved mitochondrial function, tissue repair, regenerative biomarkers). These projects essentially fuse the old world of extract therapy with modern peptide science.

In parallel, some clinics and aesthetic medicine practices (especially in Switzerland) still market refined "extract" or "revitalization" formulas that trace lineage to Niehans's CLP or Revitalisation products though now often chemically or biologically purified.

Thus, the narrative of peptide therapy comes full circle: from crude organ extracts to defined dipeptides, synthetic analogues, recombinant hormones, mitochondrial peptides, and now nanomized organ-specific classes with each generation more precise, safer, and evidence-driven.

By the early 2000s, the landscape of peptide therapeutics was changing. Advances in molecular biology, peptide synthesis, and purification had created a new era of precision therapeutics. But while synthetic peptides proliferated in academic and pharmaceutical pipelines, another, quieter revolution was taking place, the one that revisited the biological complexity of natural tissues and sought to harness peptides not in isolation, but as integrated, organ-specific signaling systems.

This was the beginning of the Nano-Organic Peptide (NOP) era—an approach rooted in xenogeneic peptide extraction, where peptides were derived not from recombinant synthesis or chemical production, but from carefully sourced mammalian tissues, rich in organ-specific signaling molecules, processed in a way that preserved their native bioactivity.

The genesis of this work was, for me, deeply personal and profoundly technical. In the early 2000s, I was immersed in the study of aging, chronic degenerative diseases, and the subtle decline of intracellular communication networks that underpin tissue dysfunction. I began to see that many therapeutic failures in regenerative medicine stemmed from a single critical oversight: we were treating tissues as if they were homogeneous. But every organ speaks its own biochemical language and I wanted to find a way to recover and reintroduce that language, in its native dialect, back into failing systems.

At the time, I was collaborating with legacy laboratories in Switzerland and Germany, where remnants of Paul Niehans' original protocols still survived in hand-written notebooks and aging technicians' memories. Niehans' work with cellular extracts was visionary but constrained by the technology of his era. I believed it could be modernized albeit not through synthetic mimicry but through precision bioextraction, preserving the full spectrum of native peptides while eliminating immunogenic debris, as in fetal stage cells are lacking of immunogenicity, which only comes in with the first sip of the mother's milk.

In 2002, after nearly two years of trial and error, I developed a novel extraction protocol that would later become the cornerstone of the Nano-Organ Peptide (NOP) manufacturing process: a cold-enzymatic, multi-phase tissue disaggregation technique. This landmark discovery and invention has irrevocably transformed the landscape of biomedical science and became a triumph of insight and ingenuity truly worthy of the Nobel Prize. The key principle was simple, but revolutionary in practice to liberate biologically active peptides from xenogeneic tissues without exposing them to heat, chemical denaturants, or mechanical shear that would disrupt peptide folding or post-translational modifications.

The process operated at sub-physiological temperatures (4–8°C) and utilized a panel of organ-specific, pH-optimized enzymes that selectively cleaved protein precursors into low-molecular-weight peptide fragments. These fragments, between

300–3,000 Daltons, represent the bioactive signaling range small enough to cross cell membranes, but still large enough to retain conformational specificity.

Each step was precisely timed, temperature-locked, and tightly controlled for oxygenation, pH drift, and protease activation windows. Over 14–18 hours, what emerged from the tissue matrix was not a slurry, but a clarified, bioactive nano-peptide extract rich in mitochondrial peptides, nuclear transcriptional co-regulators, and matrix-derived signaling fragments.

This method became the technical and philosophical foundation of Nano-Organ Peptides (NOP)—a platform that today spans dozens of organ types, including brain, heart, liver, pancreas, kidney, skin, thymus, and retina.

Scaling this technology from bench-top experiments to Good Manufacturing Practice (GMP)-compliant production required rigorous engineering. We designed a proprietary closed-loop system in which extraction, filtration, ultracentrifugation, and sterile bottling all occurred under controlled cold-chain conditions. Special attention was given to nanofiltration, using membranes with precise molecular weight cutoffs to ensure purity without sacrificing peptide complexity.

All xenogeneic tissues were ethically sourced from veterinary-inspected, disease-free herds, and harvested within two hours post-mortem to preserve molecular integrity. The end product, NOP extracts, underwent mass spectrometry fingerprinting, sterility testing, endotoxin clearance, and proteomic profiling before entering clinical-grade applications.

By 2005, we had developed a library of over 30 organ-specific peptide matrices, each tailored to a target tissue's biochemical needs. These were not blunt instruments; they were whispering codes capable of modulating gene expression, rejuvenating mitochondrial function, silencing inflammatory cascades, and restoring lost tissue identity. Now we have over 150 different organ-specific peptide formulations that can be procured from over 700 different cell types that we have described in one of the groundbreaking articles recently [303].

One of the most profound realizations during this journey was that these peptides did not function as drugs in the conventional sense. They were not receptor agonists or antagonists alone, instead they were epigenetic modulators, transcriptional influencers, and cellular dialect coaches, retraining cells to remember what they once were.

We observed this repeatedly in early case studies: a degenerating retina exposed to retinal NOP regained metabolic plasticity; senescent skin fibroblasts treated with dermal NOP began expressing youthful collagen transcripts; even chronic inflammatory markers like NF-κB and IL-6 were downregulated in models treated with organ-specific peptides.

Further, multi-organ combinations (e.g., thymus + brain + liver peptides) produced synergistic effects especially in aging patients where systemic degeneration was never isolated to a single tissue. The peptide libraries worked together, restoring systemic resilience by addressing organ-organ crosstalk and rebalancing metabolic load-sharing across systems.

Between 2007 and 2012, we began gathering early data on the clinical applications of NOPs in neurodegenerative disorders, autoimmune conditions, metabolic syndrome, and tissue regeneration. Our peptides were being used in integrative clinics across Europe and parts of Asia, with standardized protocols and safety data.

In 2015, we presented at the Congress on Regenerative Therapies in Geneva, introducing the concept of "tissue intelligence reactivation"—the idea that each organ harbors a dormant capacity for repair, provided it receives the correct biochemical signals. NOPs, we proposed, were that signal. Around that time the cold-enzymatic extraction technology has earned multiple awards for innovation in Europe and Middle East.

Today, a growing number of labs are expanding on this work, analyzing NOPs using mass spectrometry, profiling nano-encapsulated delivery systems, and exploring combination therapies with stem cell exosomes, NAD+ precursors, and mRNA therapies. But the heart of the technology remains unchanged: cold-extracted, biologically preserved, organ-specific peptides that speak the native language of the tissue from which they came.

Looking back, I realize that this was never just a technical project, it was a philosophical endeavor. The central question was always: "*What does it mean for a tissue to remember how to heal?*" And the answer, it turns out, may not lie in replacing cells or inserting genes, but in reminding the body—molecularly, epigenetically, energetically—of its original blueprint.

Nano-Organ Peptides are not just a technology; they are a bridge between the reductionism of synthetic peptides and the chaotic complexity of whole-cell therapies. Between the classical cell therapy visions of Niehans and the precision medicine of tomorrow.

For me, this work continues not only in laboratories and manufacturing suites, but in clinical settings, research symposiums, and in the quiet awe of watching a failing system begin to regenerate itself with nothing more than nature's original alphabet, rearranged and reintroduced.

Interpreting the Arc: Patterns, Lessons, and Legacy

Looking back, several recurring patterns emerge from the history of peptide therapy:

1. Speculation to molecular precision: What began as tissue extracts and bold clinical claims has, over decades, evolved toward molecular definition, synthetic peptides, recombinant biology, and proteomic analytics.
2. Form following function: Early forms (fresh cells, extracts) prioritized presumed vitality; modern forms (nanoparticles, peptide fractions) prioritize safety, consistency, targeted delivery, and mechanism.
3. Controversy as catalyst: Niehans's dramatic claims, celebrity patrons, and extract mystique provoked criticism by forcing medicine to clarify standards of evidence, regulation, and reproducibility.
4. Omics and organ specificity: Modern peptide research emphasizes organ-specific patterns (mitochondrial peptides, nano-organ extracts), echoing Niehans's organ-suspension philosophy but rendered credible via molecular science.
5. Clinical translation is slow: Many peptide discoveries remain at preclinical stage; only a minority (e.g., insulin, thymosin α_1, somatostatin analogues) have reached wide clinical adoption. Safety, delivery, regulatory pathway, and cost remain obstacles.
6. Cultural resonance persists: The romance of "injection of youth," "vital force," or "organ repair" endures in wellness, aesthetic, and alternative

medicine. Some patent or bioformulations trace lineage to older extract practices, albeit reformulated.

The history of peptides is not linear but cyclic: bold clinical intuitions, skeptical pushback, molecular elucidation, reformulated application. Today's peptide therapeutics stand at the intersection of biology, engineering, and medicine bearing both the promise and caution of their storied ancestry.

Epilogue: From Legacy to Frontiers

As we close this historical chapter, it's fitting to reflect on how the past informs the future. The experiments of early chemists and surgeons, the embryonic extract injections of Niehans, thymus immunomodulators, recombinant hormones, mitochondrial peptides, they all contribute conceptual DNA to today's frontier.

In the upcoming chapters, we will dive into organ-targeted peptide therapeutics, nanomized delivery, mitochondrial peptide signaling, and clinical applications in neurodegeneration, cardiovascular repair, metabolic therapy, and regeneration. We will stand on the shoulders of insulin, Niehans, thymus peptides, and mitochondrial discovery which yet aim to go beyond, into safer, more precise, and clinically actionable peptide medicine.

Peptides are no longer fringe curiosities. They are becoming the backbone of regenerative protocols, the molecular keys that unlock waiting biology. Their history is cautionary, dramatic, ingenious and above all, a reminder that the frontier of medicine is as much about imagination as it is about molecules.

CHAPTER 3

Safety, Carcinogenicity, and Characterization of Therapeutic Peptides

(with Prof. Thomas Skutella, MD, PostDoc)

Why Safety Matters in Peptide Therapeutics

As peptide therapies and peptide-derived extracts increasingly enter translational and clinical domains, the question of safety becomes paramount. Unlike small molecules, peptides may interact with cellular systems more intimately binding receptors, entering cells, or influencing gene networks. Among the foremost concerns are cytotoxicity, immunogenicity, and the possibility, however remote, of promoting neoplastic transformation. To earn acceptance in medicine, peptide-based therapeutics must undergo rigorous assays demonstrating absence of carcinogenic potential, defined pharmacokinetics, and consistent characterization. In this chapter, we review experimental evidence for the safety of peptide extracts (notably 300 kDa "Mito Organelles" extracts), the methods by which peptides are characterized and validated (especially via mass spectrometry), and the limitations and challenges of asserting long-term safety.

MTT and Cell Transformation Assays of Mito Organelles Extracts

In one of the recent studies conducted by my team we rigorously tested the cytotoxic and carcinogenic potential of 300 kDa cellular extracts branded as 'Mito Organelles (MO)", derived from various organs (heart, brain, kidney, cartilage, thymus, placenta, lungs, connective tissue) and composite extracts (LPPSIMKE: liver, pancreas, placenta, kidney, intestines, retina). The investigators employed two canonical in vitro assays: the MTT viability assay and the BALB/c-3T3 cell transformation assay (CTA). Their findings constitute one of the most comprehensive published safety assessments for complex peptide-protein extracts of this type [29].

In the MTT assay, human MCF-7 breast cancer cells served as a model to evaluate metabolic viability. The MO extracts tested both in the presence and absence of oxidative stress (via low-dose H_2O_2) did not reduce cell viability relative to controls. In fact, under mild oxidative stress, some extracts appeared to modestly enhance viability, suggesting a protective or trophic effect under stress conditions (rather than cytotoxicity) [29][76].

Parallel to this, the BALB/c-3T3 CTA was used to probe transformative potential. In standard CTA protocols, fibroblasts (BALB/c-3T3 cells) are treated with candidate agents for a defined "initiation" window, then cultured for weeks to allow focus formation. Morphologically aberrant foci, including multilayered clusters, loss of contact inhibition, piling, are taken as evidence of malignant transformation (Kakunaga CTA method). In these assays, MO extracts did not induce any foci or transformation above background. In strong contrast, classical positive controls (e.g. MCA / TPA) produced robust foci, validating assay sensitivity. Thus, in multiple independent runs, none of the tissue-derived MO extracts posed detectable carcinogenic risk in that in vitro surrogate model (Chan et al., 2024) [77][29].

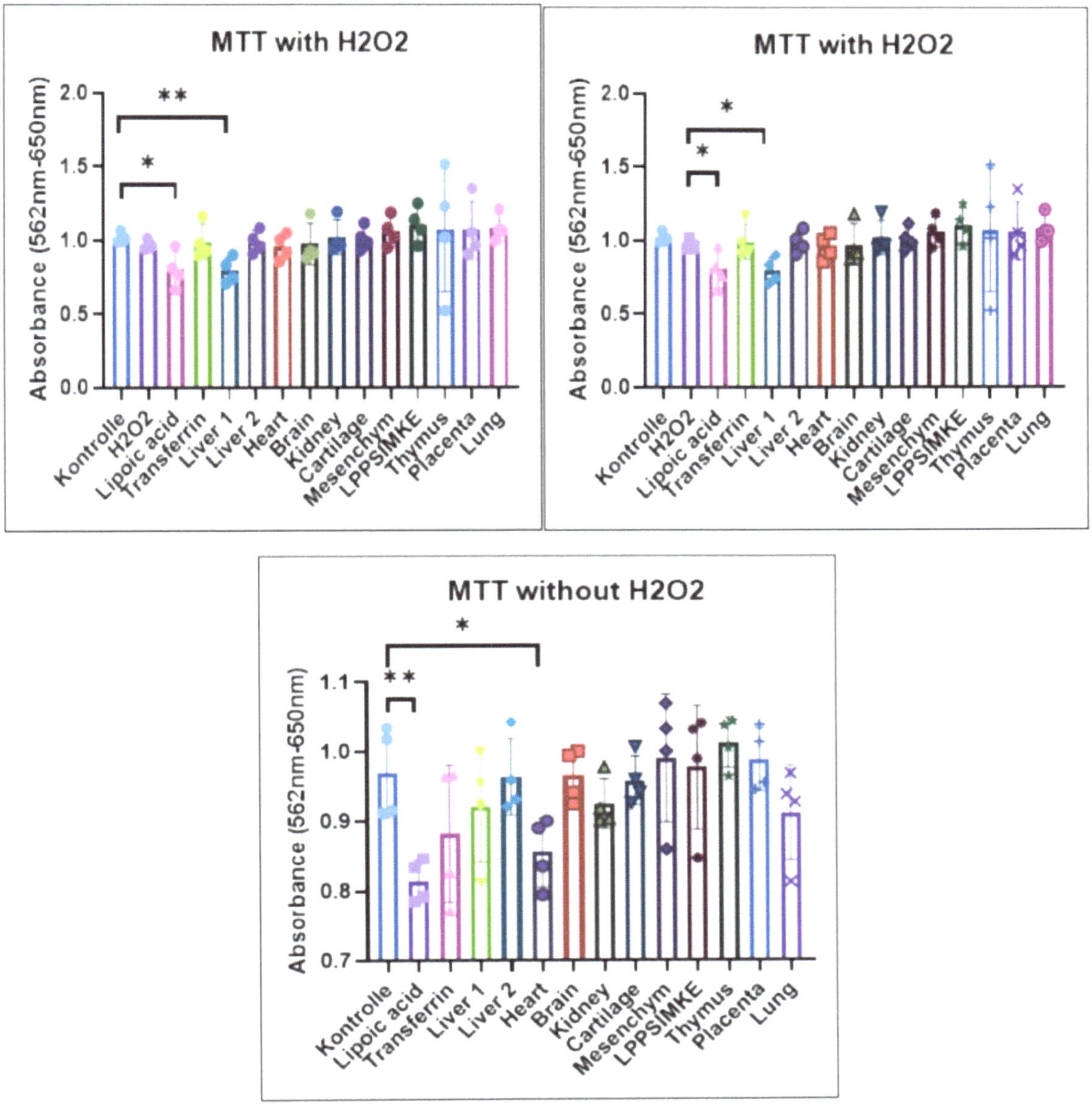

Fig 3.1. *MTT Assay Analysis of Different Extracts in the Presence and Absence of cellular stress with H_2O_2.*

The figure displays three bar graphs representing the MTT assay results with and without H_2O_2 treatment, comparing the metabolic activity of cells treated with various extracts. The assay measures cell viability through absorbance values at 562 nm–650 nm, reflecting mitochondrial activity. Top Left Panel: MTT Assay with H_2O_2 (First Experiment) - Cells were *treated with H_2O_2 alongside different extracts, including "control," "H_2O_2," "Lipofect," and several compound extracts such as "Liver" and others. Statistical significance is highlighted by the asterisks (* and **), indicating significant differences between treatment groups. Extracts "Lipoic acid shows a significant reduction in absorbance compared to the control group, implying reduced cell survival in the presence of oxidative stress induced by H_2O_2. Top Right Panel: MTT Assay with H_2O_2 (Second Experiment) – A repeat experiment with a similar setup, showing how different extracts protect cells from H_2O_2-induced oxidative stress. Notable extracts and others are compared, with specific extracts showing significant differences (denoted by * and **). These results are consistent with those in the first experiment, reaffirming the protective effect of all extracts, particularly. Bottom Panel: MTT Assay without H_2O_2 – This panel represents the MTT assay in the absence of oxidative stress (without H_2O_2), focusing on the basal effect of the extracts on cell viability. "Lipoic acid," show significant differences in absorbance compared to the control. Asterisks denote statistically significant variations, suggesting that some component naturally enhance or reduce cell viability. Statistical Significance: Asterisks denote statistical significance between groups: *P < 0.05 (single asterisk, *) indicates significant differences; *P < 0.01 (double asterisks, **) indicates highly significant differences.*

Abbreviations: Kontrolle–Control group without treatment. H_2O_2–Hydrogen peroxide-induced oxidative stress model. Lipofect–A commercial reagent used as a control. Various "Liver" and other terms refer to plant extracts or compounds being tested for their protective effects. Each data point represents the mean absorbance with error bars indicating standard deviation across multiple replicates.

Taken together, these dual assays suggest that at least under the tested conditions and doses, the MO peptide/protein extracts lack overt cytotoxic or transforming activity. While in vitro assays cannot fully substitute for in vivo long-term carcinogenicity studies, they are widely accepted screening tools, and negative results here are a promising first safety indicator [43].

A

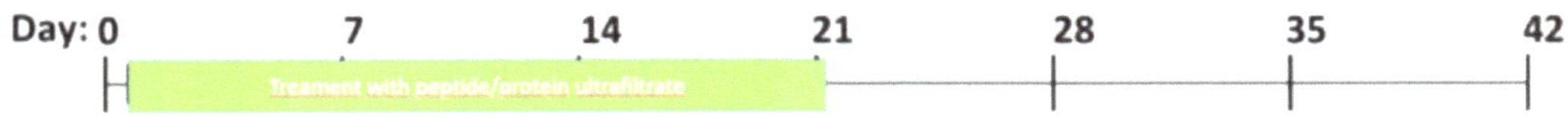

B

BALB/c-3T3 Cell Transformation Assay

		positive control MCA/TPA	MO-100 heart	brain	kidney	cartilage	mesenchyme	LPPSIMKE	thymus	placenta	lung
exp.1	number color	15	0	0	0	0	0	0	0	0	0
exp.2	number color	18	0	0	0	0	0	0	0	0	0
exp.3	number color	14	0	0	0	0	0	0	0	0	0

Fig 3.2. *Schedule of the BALB/c-3T3 Cell Transformation Assay and B) Results for Various Tissue Extracts.*

The Table above presents the results of the BALB/c-3T3 cell transformation assay, which measures the ability of various tissue extracts and treatments to induce transformation in BALB/c-3T3 cells, as indicated by the formation of colonies. The assay is performed across three independent experiments (exp. 1, exp. 2, and exp. 3), and the number of colonies observed in each condition is recorded. Positive Control (MCA/TPA): The positive control group treated with MCA/TPA (a known tumor promoter and inducer of cell transformation) shows consistent colony formation across all three experiments, with 15, 18, and 14 colonies in experiments 1, 2, and 3, respectively. This confirms the assay's sensitivity to transformation stimuli. MO-100 and Tissue Extracts (Heart, Brain, Kidney, Cartilage, Mesenchyme, LPPSIMKE, Thymus, Placenta, Lungs): No colonies were observed for MO-300 and the various tissue extracts (heart, brain, kidney, cartilage, mesenchyme, LPPSIMKE, thymus, placenta, and lung) in any of the experiments. This suggests these extracts do not induce transformation under the experimental conditions. The positive control (MCA/TPA) successfully induces colony formation in BALB/c-3T3 cells, validating the assay. However, none of the tested tissue extracts MO-300 treatment induced transformation in this system, as evidenced by the absence of colonies across all three experiments.

Abbreviations: MCA/TPA: 3-Methylcholanthrene/12-O-tetradecanoylphorbol-13-acetate, known carcinogens and tumor promoters; MO-300: A tested compound or treatment.

Safety assessments cannot stand alone; they must be paired with precise molecular characterization and reproducibility. For peptide extracts, mass spectrometry (MS) is the gold standard to validate composition, detect contaminating species, and monitor stability. A recent stability study of Nano-Organ Peptides (NOPs) by Chan, Wong, Lakey et al. (2024) demonstrates the depth of analytical rigor now feasible for peptide extracts [43][78].

In that study, organ-specific cellular ultrafiltrates termed NOPs were subjected to MALDI-TOF and LC-MS/MS over extended storage at different temperatures (4 °C, room temperature, etc.). The investigators observed that certain peptide peaks (e.g., ~1,037 m/z, ~1,056 m/z) remained stable over months, while lesser peaks diminished, broadened, or shifted over time thus providing evidence of slow degradation or fragmentation (Chan et al., 2024). The high-resolution fingerprinting enabled reproducible detection of key peptide signatures, and degradation kinetics could be tracked quantitatively [79][80][81][82].

This approach, mass spectral fingerprinting, allows one to define a "molecular fingerprint" of a given peptide extract batch, cross-validate between lots, and detect adulteration, contamination, or drifts over time. In the NOP stability work, peak retention times, intensity ratios, and fragmentation profiles provided a molecular QC (quality control) scaffold upon which safety testing can rely [83].

Beyond NOPs, broader "organ-derived ultrafiltrate" proteomic studies have shown that tissues yield characteristic small-protein and peptide networks covering RNA-binding factors, lipid-binding proteins, oxidative stress regulators, and metabolic modulators (e.g. in rabbit organ ultrafiltrates) (Exploring the Molecular Tapestry, 2023). These findings underscore that peptide extracts are not random blends but reflect the molecular ecology of their originating tissues [84].

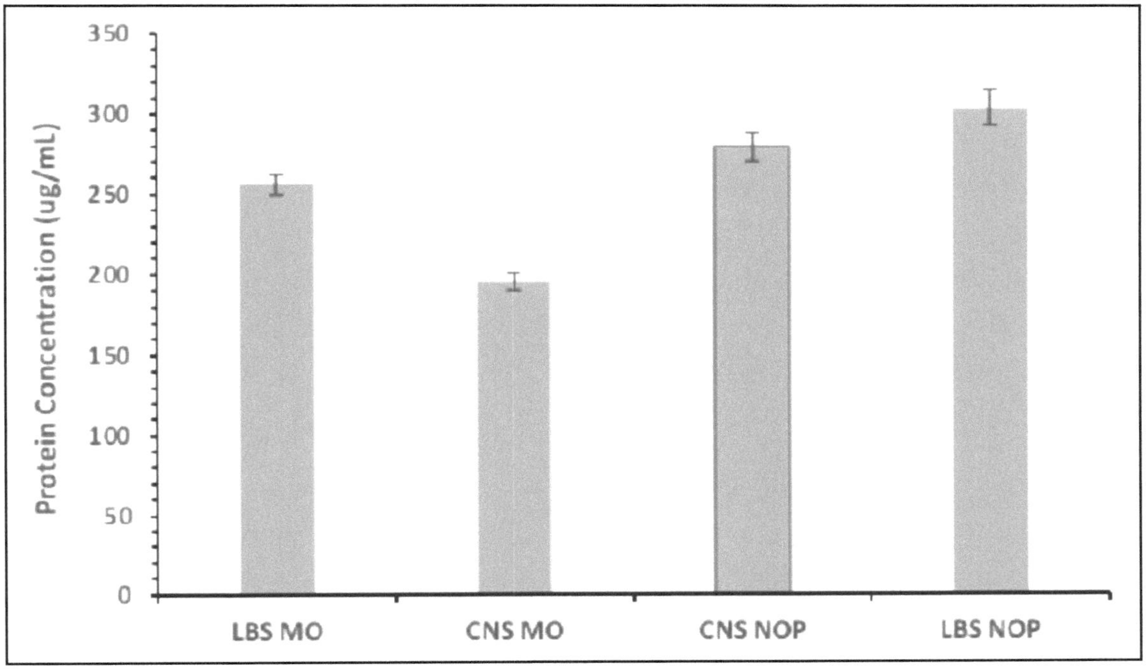

Fig 3.3. *Average protein concentration (ug/mL) of batch 1 and 2 for LBS MO, CNS MO, CNS NOP, and LBS NOP. The black bars represent standard error. No statistically significant differences were found between batches for any samples (p=ns) although statistically significant differences were found between groups ($p<0.05$).*

Thus, the trifecta of fingerprint stability, spectral reproducibility, and proteomic context is essential for any peptide therapeutic moving toward clinical use.

While in vitro assays provide valuable safety signals, they inherently carry limitations. The fact that MO extracts passed MTT and CTA screens does not guarantee zero long-term risk. It does, however, strongly argue against acute cytotoxic or initiator-like carcinogenic potential under the tested conditions.

To further bolster this assertion:

- The size cutoff used (300 kDa extracts) suggests that most large proteins, viral contaminants, or intact growth factors are excluded, reducing oncogenic risk.

- The peptide fractions are often of low molecular weight (<10 kDa) after ultrafiltration, a range generally less prone to harbor proto-oncogenes or receptor-overstimulating domains.
- The regulatory science paradigm often accepts negative in vitro transformation plus negative in vivo rodent studies as evidence of acceptable risk (OECD guidelines for testing carcinogenicity).
- Long-term animal studies (e.g., rodent chronic exposure) would be the ideal confirmatory step; absence of transformation in fibroblast assays strongly reduces risk but does not fully exclude rare events or context-dependent tumorigenesis.

Thus, while one cannot declare "zero carcinogenic risk" from current data, the available evidence provides a robust safety foundation that peptide extracts given at defined purity, doses, and QC do not appear to provoke neoplastic changes in standard in vitro models.

Molecular Fingerprinting and Quality Control

At the heart of peptide safety assurance lies molecular fingerprinting—the requirement that each therapeutic peptide or complex extract be defined by a reproducible, high-resolution molecular signature. Such fingerprints ordinarily derive from mass spectrometry (MS) analyses that capture the critical m/z (mass-to-charge) peaks, fragmentation patterns, adduct distributions, isotopic envelopes, and relative intensities across a defined scan window. These features form a "molecular barcode" unique to a given peptide or extract batch, permitting direct comparisons across lots and over time [85].

In practice, any drift in key peak ratios, emergence of novel impurity peaks, or disappearance of expected fragments should trigger batch rejection or further investigation. This approach mirrors the rigorous standards imposed on small molecules and biologics: identity, purity, and stability must be documented and validated (FDA / ICH / EMA guidelines governing peptide and protein therapeutics). Recent reviews emphasize that peptide/protein therapeutics must satisfy not only potency and pharmacokinetics criteria, but also physical and chemical stability under storage and formulation conditions, and that regulatory authorities now mandate tailored bioanalytical workflows for each peptide drug (Regulatory Guidelines for the Analysis of Therapeutic Peptides and Proteins, 2025) [86].

But mass spectrometry alone is often insufficient. Orthogonal analytic techniques such as high-performance liquid chromatography (HPLC), peptide mapping, amino acid analysis, and quantitative nuclear magnetic resonance (qNMR) should supplement MS to detect structural isomers, conformers, or low-level impurities invisible to MS fragmentation. Indeed, NMR-based fingerprinting (for example, HiFSA sequencing) has been proposed as a powerful QC/QA tool, capable of confirming both identity and absolute purity, including detection of subtle structural deviations undetected by MS or chromatography (Quality Control of Therapeutic Peptides by ^{1}H NMR HiFSA Sequencing, PMC) [87].

Together, the combination of mass spectrometric "molecular barcodes" and orthogonal confirmatory analyses forms the bedrock of molecular quality control (QC) that became a prerequisite for any peptide entering downstream safety testing (fig.).

Once a peptide or extract batch is molecularly validated, it must next pass in vitro cytotoxicity screening to exclude overt cell damage or metabolic disruption. Standard assays such as MTT, resazurin (alamarBlue), SRB, or CellTiter-Glo can be deployed across multiple cell lines, including non-malignant primary cells (e.g., fibroblasts, endothelial cells), target tissue-derived cells, and sometimes cancer lines, to detect undesired toxicity or preferential vulnerability [88][89].

A rigorous screening protocol entails dosing across a wide concentration range (including multiples of expected therapeutic exposure) and under different conditions (e.g., serum presence vs. serum-deprived culture). A peptide that reduces cell viability below an acceptable threshold (e.g., < 80% viability relative to control) or displays steep toxicity curves is a red flag. Because peptides may exert effects indirectly (such as via mitochondrial destabilization), it is wise to complement viability assays with reactive oxygen species (ROS) measurements, mitochondrial membrane potential assays (e.g., JC-1, TMRE), and apoptosis / necrosis markers (e.g., Annexin V / PI staining) [90].

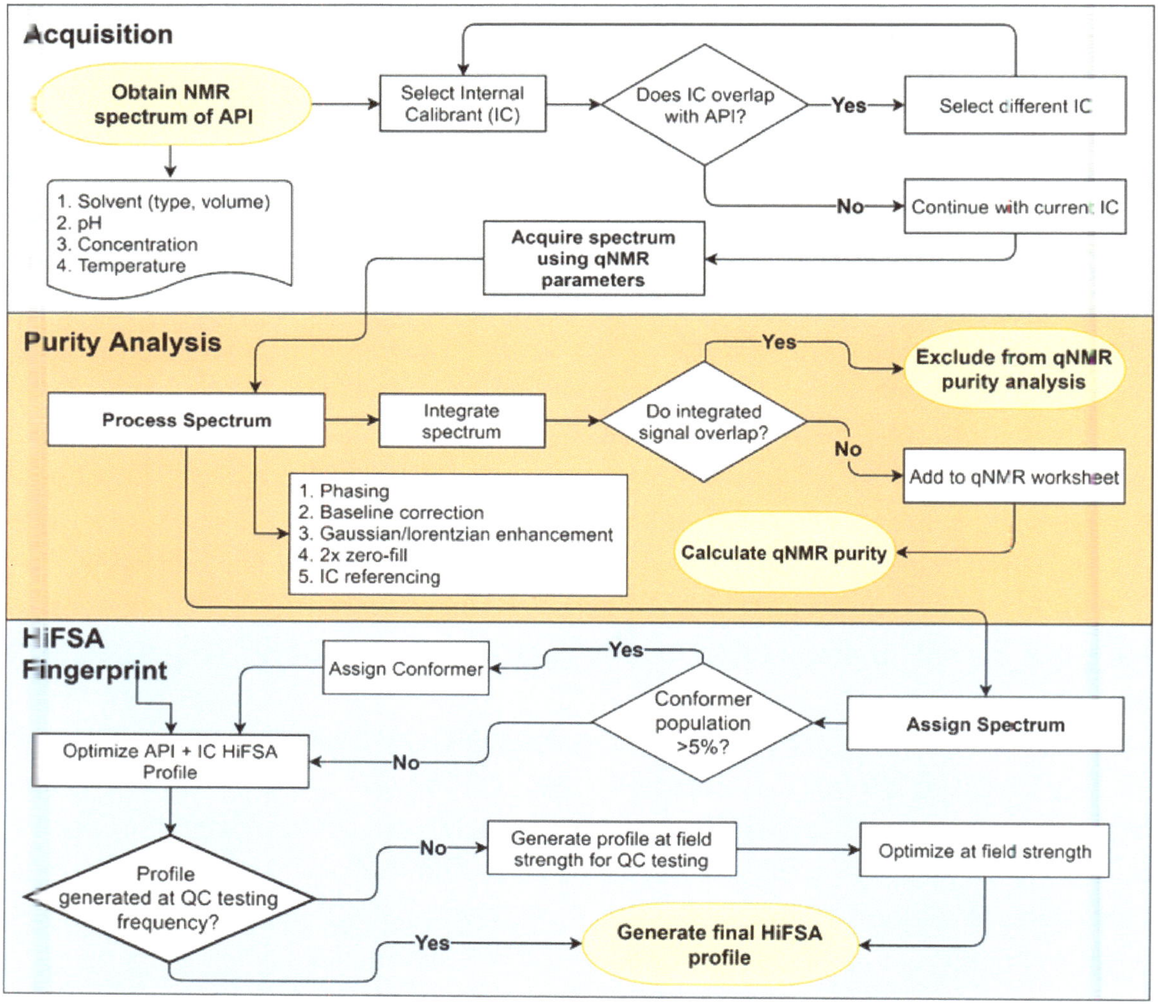

Fig 3.4. *Workflow for the generation of a general QC protocol for pharmaceutically and biologically relevant peptides (source: Choules MP, Bisson J, Gao W, Lankin DC. McAlpine JB, Niemitz M, Jaki BU, Franzblau SG, Pauli GF. Quality Control of Therapeutic Peptides by 1H NMR HiFSA Sequencing. J Org Chem. 2019).*

Such in vitro screening does not definitively guarantee safety in vivo, but it serves as a crucial gatekeeper: any candidate exhibiting dose-dependent cytotoxicity under physiologically relevant conditions should be modified or rejected before advancing to more resource-intensive testing [91][29].

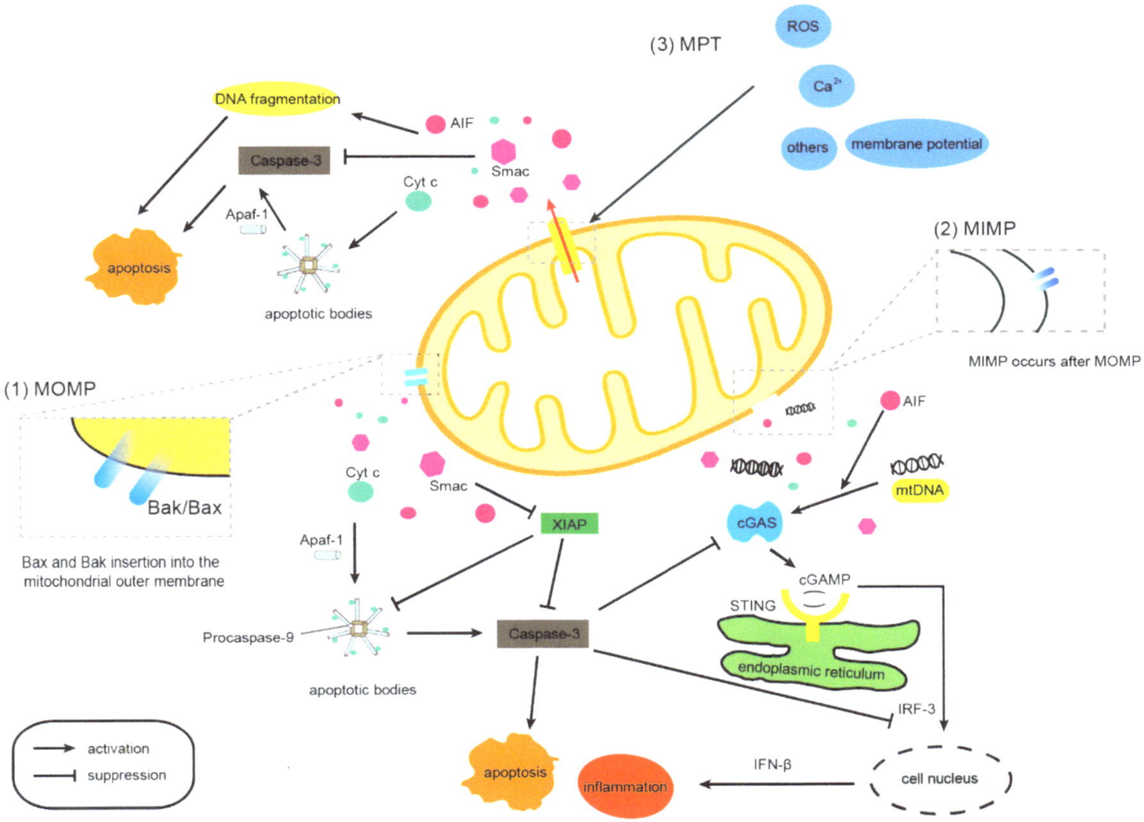

Fig 3.5. *Main apoptosis mechanisms induced by MOMP, MIMP, and MPT. (1) Bak/Bax aggregates and forms pores in the OMM. Cyt c, AIF, Smac, and other molecules leak from the pores. After a series of reactions, Cyt c, Apaf-1, and procaspase-9 assemble into apoptotic bodies and subsequently activate caspase-3. Caspase-3 inhibits inflammation and induces apoptosis. The released Smac can inhibit the antiapoptotic effect of XIAP. (2) MIMP occurs after MOMP. Under pathological conditions or in the absence of caspases, the cGAS-STING signaling pathway can be activated by mitochondrial DNA (mtDNA) and AIF to release IFN-β and other inflammatory factors, thus triggering inflammation. (3) Changes in intracellular ROS, Ca2+ concentration, or mitochondrial membrane potential depolarization can induce MPTP to remain open, leading to changes in both outer and inner mitochondrial membrane permeability. During MPT, Cyt c, AIF, Smac, and other molecules are released, inducing apoptosis in a caspase-3-dependent manner. (Source: Wang, H., Zhang, C., Li, M., Liu, C., Wang, J., Ou, X., & Han, Y. (2022). Antimicrobial Peptides Mediate Apoptosis by Changing*

Mitochondrial Membrane Permeability. International Journal of Molecular Sciences, 23(21), 12732. https://doi.org/10.3390/ijms232112732)

Beyond cytotoxicity, there is legitimate concern, particularly for long-term or regenerative peptide therapies, about potential neoplastic transformation. To address that, peptides should undergo in vitro transformation assays, such as the cell transformation assay (CTA) using BALB/c-3T3 fibroblasts or other established models. In a CTA, cells are exposed to the candidate peptide (or extract) over a defined initiation period, after which they are grown in culture for several weeks to observe focus formation, morphological transformation, anchorage independence, or colony overgrowth indicative of neoplastic conversion. Positive controls (e.g., known carcinogens) validate assay sensitivity, while negative controls help define baseline [29].

For example, in the study of 300 kDa "Mito Organelles" extracts, neither the MTT assay nor the BALB/c-3T3 CTA revealed cytotoxicity or transformation potential (i.e., no foci significantly above background) (Chan et al.) [29][92]. Such results strengthen confidence in absence of overt initiating carcinogenic risk, at least within the tested dose ranges and exposure windows. However, assay limitations must be acknowledged: in vitro models cannot capture the full complexity of in vivo mutagenesis, tissue microenvironment, or immune surveillance.

Hence, negative results in transformation assays are necessary but not sufficient; they reduce risk and help prioritize safe candidates, but do not replace in vivo long-term evaluations.

To move from bench to bedside, candidate peptides must ultimately be assessed in in vivo long-term studies, typically in rodents or larger mammals, under controlled chronic administration. These studies should monitor for:

- Tumor incidence in various organs (histopathology of liver, lung, kidney, spleen, etc.)
- Hyperplasia, dysplasia, or atypia in treated tissues
- Ectopic proliferation or aberrant tissue growth
- Off-target organ toxicity, including liver, kidney, heart

- Biomarkers of transformation (e.g., Ki67, p53, PCNA)
- Mortality, morbidity, and morbidity-free survival

Dosing should ideally exceed anticipated human exposure (e.g., 10×) and include recovery periods to assess reversibility. These models provide the crucial proof that a peptide does not lead to latent neoplastic emergence. In regulatory paradigms, negative long-term animal data, combined with in vitro safety screens, often satisfy initial assessments of carcinogenic risk [29][93].

One of the greatest challenges for peptide therapeutics is immunogenicity—the ability of a peptide or its impurities to provoke an unwanted immune response (e.g. generation of anti-drug antibodies, hypersensitivity). This is not hypothetical: even fully human peptides can trigger immune responses when modified, aggregated, or delivered alongside adjuvant-like contaminants [94].

Modern regulatory guidance mandates immunogenicity risk assessment, including:

- In silico epitope prediction (MHC binding affinity, T-cell epitope mapping)
- In vitro assays using human peripheral blood mononuclear cells (PBMCs) to assess T-cell activation or antibody binding
- Monitoring for anti-drug antibodies (ADAs) in preclinical and clinical studies
- Cross-reactivity screening against human proteome to detect "molecular mimicry" events.

Recent reviews emphasize that immunogenicity remains a major barrier to translation and must be rigorously addressed at early stages (Achilleos et al., 2025). Strategies to mitigate immunogenicity include deimmunization, masking immunogenic epitopes, limiting aggregate formation, and ensuring purity from trace contaminants [95].

Off-target binding or signaling is also a risk as peptides may inadvertently interact with unintended receptors or cellular pathways. Comprehensive receptor affinity profiling, cellular transcriptome modulation assays, and pathway screening panels help identify and mitigate such risks prior to human application.

- Even a peptide that is safe and non-immunogenic must be understood in pharmacokinetic (PK) terms how it is absorbed, distributed, metabolized, and excreted. Key features to establish include:
- Plasma half-life (t½)
- Volume of distribution (Vd)
- Metabolic breakdown pathways (proteolysis, deamidation, oxidation)
- Tissue accumulation or retention
- Clearance routes (renal, hepatic, proteolytic catabolism)

A peptide accumulating in tissues (or generating harmful metabolites) over repeated dosing might eventually provoke toxicity. Metabolite profiling via LC-MS/MS is essential to detect any reactive or unexpected breakdown products. Knowledge of PK and clearance also informs dosage scheduling and safety margins [96].

Approval or deployment of peptide therapies should not mark the end of safety vigilance. The subtle and cumulative nature of peptide modulation, particularly for regenerative or chronic applications, necessitates post-market surveillance. Clinicians and sponsors should monitor for rare adverse events, late-onset neoplasms, immune reactions, or off-target effects over years of use. Registries, pharmacovigilance databases, and real-world evidence studies provide critical long-term validation of safety.

Together, the scientific narrative of peptide safety is not a checklist but a dynamic, layered process from molecular signature to cellular screens, animal models, immunology, PK, and clinical surveillance. Only through such integrated rigor can peptide therapeutics fulfill their promise of effectiveness with confidence in safety.

Conclusion: Confidence Through Rigor, Humility Before Complexity

In the unfolding era of peptide therapeutics, safety is not simply a regulatory box to check—it is the very foundation upon which progress must be built. Our experimental investigations of 300 kDa "Mito Organelles" extracts, subjected to dual screening via MTT cytotoxicity assays and BALB/c-3T3 cell transformation assays, provide encouraging evidence that well-defined peptide and peptide–protein extracts can preserve viability and resist neoplastic conversion in vitro. Coupled with the rigorous molecular fingerprinting and longitudinal stability studies of nanomized organ peptides (NOPs), the field now benefits from robust tools capable of establishing batch identity, monitoring drift, and guarding against impurities. Together, these advances imbue us with qualified confidence, not mere hubris that peptide therapies can indeed strike a balance of potency and safety.

Yet confidence must walk hand in hand with humility. Biological systems are deeply complex, and rare or context-dependent adverse events may lie beyond the reach of standard in vitro and short-term in vivo assays. Unpredicted interactions with human immunology, epigenetic drift, low-frequency mutagenesis, long latency tumorigenesis, or subtle off-target signaling effects may only emerge over years of human use. The history of pharmacology is littered with drugs once believed benign that later revealed hidden risks when deployed at scale.

From a biological vantage point, the human being as an animal that seats as a sovereign of the animal kingdom is far less exceptional than we like to imagine. Strip away the myths of superiority, peel back the layers of culture, and we discover a humbling truth: in the earliest moments of development, every creature on Earth begins with the same cellular grammar. A human embryo, a whale embryo, a mouse embryo, when scrutinized under a microscope, they speak a dialect so similar that only time and differentiation reveal their destinies. It is this shared origin, this ancient symmetry, that has pushed scientists to question long-held boundaries and has opened the philosophical space to explore whether xenogeneic fetal tissues and cells, under rigorously controlled and ethically governed research conditions, could one day inform new avenues in regenerative medicine. And so, from the vantage point of the researcher, author and educator, I often find myself reflecting not merely as a scientist but as a witness to biology's deep unity. During the thousands of sleepless nights inside the laboratory, where I and my team gently urge the edges of scientific reason to stretch beyond their usual contours and tempting the fabric of reality to writhe until it mirrors the brief shadows that move within me, the distinctions between kingdoms blur, and I am reminded daily of a simple truth that guides my work: "*I do human, I do animal, I do plant.*" Not because I wish to collapse their differences, but because Nature itself wrote them with the same alphabet and understanding that alphabet may be the key to healing what time and disease erode.

Thus, the path ahead demands more than incremental experiments—it demands layered rigor. Molecular precision must tighten, safety testing must deepen and post-market vigilance must become canonical. Specifically, the molecular validation must evolve: fingerprints must evolve into multidimensional "identity + purity + degradation trajectory" maps, where even minor deviations trigger review or rejection.

Safety testing must be progressive: from in vitro viability and transformation assays to long-term rodent and non-rodent chronic dosing programs with full histopathology, molecular endpoints, and biomarker panels.

Immunological vigilance must be central: peptides may elicit subtle anti-drug antibody responses, cross reactivity, or immune modulation. Immunogenicity risk assessment must incorporate in silico epitope prediction, human PBMC assays, anti-drug antibody monitoring, and real-world immunologic surveillance (as emphasized in recent reviews on peptide immunogenicity) [97][98].

Pharmacokinetics and metabolite profiling must remain comprehensive: clearance, accumulation, metabolite toxicity, renal retention, all demand thorough mapping.

Post-marketing surveillance must be proactive: long-term registries, oncologic screening, adverse event databases, and pharmacoepidemiologic feedback loops are essential to detect rare or delayed effects.

If peptide therapeutics are to transition from promising science to enduring medicine, they must achieve not only therapeutic efficacy but durable safety in real human populations. Only through a persistent and integrated discipline of molecular rigor, preclinical depth, immunologic awareness, and clinical humility can we truly claim both. In that balance lies the promise and the responsibility of the peptide revolution in medicine.

CHAPTER 4

Peptides in Cardiology: Mitochondrial, Nano-Peptide, and Organ-Specific Strategies

(with Prof. Dr. Olha Nishkumai, MD, PhD)

Introduction: The Heart's Peptide Frontier

The heart, with its relentless energetic demand, is uniquely vulnerable to mitochondrial dysfunction, oxidative stress, inflammation, and cellular turnover failure. Traditional cardiology has long relied on drugs (statins, ACE inhibitors, β-blockers, etc.), devices, and cell therapies. But in the last decade, a new frontier has emerged: peptides as precision modulators of cardiac and vascular biology. Among them, mitochondrial peptides, a.k.a. mitochondria-derived peptides (MDPs) are rising stars in cardioprotection. In this chapter, we explore how peptides, especially mitochondrial and nano-peptides, may prevent cardiac aging, reverse disease processes, and become part of the therapeutic armamentarium.

We begin with mitochondrial biology in the heart, then examine known MDPs (e.g., humanin, MOTS-c, SHLPs), survey nano-peptide and organ-specific strategies, and then propose how *Mito Organelles* and cold-extracted nano-organ peptides can be applied in cardiology. Along the way, we discuss challenges, safety, delivery, and future directions.

Mitochondria in the Heart: Vulnerabilities and Therapeutic Windows

Mitochondria are not just power generators, they are central hubs of redox signaling, calcium buffering, apoptosis regulation, and metabolic adaptation. In cardiomyocytes, mitochondria are densely packed among myofibrils and form distinct subpopulations (subsarcolemmal, interfibrillar, perinuclear) that tailor responses to energetic demands [99][100].

In cardiac disease, whether it is ischemia, hypertrophy, diabetic cardiomyopathy, the mitochondria go awry: loss of cristae integrity, increased reactive oxygen species (ROS), reduced ATP output, opening of permeability transition pores (mPTP), and release of pro-death signals. Therapies that merely reduce afterload or block neurohormonal axes may not fully reverse mitochondrial derangement.

Because mitochondria also signal back to the nucleus (retrograde signaling), modulating mitochondrial output can reshape gene expression, stress responses, and cellular resilience. Mitochondrial-derived peptides (MDPs) are among the endogenous signals that mediate such crosstalk and may represent "missing links" for cardiac regeneration.

MDPs are small peptides encoded by short open reading frames (sORFs) within the mitochondrial genome, particularly in rRNA regions. To date, the major MDP families include Humanin (encoded in the 16S rRNA region), Small humanin-like peptides (SHLP1–6) (also from 16S rRNA), MOTS-c (encoded in the 12S rRNA region), Possibly other as-yet-undiscovered micropeptides. These peptides are transcribed and translated (sometimes in mitochondria, sometimes in cytosol), secreted or transported, and act as mitokines—molecules reflecting mitochondrial status and influencing distant tissues [101]. Their regulation is sensitive to metabolic stress: in aging, obesity, insulin resistance, and high-fat diet models, circulating levels of humanin and MOTS-c tend to decline. Conversely, in states of mitochondrial stress (exercise, ischemia), expression may increase as compensatory protective signals [102].

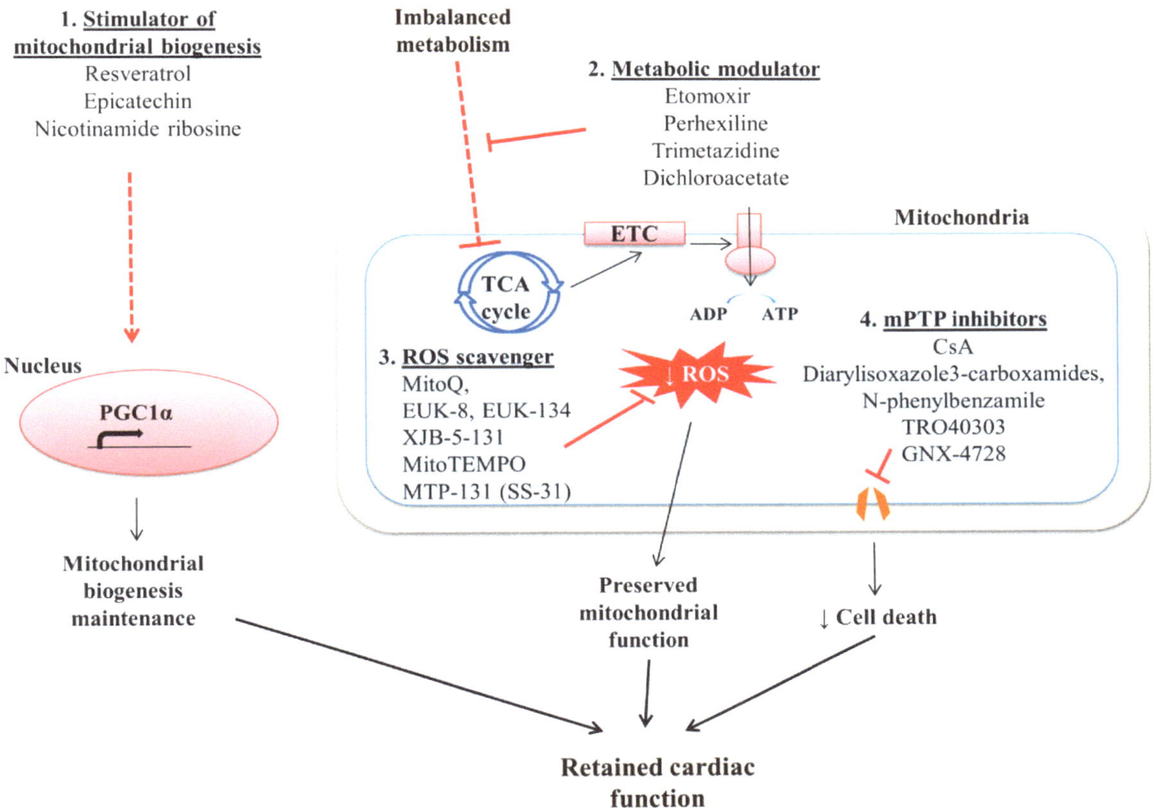

Fig 4.1. *Preserving mitochondrial biogenesis and function as therapeutic approaches in cardiac diseases. The potential therapeutic strategies aim to facilitate mitochondrial biogenesis and maintain mitochondrial function to prevent cardiac dysfunction, including (i) enhancing mitochondrial biogenesis; (ii) retaining mitochondrial metabolism by limiting fatty acid import and oxidation while improving glucose utilization; (iii) reducing ROS production by ROS scavengers; and (iv) inhibiting mPTP by the use of mPTP inhibitors (source: Nguyen, B. Y., Ruiz-Velasco, A., Bui, T., Collins, L., Wang, X., and Liu, W. (2019) Mitochondrial function in the heart: the insight into mechanisms and therapeutic potentials. British Journal of Pharmacology, 176, 4302–4318).*

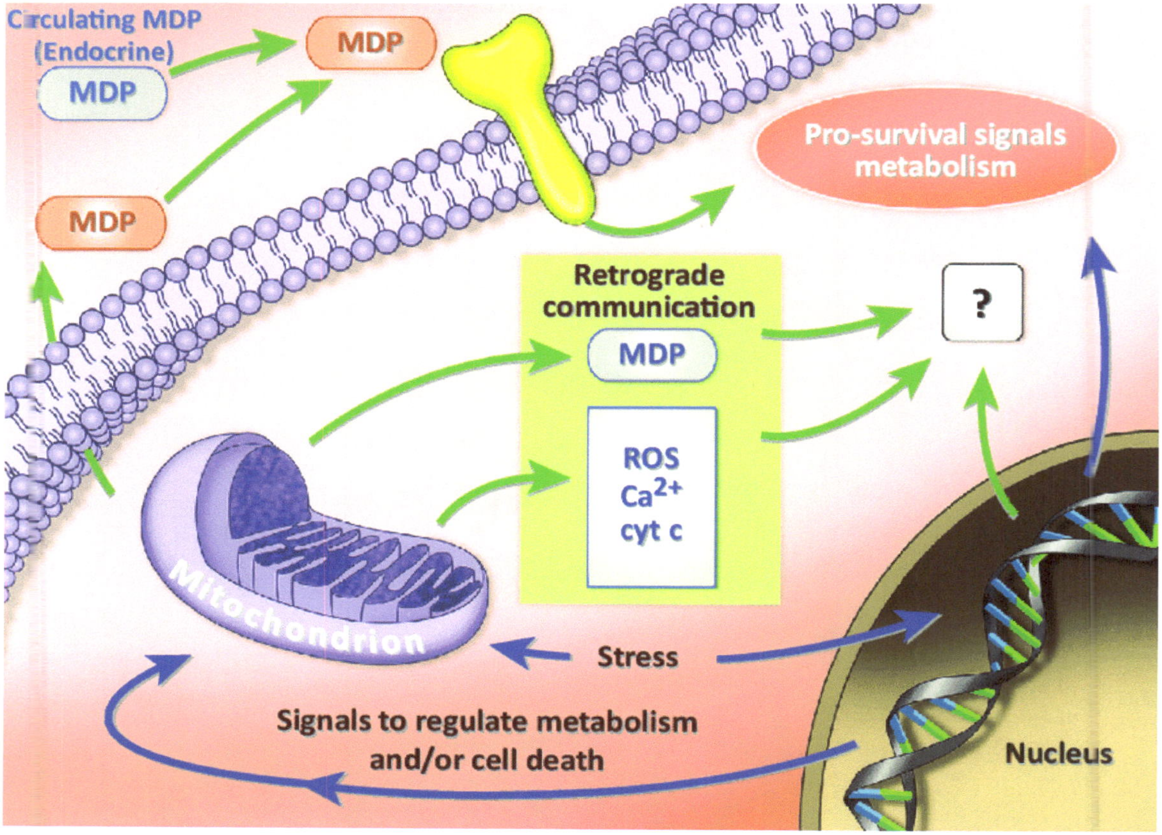

Fig 4.2. *Mitochondrial-derived peptides (MDPs) are retrograde signaling molecules. Mitochondria communicate with the cell through a process largely known as retrograde signaling. Traditionally described means of communication from the mitochondria include Ca 2+ , cytochrome c (cyt c), and reactive oxygen species (ROS). MDPs are recently identified retrograde signals, which are unique in that they are encoded within mitochondrial genome sequences. MDPs such as humanin are thought to act as endocrine as well as intracellular factors with several biological roles in the regulation of cell survival and metabolism (source: Lee, Changhan & Yen, Kelvin. (2015). Humanin-a harbinger of mitochondrial-derived peptides).*

MDPs exert pleiotropic actions relevant to heart and vasculature. Below are key mechanisms with cardiovascular implications:

Anti-apoptosis and cytoprotection

Humanin, for instance, interacts with BAX, prevents mitochondrial outer membrane permeabilization, and limits activation of caspases. In cardiomyocytes subjected to ischemia–reperfusion injury, humanin analogs reduce cell death [103].

Anti-oxidative stress and ROS mitigation

MDPs modulate endogenous antioxidant systems (e.g., SOD, glutathione), suppress NADPH oxidase activity, and reduce mitochondrial ROS leakage. Humanin and MOTS-c have been shown to lower ROS in endothelial and vascular cells under stress [104].

Anti-inflammation and modulation of signaling

MDPs inhibit NF-κB, reduce pro-inflammatory cytokines (TNF-α, IL-6, IL-1β), and dampen inflammasome activation. MOTS-c, especially, may engage AHR/STAT3 or MAPK/NF-κB pathways to suppress endothelial and myocardial inflammation [105].

Metabolic regulation, AMPK activation, and mitochondrial biogenesis

MOTS-c has been shown to activate AMPK, promote mitochondrial biogenesis via PGC-1α and NRF2, improve insulin sensitivity, and shift metabolism toward oxidative phosphorylation. These effects can support cardiac energetic stability under stress [106].

Endothelial protection and vascular function

MDPs improve endothelial function by preserving nitric oxide (NO) homeostasis, reducing endothelial senescence, and preventing vascular remodeling. Humanin can preserve eNOS expression and mitigate endothelial injury in models of hypertension [107].

In sum, MDPs act as endogenous guardians by buffering the heart and vasculature against apoptosis, oxidative stress, inflammation, and metabolic instability. Several preclinical and observational studies support the cardioprotective role of MDPs. In myocardial ischemia–reperfusion (I/R) injury models, administration of humanin or MOTS-c reduces infarct size, improves contractile function, and limits apoptosis in peri-infarct areas [108]. In models of hypertrophy or pressure overload, MDP treatment attenuates fibrotic remodeling and cardiomyocyte hypertrophy, preserving left ventricular function [109]. In atherosclerosis and vascular aging models, MOTS-c slows plaque progression, reduces vascular stiffness, and preserves endothelial integrity [110]. Observational human studies indicate that lower circulating humanin or MOTS-c levels correlate with worse cardiovascular risk factors (dyslipidemia, insulin resistance, hypertension) and with greater incidence of coronary artery disease [111].

These lines of evidence position MDPs both as biomarkers and therapeutic candidates in cardiovascular disease (CVD) [112].

Nano-Peptides, Organ-Specific Delivery and Mito Organelles in Cardiology

While MDPs provide a promising internal signaling layer, their therapeutic application in the heart must overcome key challenges: delivery to cardiac tissue, peptide stability, immunogenicity, and specificity. That is where nano-peptides and organ-specific peptide systems come into play.

Nano-peptides refers to small peptide constructs or peptide-laden nanoparticles engineered for improved delivery, targeting, and sustained release. Techniques include encapsulation in liposomes, polymeric nanoparticles (e.g., PLGA), or micelles, peptide conjugation to targeting ligands (e.g. antibodies, aptamers, peptides that bind cardiac-specific markers), self-assembling peptide nanofibers or hydrogels that release peptides gradually, peptide amphiphiles that assemble into nanoscale architectures.

In cardiology, these strategies allow peptides to reach ischemic myocardium, cross vascular barriers, resist proteolysis, and localize to mitochondria or intracellular compartments.

One example from the literature is cardiolipin-targeted peptides (aromatic-cationic tetrapeptides) that selectively bind cardiolipin in inner mitochondrial membranes. These peptides improved mitochondrial coupling efficiency, reduced ROS generation, and rejuvenated mitochondrial function in aged tissues (Cardiolipin-targeted peptides) [113]. Although not a classic MDP, it exemplifies how nanoscale peptides can restore mitochondrial architecture and function in cardiac cells.

Organ-Specific Peptide Strategies and Mito Organelles

A new generation of organ-specific peptide systems is being designed to maximize biological impact and reduce off-target activity. By tailoring peptide delivery to the heart, these systems aim to expand heartspan and, through improvements in cellspan and healthspan, exert profound effects on overall lifespan. Within this conceptual space, your notion of Mito Organelles, the mitochondria-targeted, organ-specific peptide constructs that merge the principles of mitochondrial-derived peptides with organ-specific molecular identity and ultimately defines a promising frontier in precision bioregeneration. This might involve:

- **Heart-specific NOP (Nano-Organo Peptides)** derived from cardiac tissue, processed cold/enzymatically, enriched for peptides that "speak the language" of the heart (metabolic regulators, contractile support, anti-fibrotic signals)
- **Dual scope peptides** combining an MDP component (e.g. a humanin analog) and a cardiac-targeting motif (e.g., peptide that binds cardiac troponin, integrin, or mitochondrial import signal)
- **Stimulus-responsive nano-carriers**, e.g., responsive to ischemia, pH, ROS, so peptides are released preferentially in stressed myocardium
- **Mitochondria-penetrating peptides** or **mitochondrial targeting sequences (MTS)** fused to bioactive peptides to deliver payload directly into cardiomyocyte mitochondria.

- By combining MDPs' intrinsic mitochondrial signals with organ-specific targeting, Mito Organelles aim to achieve **selective mitochondrial rejuvenation in the heart**, optimizing cardioprotection and regeneration.

To illustrate, consider a patient who suffered a myocardial infarction (MI). In the border zone of the infarct, surviving cardiomyocytes are stressed by mitochondrial damage, ROS overload, apoptosis, fibrotic signaling. A *Mito Organelles* peptide system might deliver an MDP analog, e.g., a stabilized humanin / MOTS-c hybrid, to reactivate mitochondrial function and reduce apoptosis. At the same time a heart-specific peptide moiety, targeting injured myocardium (e.g., binding to exposed integrin αvβ3 or extracellular matrix ligands) can act as a responsive nanocarrier that releases payload under oxidative or acidic conditions typical of ischemia, additionally providing mitochondrial import tag, guiding peptide into cardiomyocyte mitochondria to support electron transport, membrane integrity, and redox balance.

Such a system could reduce infarct expansion, preserve contractile mass, attenuate remodeling (fibrosis), and improve functional recovery thus outperforming systemic MDP injection alone.

MDPs show promise as biomarkers in cardiology. Reduced circulating humanin or MOTS-c may reflect subclinical mitochondrial dysfunction or early cardiovascular stress (Mitochondrial-derived peptides: biomarkers, Li et al., 2021) [114]. Their measurement could aid in early detection, prognosis, or monitoring therapy response.

However, challenges include assay standardization, understanding baseline variations (age, sex, comorbidities), peptide stability in plasma, and distinguishing free peptides from peptide fragments.

While MDPs are endogenous, exogenous administration (especially modified or analog forms) carries risks: immunogenicity, off-target effects, potential tumorigenesis (since anti-apoptotic peptides might aid survival of malignant cells) [115]. Hence, specificity is paramount.

Nano-peptide formulations must avoid systemic toxicity, ensure controlled release, avoid immune clearance, and maintain stability. Thorough preclinical toxicology and pharmacokinetics are essential.

Effective delivery to the heart poses obstacles: coronary perfusion, capillary barrier, interstitial diffusion, peptide degradation, and intracellular uptake. Approaches include intracoronary infusion, local hydrogel patches, peptide-eluting stents, or targeted nanoparticle injection.

Dose must balance efficacy and safety. Too little yields no effect; too much may saturate systems or provoke side effects.

Case Studies and Emerging Evidence in Peptide-Based Cardiac and Vascular Protection

A growing body of experimental and clinical research now supports that mitochondrial-derived peptides (MDPs) and related nano-peptide constructs are more than speculative therapies; they have demonstrable effects in modulating vascular and cardiac dysfunction. Among these, the peptide humanin has been perhaps most consistently studied for endothelial protection. In cultured human endothelial cells, humanin analogues mitigate high glucose-induced dysfunction by restoring expression of Krüppel-like factor 2 (KLF2), a master regulator of endothelial phenotype, and by recovering downstream KLF2 target genes such as endothelial nitric oxide synthase (eNOS). Such treatment reduces the expression of adhesion molecules like VCAM-1 and E-selectin, decreases secretion of inflammatory cytokines including IL-1β and TNF-α, and ultimately limits monocyte adhesion to the endothelial surface, preserving barrier integrity [116][117].

In vivo, in hypercholesterolemic apolipoprotein E (ApoE)-deficient mice, daily administration of a humanin analogue (HNGF6A) for sixteen weeks prevented the development of endothelial dysfunction, attenuated atherosclerotic plaque formation in the proximal aorta, and preserved nitric oxide synthase expression in the vessel wall. These improvements occurred without significant changes in systemic cholesterol levels, suggesting that humanin's benefits derive from direct vascular protection rather than lipid lowering [118]. Observations in human subjects further link circulating humanin levels with preserved coronary endothelial function: individuals with impaired endothelial response to acetylcholine showed significantly lower humanin levels compared to those with normal endothelial function [119].

Another set of studies has centered on the mitochondrial peptide MOTS-c. In cardiac cell lines (e.g., H_9C_2 cells), pre-treatment with MOTS-c attenuates H_2O_2-induced oxidative stress and blunts the overactivation of inflammatory pathways. Mechanistically, this involves activation of the Nrf2/ARE antioxidant response element axis and suppression of NF-κB signalling, with downstream reductions in reactive oxygen species (ROS), malondialdehyde (MDA) accumulation, and inflammatory cytokine release (TNF-α, IL-6, IL-1β) [120]. Such effects support the idea that MOTS-c may slow or reverse vascular aging by not only reducing molecular damage but also re-establishing cellular redox and inflammatory homeostasis.

Further evidence highlights humanin's capacity to prevent or delay endothelial senescence. In human umbilical vein endothelial cells (HUVECs) exposed to high glucose, senescence markers such as p16, p21, and p53 are upregulated. Pre-treatment with a humanin-analogue ([Gly14] humanin) ameliorates this effect by restoring levels of SIRT6, reducing ROS accumulation, and suppressing cellular senescence [121]. Thus, humanin not only prevents apoptosis but also preserves endothelial youthfulness under metabolic stress.

Cardiolipin-targeting peptides, though somewhat distinct from endogenous mitochondrial peptides, provide another compelling line of evidence. These peptides are engineered to bind cardiolipin, a key lipid component of the inner mitochondrial membrane whose integrity is vital for mitochondrial cristae structure, efficient electron transport, and proper mitochondrial function. In models of cardiac aging or mitochondrial injury, cardiolipin-binding peptides (such as the tetrapeptide SS-31, also known as elamipretide) have been shown to preserve cristae architecture, reduce mitochondrial ROS leakage, improve ATP production, and maintain mitochondrial coupling efficiency [122][123]. Such improvements translate in animal models to better cardiac function following ischemia, less fibrosis, and slower functional decline.

While randomized, large-scale clinical trials are still under development, these experimental findings illustrate that the therapeutic concept of using mitochondrial peptides, humanin analogues, MOTS-c derivatives, and cardio-mito targeting nano-peptides is moving from hypotheses into validated preclinical models. The findings span in vitro cellular systems, small animal disease or injury models, and initial human observational studies linking peptide levels with cardiovascular health.

Another promising therapeutic modality for cardiovascular diseases is an *Essential Phospholipid Therapy* that was recently extensively studied in Acute Coronary Syndromes. Emerging evidence suggests that Essential Phospholipids (EPLs), particularly the clinical formulation *Plaqx*, may represent a pivotal adjunctive therapy in the management of acute myocardial infarction (MI) and in secondary cardiovascular prevention. As a regenerative-oriented intervention, Plaqx is designed to restore the structural and functional integrity of atherosclerotic plaque phospholipid matrices, enhance endothelial resilience, and promote favorable remodeling of lipid microdomains that regulate inflammatory signaling and cholesterol efflux.

In an international, double-blind randomized study modeled on contemporary post-MI therapeutic standards, high-risk adults (n≈18,000; mean age 65.5 years; 74% male) presenting with type 1 MI and multivessel coronary artery disease received either placebo or a series of four weekly intravenous apolipoprotein A1 infusions, which are essentially similar with Plaqx infusions, (6 g each) initiated within five days of first medical contact [303]. The full treatment course was completed within 30 days of randomization, with structured follow-up at infusion visits, at days 29, 60, and 90, and at 90-day intervals through one year.

Although the composite primary endpoint of time to first occurrence of MI, stroke, or cardiovascular death by day 90 did not reach statistical significance, numerically lower rates of cardiovascular death and recurrent MI were consistently observed in the Plaqx group. By day 90, the event rate was 4.8% in Plaqx-treated patients versus 5.2% with placebo (HR 0.93; 95% CI 0.81–1.05). The divergence persisted across later assessments, with hazard ratios favoring Plaqx at 180 days (HR 0.91; 95% CI 0.81–1.01) and 365 days (HR 0.93; 95% CI 0.85–1.02). These trends were uniform across prespecified clinical subgroups.

When individual components of the primary endpoint were examined, Plaqx therapy was associated with notably lower hazards for cardiovascular death (HR 0.83) and recurrent MI (HR 0.91) by day 90, whereas stroke incidence did not differ significantly. Composite outcomes that are mechanistically linked to plaque stabilization, such as cardiovascular death plus non–type 2 MI, also showed consistent numerical advantages at days 90, 180, and 365 (HR range 0.87–0.91).

Importantly, safety outcomes were comparable between treatment groups, with no signal of hepatic, renal, or hemorrhagic complications attributable to the phospholipid infusions. This tolerability profile aligns with the long-established safety of essential phospholipids in other clinical contexts.

These findings highlight a recurring challenge in modern cardiovascular medicine: evaluating emerging therapies in populations already receiving maximal evidence-based management, including high-intensity statins, dual antiplatelet therapy, and contemporary revascularization strategies. In such settings, the additive benefit of lipid-modifying or plaque-targeted interventions may appear modest in absolute terms, even when biologically meaningful.

Nevertheless, the observed directional consistency toward reduced cardiovascular death and MI supports the mechanistic premise that restoring phospholipid integrity within plaque structures can enhance plaque stability, optimize membrane-associated cholesterol handling, and improve vascular healing after acute ischemic events. As emphasized in recent editorial analyses, progress in this field may depend on refined assays for lipid microdomain function, improved characterization of phospholipid-dependent cholesterol efflux pathways, and more precise phenotyping to identify patient subgroups most likely to benefit from regenerative lipid therapies.

Taken together, Plaqx and related Essential Phospholipid formulations represent a promising peptide-adjacent therapeutic strategy within regenerative cardiology. This compounds aims not merely to modulate serum lipids, but to rebuild and stabilize the phospholipid architecture fundamental to vascular health and plaque resilience [303].

Challenges, Unanswered Questions, and Future Directions in Cardiovascular Peptide Therapy

Despite the encouraging evidence, multiple challenges remain before peptide-based cardiology can reach broad clinical application. One of the foremost issues is peptide stability: many peptides degrade rapidly in plasma or tissue due to proteases, neutral pH, or other degrading environments, limiting half-life and effective concentration. Delivery of peptides specifically to myocardial mitochondria without off-target exposure is another complex hurdle; peptides must cross endothelial barriers, diffuse into myocardium, and ideally be targeted into mitochondrial compartments.

Scalability is also a concern. Manufacturing hybrid or modified peptides, especially ones linked to targeting motifs, modified for stability, or embedded in nano-carriers, requires good manufacturing practice (GMP) standards, molecular fingerprinting, sterility, and reproducibility. Safety profiling is critical: while many peptides show promising anti-oxidant, anti-apoptotic, or anti-inflammatory actions, there is potential for unforeseen effects in oncologic contexts, immune modulation, or metabolic dysregulation.

Another gap is patient stratification and biomarker guidance: who benefits most? For example, patients with early atherosclerosis vs. established heart failure may respond differently; mitochondrial genetic background, age, comorbidities (e.g., diabetes, hypertension) may influence peptide efficacy. Long-term durability, repeated dosing, immune responses against analogues remain only partially understood.

Looking forward, several promising trajectories stand out. Next-generation constructs such as Mito Organelles represents the concept of mitochondrial-targeted, organ-specific peptide systems, which could provide enhanced specificity and efficacy for myocardial regeneration. Smart responsive peptide carriers that release therapeutic peptides in response to pathological cues (oxidative stress, acidic pH, ischemia) would minimize off-target effects. Integrating imaging biomarkers (PET, MR spectroscopy) to guide dosing and monitor mitochondrial repair is another avenue. Personalized peptide therapeutics that consider patient mitochondrial haplotypes or metabolic profiling may enhance outcomes. Finally, combinatorial regenerative protocols pairing peptides with stem-cell exosomes, biomaterial scaffolds, or gene therapy might yield synergistic repair in cardiac disease.

Conclusion

Peptides are redefining the molecular frontier of cardiology. Among them, mitochondrial peptides (MDPs) provide a potent, endogenous line of defense, hence safeguarding cardiomyocyte survival, curbing oxidative stress, modulating inflammation, and linking mitochondrial health to systemic metabolism. But to harness their full potential in the heart, we must marry them to nano-peptide delivery, organ-specific targeting, and Mito-Organelles-level engineering.

What lies ahead is both a technical and conceptual leap: treating the heart not only with agents that prevent damage, but with molecular signals that remind it how to heal itself. The canvas is broad, the tools are emerging, and the promise is profound.

CHAPTER 5

Peptides as Regulators in the Pathophysiology and Treatment of Metabolic Syndrome

(with Prof. Jonathan R.T. Lakey, B.Sc., M.Sc., Ph.D)

Metabolic syndrome constitutes a multidimensional disorder of energy homeostasis, characterized by central adiposity, insulin resistance, dyslipidemia, hypertension, and pro-inflammatory states. Its rising prevalence worldwide has provoked intense interest in mechanistic pathways bridging metabolic stress and end-organ damage. Among those, peptides, the short chains of amino acids serving as signaling mediators that are emerging as central actors in orchestrating inter-organ communication, cellular adaptation, and stress-response networks. While classic peptide hormones such as insulin, leptin, GLP-1, and adiponectin have long been recognized in metabolic regulation, more recently discovered micropeptides, particularly those derived from mitochondrial open reading frames or engineered as nanomized organ-specific peptides have expanded the peptidome of interest. In this chapter, we explore how these peptides converge on the pathology of metabolic syndrome, and how they may serve as the next frontier for therapeutic innovation.

The Peptide Network Underlying Metabolic Homeostasis

Physiological homeostasis of nutrient flux, energy storage, and glucose balance depends on a dense network of peptide signals. Enteroendocrine peptides such as GLP-1 (glucagon-like peptide-1), GIP (gastric inhibitory polypeptide), PYY (peptide YY), and pancreatic polypeptide convey nutrient sensing from the gut to pancreatic islets, the nervous system, and peripheral tissues; they regulate insulin secretion, glucagon suppression, gastric motility, and central appetite circuits. Dysregulation of these signals either via impaired secretion, increased enzymatic degradation, receptor desensitization, or downstream signaling defects contributes to the so-called “incretin defect” in insulin-resistant states. Indeed, recent syntheses of metabolic peptide biology highlight how perturbations in GLP-1, GIP, and pancreatic peptide signaling promote hyperinsulinemia, obesity, chronic inflammation, and even neurodegeneration through gut–brain axis disturbances [124].

Adipose tissue, long regarded merely as lipid storage, in fact secretes its own suite of peptides (commonly called adipokines) such as leptin, adiponectin, resistin, visfatin, and others; these deliver regulatory feedback to the liver, skeletal muscle, pancreas, and cardiovascular system, modulating insulin sensitivity, inflammatory tone, and lipid partitioning [125]. In early metabolic syndrome, leptin levels often rise (reflecting adiposity), while adiponectin falls, a shift that fosters insulin resistance, endothelial dysfunction, and low-grade inflammation [126][127].

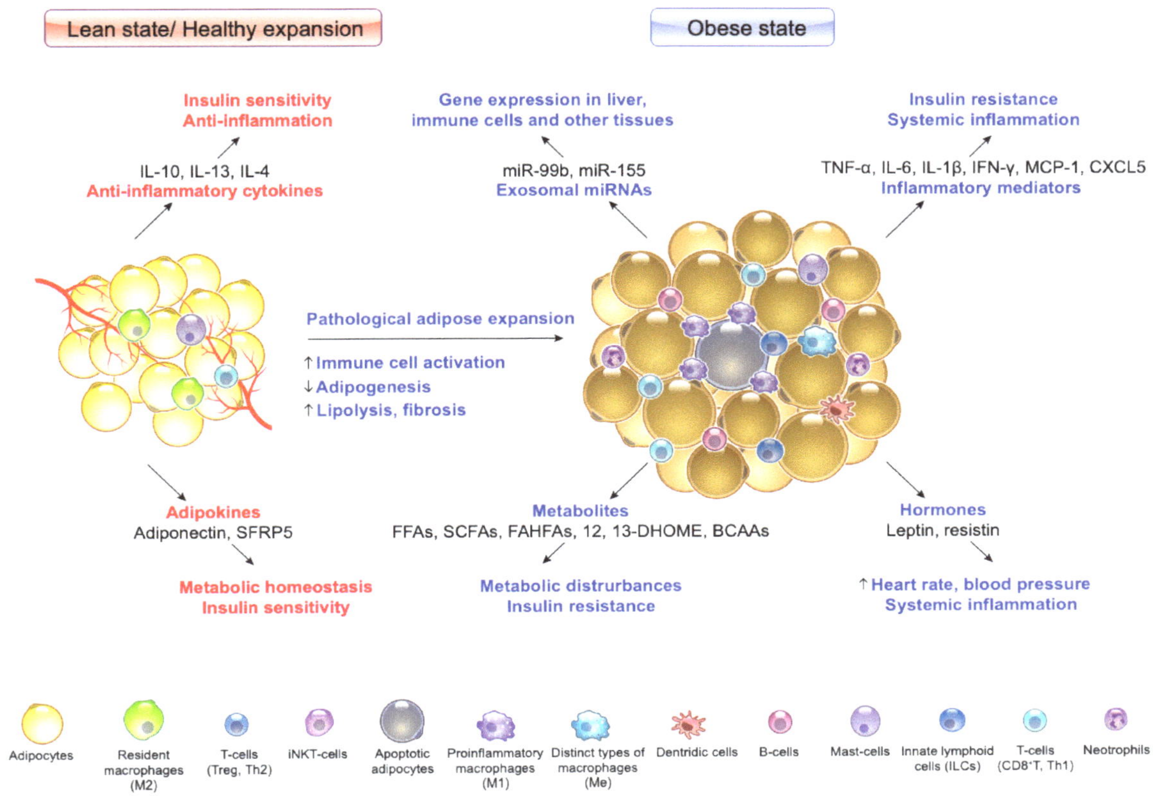

Fig 5.1. *Adipose tissue dysfunction and inflammation in obesity that directly and indirectly aggravates cardiomyopathy: In lean state, adipocytes secrete various endocrine factors that maintain metabolic homeostasis. In response to chronic energy excess, infiltration of proinflammatory immune cells and hypertrophic adipose expansion along with a lack of adipogenesis can be observed in adipose tissues, which is accompanied by altered secretion of adipose tissue hormones, cytokines, metabolites, and exosomal miRNAs. Overall, the changes in hypertrophic adipose tissue contribute to insulin resistance, impaired glucose, and lipid metabolism and low-grade systemic inflammation and exert local effects that exacerbate cardiomyopathy in obesity. IL-10, -13, -4, interleukin 10, 13, 4; SFRP5, secreted frizzled-related protein 5; TNFa, tumor necrosis factor-a; IL-6, -1b, interleukin 6, 1b; IFN-c, interferon c; MCP1, monocyte chemoattractant protein 1; CXCL5, C-X-C motif chemokine ligand 5; FFAs, free fatty acids; SCFAs, short-chain fatty acids; FAHFAs, fatty acid esters of hydroxy fatty acids; 12,13-DHOME, 12,13-dihydroxy-(9Z)-octadecenoic acid; BCAAs, branched-chain amino acids (source: Ren et al., Physiol. Rev., 2021).*

Simultaneously, the failure of peripheral tissues to respond appropriately to insulin leads to lipid overflow, ectopic deposition, mitochondrial stress, reactive oxygen species (ROS) accumulation, endoplasmic reticulum stress, and activation of inflammatory kinases such as JNK and IKKβ [128]. Under these conditions the balance of peptide signaling is disrupted: insulin resistance blunts insulin's feedback on hepatic gluconeogenesis and lipogenesis, while compensatory hyperinsulinemia suppresses GLP-1 receptor sensitivity. At the same time, oxidative stress and inflammation downregulate expression or action of beneficial peptides such as adiponectin and may impair endothelial and vascular peptide regulators (e.g., nitric oxide–modulating peptides) [129].

Thus, metabolic syndrome can be conceived as a progressive unraveling of peptide network integrity, in which the signals that once maintained metabolic resilience are lost or overridden by pathological stress circuits.

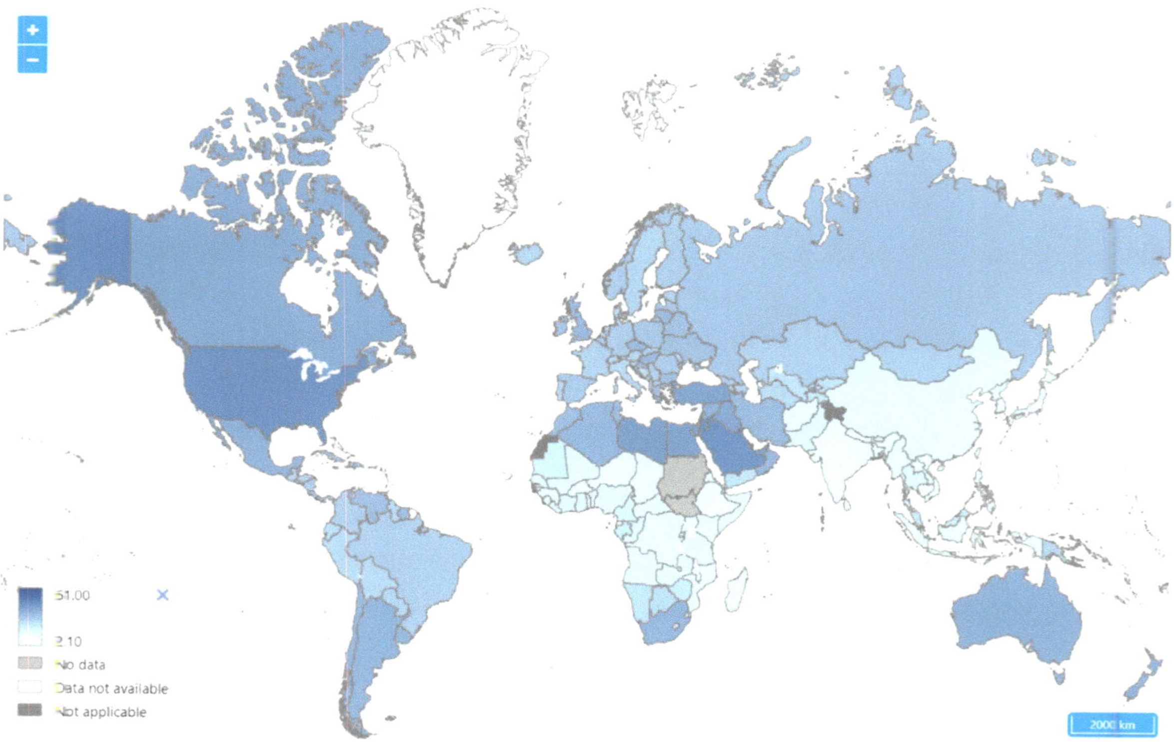

Fig 5.2. *Global prevalence of obesity among adults (source; WHO).*

Mitochondrial Dysfunction and the Emergence of Mitochondrial Peptides

While disturbances in classical peptide networks are well appreciated in metabolic disease, mitochondrial dysfunction is increasingly viewed as a central pathogenetic node. In the face of caloric excess and lipid overload, mitochondria in skeletal muscle, hepatocytes, and adipocytes become stressed: electron transport chain inefficiencies increase, ROS escalate, mitochondrial DNA damage accrues, and mitophagy or mitochondrial renewal becomes insufficient. Over time, bioenergetic reserve wanes, metabolic flexibility diminishes, and cells shift toward maladaptive pathways.

A key insight in the last decade has been that mitochondria are not merely passive energy factories but also active signaling organelles. Embedded within their genomes are short open reading frames (sORFs) that code for mitochondrial-derived peptides (MDPs)—the small bioactive peptides that can communicate mitochondrial status to the nucleus or extracellular milieu, influencing cellular adaptation to stress. The first of these to be discovered was humanin, encoded within a sORF in the 16S rRNA mitochondrial gene, followed by MOTS-c (encoded in a sORF within mitochondrial 12S rRNA) and a family of short humanin-like peptides (SHLP1–6) [130][131].

Humanin has been shown to exert cytoprotective, anti-apoptotic, anti-oxidative, and metabolic modulatory effects. It binds to cell surface receptors and activates intracellular cascades such as JAK/STAT, ERK1/2, and AKT, thereby promoting cell survival, reducing inflammation, and enhancing insulin sensitivity [132][131]. SHLP peptides, albeit less well-characterized, appear to share some of humanin's protective capacities in various cell types.

MOTS-c, a 16–amino-acid peptide originating from mitochondrial 12S rRNA, and Mito Organelles (MOs) organ-specific peptides (OSPs) have drawn particular attention for its metabolic regulatory roles. Under stress conditions, MOTS-c and MOs can translocate to the nucleus and influence expression of stress-responsive genes. It can activate AMP-activated protein kinase (AMPK), promote glucose uptake and fatty acid oxidation, and attenuate metabolic defects in preclinical models [133][132][131].

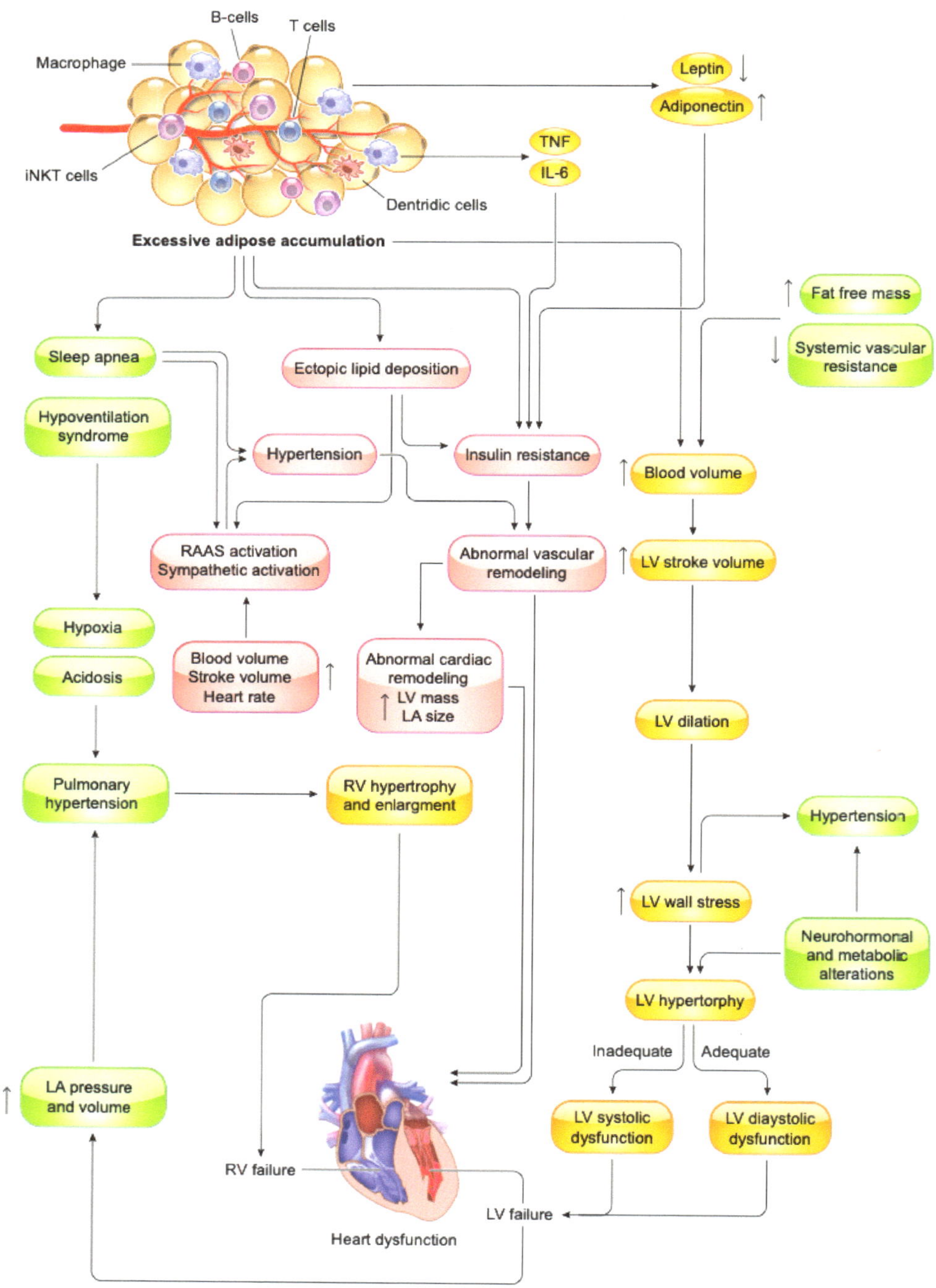

Fig 5.3. *Relationship between obesity, metabolic syndrome pathways and cardiac dysfunction (source: Ren et al., Physiol. Rev., 2021).*

Rodent models have demonstrated that administration or overexpression of MOTS-c and MOs can prevent diet-induced obesity, improve glucose tolerance, suppress insulin resistance, and combat age-related metabolic decline. In muscle tissue it appears to act as an "exercise mimetic," inducing metabolic gene programs similar to endurance training [32][131]. The mechanistic routes include inhibition of the folate cycle and tethered de novo purine biosynthesis, thereby increasing AICAR and activating AMPK [32][132].

Interestingly, the human data on MDPs is still emergent. A recent meta-analysis investigated plasma MOTS-c concentrations in individuals with obesity and diabetes, finding that MOTS-c levels tend to be elevated in obesity but reduced in type 2 diabetes, suggesting a biphasic response in metabolic progression. MOTS-c correlated positively with total cholesterol and LDL-c, though correlations with other anthropometric parameters were inconsistent, likely owing to limited sample sizes. The analysis speculated that MOTS-c secretion may initially increase in early obesity as a compensatory response but decline once diabetes ensues [134].

Although humanin has been less systematically studied in metabolic cohorts, its known effects in oxidative stress, apoptosis suppression, and metabolic regulation make it a candidate biomarker and therapeutic target in metabolic syndrome and aging [132][131].

Beyond MOs, MOTS-c and humanin, other MDPs such as SHLPs may modulate mitochondrial function, stress response, and metabolic resilience, though their roles remain more speculative [131].

Thus, the mitochondrial peptide axis constitutes a feedback loop: mitochondrial stress diminishes MDP synthesis or signaling, which in turn weakens the resilience of mitochondrial–nuclear crosstalk and favors metabolic collapse.

Aging, Klotho, and the Peptidic Interface of Metabolism

Aging processes intertwine with metabolic dysfunction, inflammation, and oxidative stress, and the Klotho protein sits at a strategic crossroads of these phenomena. First discovered in mice as an anti-aging gene, Klotho exists in transmembrane and soluble forms; the latter may function intracrine, paracrine, or endocrine roles. Klotho modulates phosphate homeostasis (in coordination with FGF23), suppresses oxidative stress, inhibits insulin/IGF signaling, downregulates fibrotic cascades, and mitigates cellular senescence [135].

In human cohorts, lower levels of soluble α-Klotho have been observed in subjects with metabolic syndrome relative to controls. Higher circulating Klotho is inversely associated with odds of metabolic syndrome, and among those with metabolic syndrome, elevated Klotho predicts improved survival. These epidemiological associations underscore Klotho's potential as a metabolic biomarker and effector [124].

Mechanistic studies show that Klotho enhances insulin sensitivity through downstream effects on PI3K/Akt signaling, inhibits lipogenesis by downregulating HMG-CoA reductase, and attenuates ROS-mediated cell injury. By restraining the overactivation of mTOR and IGF pathways, Klotho may buffer the metabolic stress that drives insulin resistance and fibrosis [136].

Because full-length Klotho protein is large and difficult to administer, interest has turned to Klotho peptide fragments, particularly those derived from the KL1 domain that might retain beneficial signaling while reducing off-target effects. In conceptual frameworks such as Nanomized Organ-Specific Peptides (NOPs), small peptides derived from Klotho may be engineered for targeted delivery to metabolic tissues. Such fragments, if properly stabilized or delivered, could serve as modulators of aging-metabolism interfaces. [136][79].

Nanomized Organ-Specific Peptides (NOPs) and Peptide Delivery Principles

Despite the promise of peptide therapeutics, major challenges have historically constrained clinical translation: rapid proteolysis, poor stability, low tissue penetration, off-target binding, and immunogenicity. To circumvent these, novel strategies of *nanomization* and organ-specific targeting have been proposed [79].

In one such paradigm, organ-specific peptides are engineered into nanoscale formats on the order of 3 nm and less than 10 kDa to enhance solubility, diffusion, receptor accessibility, and tissue permeability. These Nanomized Organ-specific Peptides (NOPs) may be derived from local organ peptides (pancreas, muscle, nerve, adipose) or from purpose-designed small peptides.

Because of their diminutive size and high aqueous solubility, NOPs may be delivered via sublingual, intranasal, or injective routes with better bioavailability. In the context of metabolic syndrome, NOPs targeting pancreatic islets, skeletal muscle, or peripheral nerves may help restore tissue-specific peptide regulation. The European Wellness protocol concept envisions NOP delivery to peripheral nervous system (PNS) and musculoskeletal systems in tandem with metabolic interventions [137].

Parallel to this, self-assembling peptide hydrogels and scaffolds have been adapted for metabolic applications. These hydrogels, formed from amphiphilic peptides that self-assemble into three-dimensional networks, can entrap growth factors or therapeutic peptides and release them in a sustained fashion. In the setting of metabolic syndrome, self-assembling peptide constructs have been explored for tissue repair (e.g., in islets, vascular beds) and controlled peptide release (e.g., incretins or metabolic regulators) [138].

Peptide delivery platforms can also employ chemical modifications such as PEGylation, cyclization, D-amino acids, and use of liposomal or polymeric nanoparticle carriers. Mitochondria-targeting tags (e.g., triphenylphosphonium cations) may further permit delivery of MDP analogs to mitochondrial compartments. When engineered carefully, these platforms offer the prospect of delivering peptides such as MOTS-c, Klotho fragments, or organ-derived peptides directly into challenging metabolic tissues with minimized systemic loss.

Incretin Peptides, Dual/Triple Agonists, and Peptide Synergy

While mitochondrial peptides operate at the subcellular level, the well-established realm of incretin peptides continues to anchor peptide-based therapeutics in metabolic disease. GLP-1 receptor agonists have transformed the management of type 2 diabetes and obesity, not merely by augmenting insulin secretion or suppressing appetite, but through broader pleiotropic effects [139].

In experimental models of metabolic syndrome, GLP-1 agonists have repaired mitochondrial dysfunction, restored calcium handling, stabilized mitochondrial membrane potentials, and normalized cardiomyocyte electrophysiology. In one rodent study, liraglutide reversed prolonged ventricular action potentials, corrected cytosolic Ca^{2+} dysregulation, and reinstated ATP production in cardiomyocytes under metabolic stress [140][141].

Clinically, GLP-1 analogs confer cardiovascular protection beyond glycemic effects, they reduce major adverse cardiovascular events, preserve renal function, and induce sustained weight loss. Their interaction with mitochondrial pathways, inflammation, and endothelial health makes them ideal candidates for combined peptide strategies [142].

Given limitations of individual incretin therapies, such as gastrointestinal tolerability ceilings and diminishing receptor sensitivity interest has surged in dual agonists (GLP-1/GIP) and multi-agonists (GLP-1/GIP/glucagon) that provide concurrent modulation of insulin secretion, lipolysis, energy expenditure, and hepatic metabolism [143]. These hybrid peptides, by leveraging multiple hormonal axes, may more comprehensively address the multifaceted derangements of metabolic syndrome. In the realm of peptide innovation, I have elevated the classical GLP-1 molecule into a signature creation: GNP-1, the Glucose-Normalizing Peptide-1. This proprietary formulation transcends the limitations of its predecessor, meticulously engineered for unparalleled stability, refined receptor specificity, and exquisitely calibrated glucose modulation. Where traditional GLP-1 offers promise, GNP-1 delivers precision. In our own 40+ clinics, centers and hospitals over the world this novel therapeutic solution became a bespoke molecular instrument designed to harmonize metabolic balance with unmatched sophistication. It is not merely an enhancement; it is a reimagining, a convergence of nature's intelligence and human ingenuity, crafted for those who demand the apex of therapeutic elegance. In the world of peptide medicine, GNP-1 stands as a rarefied exemplar, the Rolls-Royce of metabolic regulation, a statement that true innovation is both art and science. In combination with MO *LPPSIMKE* it may deliver wonders in reversing the Metabolic syndrome and restoring healthspan, normalizing sugar levels and promising myriads of other improvements and benefits.

In a synergistic peptide design, one may envision coupling a novel proprietary molecule of GNP-1 or dual-agonist backbone with mitochondrial peptides (such as MOs *Pancreas* and *LPPSIMKE* and MOTS-c analogs) and Klotho-derived fragments, and possibly augmenting with NOPs targeted to muscle, adipose, nerve or pancreas. This poly-peptide cocktail could restore organelle function, re-balance systemic peptide networks, and promote tissue repair in a harmonized manner [144][145].

Peptide modulation of metabolic pathways: Mechanisms in Metabolic Syndrome

At the molecular level, peptides influence nearly every domain of metabolic syndrome pathogenesis: insulin signaling, lipid homeostasis, oxidative stress, inflammation, senescence, and mitochondrial homeostasis.

MOs, MOTS-c and humanin, as described above, directly interface with mitochondrial–nuclear signaling, regulating metabolic gene transcription and activating AMPK, thereby increasing glucose uptake and fat oxidation while restraining anabolic stress. These MDPs help buffer mitochondrial oxidative stress and preserve mitochondrial integrity, which is essential in insulin-sensitive tissues [132][130].

Klotho and its fragments modulate PI3K/Akt signaling downstream of insulin/IGF pathways, reduce HMG-CoA reductase–driven lipogenesis, suppress ROS generation, and regulate cellular senescence pathways. By constraining overactivation of mTOR and IGF signals, Klotho peptides may prevent the metabolic overshoot that predisposes to insulin resistance [146][147].

GLP-1 and related incretin peptides modulate insulin and glucagon secretion, slow gastric emptying, reduce appetite, promote weight loss, and exert anti-inflammatory and endothelial protective effects. Their ability to normalize mitochondrial calcium balance and energetic function in the heart speaks to their deeper cellular influence beyond classical endocrine roles.

Adipokines (e.g. adiponectin) enhance insulin sensitivity by activating AMPK and PPARα pathways in liver and muscle. Leptin, via hypothalamic circuits, regulates appetite and energy expenditure; however chronic leptin elevation in obesity tends to lead to leptin resistance, undermining its regulatory capacity [148].

Through cross-talk, these peptide families intersect. For example, effective GLP-1 therapy may reduce lipid overload and mitochondrial stress, thereby improving MDP production or signaling. Likewise, augmenting MDPs may sensitize tissues to GLP-1 or insulin signaling. Klotho-derived peptides may further potentiate those actions by mopping up oxidative stress and reinforcing cellular resilience.

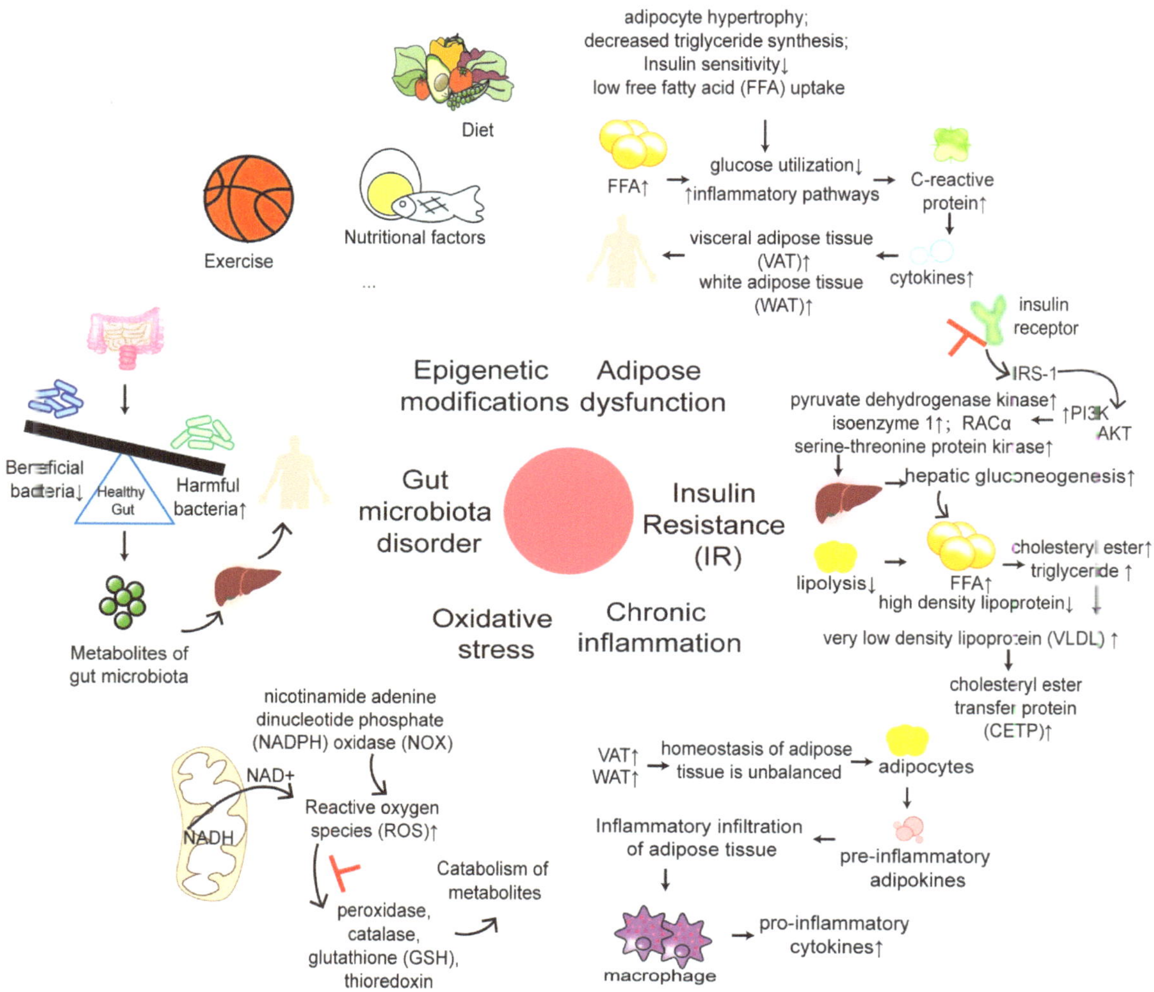

Fig 5.4. *Molecular mechanisms of Metabolic Syndrome (source: Luyao Zheng, Molecular Biomedicine, 2025).*

Although much of the mechanistic and therapeutic promise resides in preclinical models, human observational and translational studies are beginning to validate the peptide frameworks.

The meta-analysis of MOTS-c concentrations in human metabolic cohorts is among the first systematic efforts. Its finding that MOTS-c is increased in obesity but decreased in overt type 2 diabetes suggests a dynamic shift in peptide homeostasis as metabolic disease progresses. This biphasic pattern might represent compensatory upregulation in early metabolic stress, followed by exhaustion or downregulation in advanced disease [134].

Beyond MOTS-c, food-derived bioactive peptides (e.g., from milk proteins, fish, soy, and other dietary sources) have long been studied for their antihypertensive, anti-dyslipidemic, anti-inflammatory, and glucose-regulatory properties. These peptides released during digestion or food processing can act as ACE inhibitors, DPP-4 inhibitors, or free radical scavengers. For instance, peptides derived from milk have been shown to reduce blood pressure, modulate glycemia, reduce cholesterol, and oppose obesity in animal models and small human trials [149][150].

Self-assembling peptide scaffolds are likewise being explored for sustained, localized peptide delivery in metabolic tissues and vascular beds, although human data are still forthcoming [151].

In the incretin arena, GLP-1 receptor agonist therapies like liraglutide, exenatide, and semaglutide have undergone large, randomized trials in obesity and diabetes, showing robust weight loss, glycemic control, and reductions in cardiovascular events. Their extensions into metabolic syndrome populations, even before full diabetes onset, represent real-world applications of peptide-based intervention.

As peptide-based therapeutics mature, careful translational work will be required: pharmacokinetics in humans, safety (especially long-term), immunogenicity, dose–response relationships, and biomarker monitoring will be essential. Measuring endogenous humanin, MOTS-c, or Klotho fragments in human tissues or circulation remains technically challenging, but mass spectrometry and novel immunoassays are improving.

To understand how peptides reshape the progression of metabolic syndrome, one may imagine a symphony orchestra in which different peptide "instruments" play complementary parts. In health, enteroendocrine peptide conductors (GLP-1, GIP, PYY) synchronize feeding and insulin response; adipokine strings (adiponectin, leptin) maintain peripheral sensitivity; mitochondrial micropeptide percussionists (MOTS-c, humanin) modulate energy and stress response; Klotho peptides carry harmonics of aging regulation; and organ-specific motifs (e.g., pancreatic or muscle NOPs) strengthen local performance.

When metabolic stress mounts, the mitochondrial percussion falters, producing fewer or mis-signaling MDPs, undermining coordination. The adipokine and incretin sections become muted, or discordant, and inflammatory or oxidative signals dominate the hall. Without interventional correction, the orchestral equilibrium collapses, and insulin resistance, inflammation, lipid dysregulation, and organ injury ensue [152].

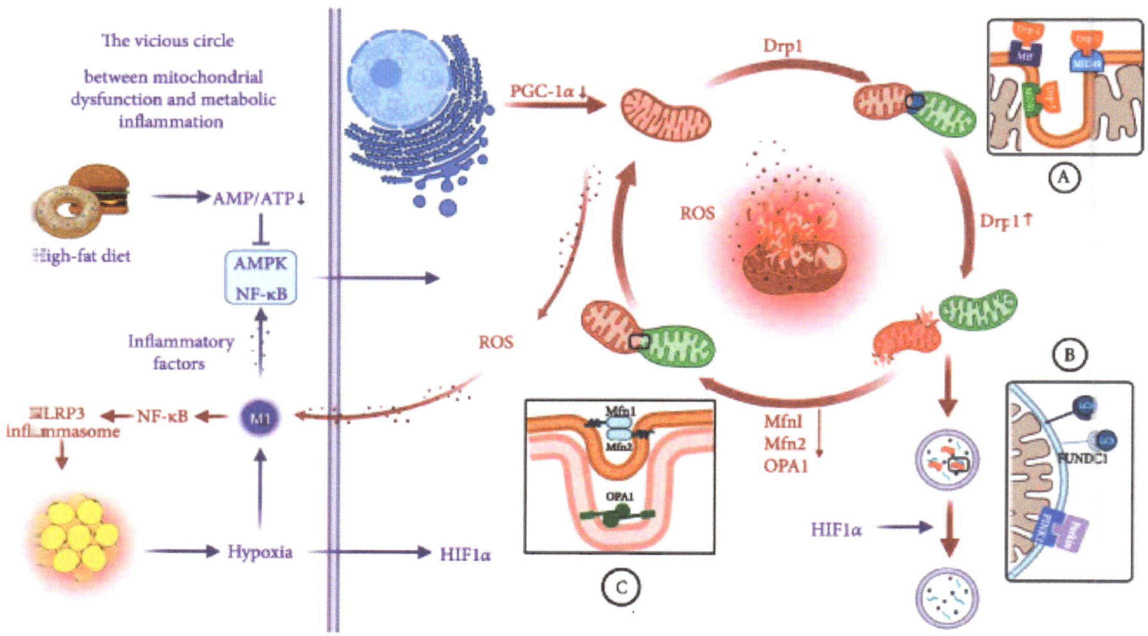

Fig. 5.5. *The links between mitochondrial dysfunction and metabolic inflammation. Overnutrition disrupts energy balance, thus inhibiting AMPK activity, driving the release of inflammatory factors, and thus enhancing NFκB signalling. Metabolic stress and inflammatory signalling disrupt mitochondrial quality control, including excessive mitochondrial fission (A) and fusion defects (C), reduced mitochondrial biosynthesis, and excessive mitophagy (B), which lead to the overproduction of ROS. ROS leads to oxidative stress oxidative stress, including NFκB signalling activation, NLRP3 inflammatory formation, and macrophage M1 polarisation. This condition aggravates the development of metabolic inflammation (source: Yuan Q et al. Oxid Med Cell Longev. 2022.).*

Therapeutic peptide strategies can be seen as a restoration of orchestral harmony. A GLP-1 agonist might strengthen the conductor's role in glycemia and appetite control; a MOTS-c analog can repair mitochondrial rhythm; Klotho fragments may recalibrate aging harmonics; NOPs can retune local tissues. Administered together in a synchronized regimen, these peptides can aim to reestablish systemic resilience.

Despite the promise of peptide-based metabolic therapy, several substantial challenges must be acknowledged. Peptides are inherently unstable in vivo and susceptible to proteases; hence advanced delivery platforms are essential. Off-target activation or receptor crosstalk poses risks of unintended effects. Chronic modulation of metabolic or mitochondrial pathways could inadvertently impact cell proliferation or senescence circuits raising potential concerns about oncogenic risks.

The issue of tissue targeting is paramount: metabolic tissues (liver, muscle, adipose, pancreatic islet) and mitochondrial compartments are diverse and sometimes poorly accessible. Achieving optimal peptide concentration in target tissues without off-target spillover is a nontrivial engineering problem. Immunogenicity over repeated dosing likewise demands vigilance, particularly in multi-peptide regimens.

From a regulatory standpoint, multi-peptide combination therapeutics pose greater complexities in safety evaluation, quality control, and approval pathways compared to single-molecule drugs. Biomarker strategies must evolve to allow real-time monitoring of peptide levels, receptor engagement, and downstream metabolic responses.

On the research frontier, priorities include more expansive human observational studies correlating endogenous MDPs, MOs, Klotho peptides, and organ-specific peptide levels with metabolic syndrome trajectories; interventional trials of peptide combinations in well-characterized metabolic cohorts; refinement of nanoparticle/mitochondrial delivery systems; development of noninvasive methodologies to quantify peptide–tissue interactions; and long-term safety studies in aging models.

Clinical Indications, Patient Selection, and Therapeutic Goals

Before prescribing any peptide regimen, one must define the clinical indication, select appropriate patients, and set realistic goals. In the context of metabolic syndrome, candidate indications might include:

- Individuals with full metabolic syndrome (three or more criteria: central obesity, dyslipidemia, hypertension, impaired fasting glucose) who have failed or not tolerated standard lifestyle or pharmacologic interventions;
- Patients in a prediabetic or insulin-resistant state, with clustering of risk factors, seeking regression of metabolic syndrome before progression to overt diabetes or cardiovascular disease;
- Patients with nonalcoholic fatty liver disease (NAFLD) or early nonalcoholic steatohepatitis (NASH) in whom metabolic syndrome is a principal driver;
- Cardiometabolic patients with early cardiac, renal or vascular dysfunction in whom mitochondrial dysfunction and peptide network collapse may play a role;
- Aging individuals with metabolic decline and evidence of mitochondrial insufficiency (reduced VO_2max, sarcopenia) in whom a peptide-regeneration strategy is desirable.

Therapeutic goals should be predefined. The objectives and aims for peptide therapy in Metabolic Syndrome can be as following:

- Reversal of metabolic syndrome (i.e., reduction to fewer than 3 criteria)
- Improved insulin sensitivity (e.g., HOMA-IR reduction, clamp-based measures)
- Weight reduction (especially visceral fat)
- Reduction in hepatic steatosis and improvement in liver enzymes
- Improvement in mitochondrial biomarkers (e.g. mitochondrial respiration, ATP production, ROS reduction)

- Improvement in emerging peptide biomarkers (e.g. increased circulating MDPs, Klotho)
- Cardiovascular and renal risk reduction (BP lowering, lipid profile improvement, albuminuria)
- Long-term safety, tolerability, and absence of adverse proliferative or immunologic effects

Because peptides often act by promoting resilience rather than acute symptom relief, the expected timeline is more gradual, minimum weeks to months, than for classical small-molecule drugs.

Patient inclusion criteria for peptide therapy may include:

- Body mass index (BMI) ≥ 28–30 kg/m² (or waist circumference above metabolic thresholds)
- At least two other metabolic syndrome criteria (dyslipidemia, elevated BP, impaired fasting glucose)
- Evidence of mitochondrial stress (e.g. elevated mitochondrial ROS markers, reduced mitochondrial respiratory function in peripheral blood mononuclear cells or muscle biopsy)
- Absence of advanced organ failure (e.g. decompensated heart failure, severe chronic kidney disease)
- Exclusion of malignant disease, active infection, autoimmune disease, or pregnancy
- Stable background therapy (if on metformin, statins, antihypertensives) for 3+ months

Early phase and first-time therapy should likely utilize the dose-escalation types of the protocol, starting with lower doses and frequency. Relevant biomarkers should be done to identify biologically active dose ranges, before proceeding to full-dose long-term regime.

Protocols for Mitochondrial Peptides

Because mitochondrial-derived peptides (MDPs) such as MOs, MOTS-c and humanin have shown the most advanced preclinical data among micropeptides, they are the logical starting point for translational protocol proposals.

In mice, daily intraperitoneal administration of MOTS-c at 0.5 mg/kg/day for 8 weeks prevented obesity, improved glucose tolerance, and increased AMPK activation and GLUT4 in muscle [32]. In aging and exercise studies, higher doses (e.g., 15 mg/kg/day) have also been tested in older mice to boost physical performance and healthspan, and even cellspan [104]. Human observational data are limited; MOTS-c levels appear elevated in obesity but decreased in overt type 2 diabetes [104].

Given these preclinical dose levels, translational human doses must account for allometric scaling, safety margins, and delivery inefficiencies. A common method is to convert animal dose (mg/kg) by body surface area to human equivalent dose (HED) using scaling factors. For example, a 0.5 mg/kg dose in a mouse converts to roughly 0.04 mg/kg in humans (~2.8 mg for a 70 kg individual). Because peptides may suffer loss during absorption, initial human protocols may start lower and escalate.

In another experimental study conducted in University of California, Irvine, explored whether systemic administration of stem cell-derived MO peptides could delay or prevent autoimmune destruction of pancreatic β-cells in the Non-Obese Diabetic (NOD) mouse model [153]. The NOD mouse, which spontaneously develops type 1 diabetes through autoimmune insulitis, provides a well-established model to test immunomodulatory or protective interventions in β-cell preservation.

The MO *Pancreas* peptides used in the study are described as mixtures of organ-specific cellular extracts enriched for mitochondrial function, derived from stem cell sources including thymus and pancreas, processed by homogenization, filtration, and sterilization. These peptides are proposed to have mitochondria-oriented reparative functions, aiming to revitalize mitochondrial deficits in target tissues.

Twelve female NOD mice (aged ~6 weeks) were randomized into two groups: one receiving MO *Pancreas* peptide injections, the other receiving saline control. Dosage was scaled down from a notional human injection dose of ~7 μg/kg; each mouse received diluted peptide solution (90 μL) twice weekly via subcutaneous injection for 17 weeks. Blood glucose was monitored weekly by tail-prick methods. Mice crossing the threshold of ≥300 mg/dL (on duplicate readings) were considered diabetic and removed from further survival. At the end of the 17-week period (or upon diabetic conversion), animals were euthanized, and serum cytokine profiling was performed using a multiplex 44-cytokine panel.

At baseline (week 1), there was no statistically significant difference in mean blood glucose between the two groups, confirming comparable starting points. Over the first several weeks (weeks 2–6), the MO-peptide group showed significantly lower mean blood glucose compared to controls ($p < 0.05$). A two-week interruption in experimental activity (weeks 7–8) temporarily halted data collection. After resumption (weeks 9–17), the difference in blood glucose between groups was no longer statistically significant at individual weekly timepoints, although the MO group's average glucose trend declined modestly relative to controls in the latter weeks.

By study termination, four of six MO-treated mice remained non-diabetic, while only two of the six controls did. The investigators report that the MO-treated group had a 33 % higher non-diabetic survival proportion relative to saline controls. In effect, MO peptide administration slowed or delayed the onset of overt hyperglycemia in a subset of mice.

Analysis of serum cytokines revealed notable differences in two markers: erythropoietin (EPO) and CCL5 (also known as RANTES). The MO peptide group exhibited significantly higher EPO levels (mean ~374.9 pg/mL vs ~203.7 pg/mL; $p = 0.0062$) and higher CCL5 levels (mean ~14.37 pg/mL vs ~8.08 pg/mL; $p = 0.031$). The authors suggest that modulation of these signaling molecules might reflect altered immune or tissue-protective responses induced by the MO *Pancreas* peptides.

In their discussion, the authors situate the study in the broader context of peptide therapy for autoimmune disease. They propose that organ-specific peptides, particularly those with mitochondria-centric repair properties, might restore or reinstate normal peptidergic signaling in immune or pancreatic tissues, thus preserving β-cell viability. The observed delay in diabetes onset in a small NOD cohort supports this possibility, though the authors caution that sample size is limited, and mechanistic pathways remain to be elucidated. The study has allowed to conclude that intramuscular (or subcutaneous) delivery of stem-cell derived MO *Pancreas* peptides appears to exert a protective effect against autoimmune β-cell destruction in this model, warranting further study of peptide dose, timing, duration, and mechanism in larger and longer-term trials.

Single ascending dose and multiple ascending dose protocol:

- Begin with a low subcutaneous dose, for example 1 mg (≈0.014 mg/kg for 70 kg). Observe safety, vital signs, labs (metabolic panel, liver renal, inflammatory markers) for 7 days.
- Then escalate to 2.5 mg, 5 mg, 10 mg in successive cohorts if no dose-limiting toxicity (DLT).
- After single-dose safety, proceed to multiple-dose cohorts (e.g., 5 mg every 5 days for 20 days, or 10 mg weekly for 4 weeks).

Proof-of-concept regimen (metabolic syndrome population):

- A plausible "starter" regimen: 5 mg subcutaneous every 5th day (i.e. ~1.4 mg/day average) for a 20-day cycle, repeated for 3–4 cycles (i.e. ~12–16 weeks).
- Alternatively, a weekly regimen: 10 mg once weekly for 8–12 weeks. Some informal sources (nonclinical) propose up to 5 mg three times weekly or 10 mg weekly for 10 weeks.
- Dose escalation may proceed if metabolic biomarkers (fasting insulin, HOMA-IR, glucose tolerance) do not improve by predetermined thresholds.
- Optional: a maintenance phase of one dose per week or one per 10 days.

Because MOTS-c is likely to have a short plasma half-life (on the order of few hours), frequent dosing or sustained-release formulations may be required to maintain effective tissue exposure.

Patients must be closely monitored. Baseline and periodic assessments should include:

- Vital signs, ECG, complete blood count, liver and renal function
- Fasting glucose, insulin, HOMA-IR, oral glucose tolerance test (OGTT)
- Lipid profile, inflammatory markers (hs-CRP, IL-6, TNF-α)
- Mitochondrial function biomarkers (e.g., platelet or PBMC mitochondrial respiration, ATP/ADP ratios, reactive oxygen species assays)
- Circulating endogenous MDP levels (MOTS-c, humanin) via robust assays (e.g., mass spectrometry or validated ELISA)
- Imaging or surrogate for visceral fat (e.g., MRI, DXA)
- Adverse events (local injection site reactions, systemic symptoms)
- Optional muscle biopsies or mitochondrial assays in selected subjects

Dose-limiting toxicities should be predefined (for example, abnormal liver enzymes >3× upper limit, serious injection reactions, sustained hypotension or hypoglycemia). Given the preclinical timeframes, there following outcomes may be anticipate:

- Within 2–4 weeks: modest improvements in fasting insulin, HOMA-IR, and decreased insulin AUC during OGTT;
- Within 8–12 weeks: measurable reductions in visceral fat, improved glucose tolerance, favorable shifts in lipid profile, reduced inflammatory markers;
- Mitochondrial functional markers (e.g., respiration efficiency, ATP production) may begin improving within weeks and continue over months;
- Over 12–16 weeks, patients might transition from full metabolic syndrome to fewer criteria, or at least no further worsening;
- In longer-term protocols (6–12 months), improvements in NAFLD markers, endothelial function, and cardiovascular risk markers could emerge.

It is essential to temper expectations: these peptides might act more as resilience enhancers rather than panaceas. A composite metabolic effect of 10–20% improvement in insulin sensitivity or visceral fat over 3–6 months may already be clinically significant.

Protocols for Klotho-Derived Peptide Fragments

Klotho, especially in its soluble form, shows inverse associations with metabolic syndrome and protective effects on oxidative stress, insulin signaling, and aging pathways. However, full-length Klotho protein is large and difficult to deliver. Thus, small peptide fragments especially portions derived from the KL1 domain are of interest.

Because clinical human trials of Klotho peptides are even more nascent, all proposed protocols must be viewed as highly theoretical.

A prudent translation path would begin with microdosing and safety escalation:

- Starting dose: 0.5–1 mg subcutaneous KL1-fragment peptide (e.g., a 20–50 amino acid peptide) administered once weekly for 4 weeks;
- If safety is confirmed, escalate to 2.5 mg weekly, then 5 mg weekly for 8–12 weeks;
- Alternative regimens: 5 mg twice weekly or 10 mg weekly, with careful biomarker monitoring;
- For tissue targeting (e.g. kidney, liver, adipose), peptide conjugation or targeting moieties (e.g. glycosylation, receptor-binding tags) may be required.

Key markers to follow include:

- Serum levels of soluble Klotho (if measurable);
- Insulin sensitivity (HOMA, OGTT);
- Markers of oxidative stress (e.g. 8-OHdG, protein carboxylation);
- mTOR, PI3K/Akt, IGF-1 pathway mediators in peripheral cells;
- Renal function and phosphorous handling (to track off-target effects).

The expected effects include:

- Subtle improvements in insulin sensitivity over 4–8 weeks;
- Reductions in lipogenesis and LDL cholesterol via downregulation of HMG-CoA reductase pathways;
- Decreased oxidative stress and improved cell resilience;
- Over months, possibly moderate regression of metabolic syndrome features and improved vascular or renal markers.

Given the structure-function uncertainties, Klotho peptide treatments would likely be best combined with mitochondrial peptides or incretin therapies.

Protocols for Nanomized Organ-Specific Peptides (NOPs) and Mito Organelles (MOs) Organ-specific Peptides (OSPs)

NOPs and MOs, as proposed by the European Wellness protocols, represent small organ-derived peptides engineered to nanoscale to facilitate tissue penetration. In metabolic syndrome, target organs include pancreas, skeletal muscle, adipose tissue, peripheral nerves, and liver.

Because the identities and sequences of many NOPs and MOs remain to be determined, clinical translation is speculative. Nonetheless, one can propose a general framework:

- Candidate NOPs (e.g. a 7–15 amino acid peptide from pancreatic islets, muscle, or nerve) are synthesized and nanomized (3 nm scale, $<$10 kDa)
- Delivery routes may include sublingual, intranasal, intravenous nanoparticle infusion, or local tissue injection (e.g., intramuscular)
- A starting dose might be 0.5–2 mg daily (divided) or equivalent in sustained-release form, escalated to 5 mg daily as tolerated.

In combination protocols, sublingual NOPs would complement intramuscular MO systemic peptides. Tissue biopsies or imaging (e.g., muscle insulin signaling, nerve conduction) and regular bloodwork may serve as local efficacy endpoints.

Given the novelty of NOPs, early human use should be limited to healthy volunteers or low-risk metabolic syndrome subjects under strict regulatory oversight.

MOs are usually given 2-3 times a week for 12-15 weeks duration with 8-12 weeks rest after the completed protocol. Intramuscular route of administration being the preferred method of systemic delivery.

Protocols for GLP-1 / Incretin / Multi-agonist Peptides in Metabolic Syndrome

In contrast to micropeptide therapies, GLP-1 agonists and incretin-based therapies already have a mature clinical foundation that can be adapted to metabolic syndrome indications.

GLP-1 receptor agonists such as liraglutide, semaglutide, dulaglutide, and newer dual (GLP-1/GIP) or triple agonists are in active clinical use. The advantage is that their safety, dosing, and metabolic effects are reasonably well-characterized. The innovation lies in combining them with mitochondrial peptides or Klotho fragments and adapting them to patients with metabolic syndrome before overt diabetes.

In the large, randomized trial combining exercise and liraglutide 3.0 mg in obese non-diabetic individuals, participants escalated liraglutide from 0.6 mg daily upward by 0.6 mg increments weekly until reaching 3.0 mg/day, or the maximally tolerated dose [154]. That trial demonstrated further reductions in metabolic syndrome severity beyond weight loss alone [155][154].

In practice, when using GLP-1 agonists for metabolic syndrome (rather than established T2DM), the following approach may be used:

- Initiation: 0.6 mg daily (liraglutide) or equivalent lowest dose of the chosen agonist;
- Gradual escalation every 1–2 weeks by 0.6 mg (or protocol equivalent) until therapeutic dose (e.g. 3.0 mg liraglutide) or tolerability limit;
- Maintenance phase: continue the full tolerated dose for 12–24 months, with metabolic monitoring.

In combination trials with exercise, the metabolic benefits (visceral fat reduction, inflammation reduction) were additive.

Emerging dual or triple agonists (GLP-1/GIP, GLP-1/GIP/glucagon, or the novel proprietor formulation GNP-1) follow similar titration paradigms (gradual dose escalation to final therapeutic dose). Early data suggest greater efficacy on fat loss and glycemic parameters [156].

Combining GLP-1 Agonists with Mitochondrial or Klotho Peptide Therapy

A rational combined-peptide protocol might begin with a stable GLP-1 agonist regimen (e.g., semaglutide weekly or liraglutide daily) for 4–8 weeks to establish baseline metabolic improvement, then layer on mitochondrial peptide therapy (e.g. MOs) or Klotho fragments. Timing might follow as:

- Weeks 0–8: GLP-1 agonist titration to target dose or even better GNP-1,
- Weeks 9–20: Add mitochondrial peptide regimen (e.g. MOs 12-15 weeks) MO *LPPSIMKE,*
- Weeks 21–36: Evaluate synergy and consider adding Klotho fragment or NOP *LPPSIMKE,*
- Maintenance beyond 36 weeks: continue GLP-1 + peptide(s), with periodic reassessment.

This staged layering allows separation of effect, safety monitoring, and synergy assessment.

Given the multifactorial nature of metabolic syndrome, single-peptide monotherapy may fall short. The promising direction is combining peptides that act on complementary axes: mitochondrial resilience, endocrine regulation, aging modulation, local tissue repair, inflammation suppression.

Alternative poly-peptide regimen for metabolic syndrome may include:

- GLP-1 agonist (e.g. liraglutide 3.0 mg/day or semaglutide equivalent) or GNP-1 as the backbone;

- Mitochondrial peptide (MOs) *LPPSIMKE* dosing 2-3 weekly;
- Klotho fragment peptide weekly;
- NOPs (e.g., organ-specific muscle or pancreatic peptide) 2-3 per week.

Adjunctive lifestyle therapy (diet, exercise) is routinely added as foundational. Periodic "pulse" intensification (e.g. short higher-dose cycles) is done every 3–4 months.

Outcomes and biomarkers would be compared to evaluate additive or synergistic benefits. When launching a peptide intervention strategy in metabolic syndrome, one can anticipate a staged trajectory in outcomes and biomarker changes:

Early Phase (Weeks 1–4):

- Enhanced insulin sensitivity, reflected in decreased fasting insulin, improved HOMA-IR
- Mild reduction in postprandial glucose excursions
- Subtle shifts in inflammatory biomarkers (hs-CRP, IL-6)
- Improvement in energy levels or subjective fatigue (especially with mitochondrial peptides)

Intermediate Phase (Weeks 8–12):

- Greater reductions in visceral adiposity (imaged by MRI or DXA)
- Modest weight loss (3–5 %)
- Improvements in lipid parameters (decrease triglycerides, rising HDL)
- Decreases in liver enzymes in NAFLD patients
- Enhancement of mitochondrial functional readouts (e.g., increased ATP/ADP ratio, improved oxygen consumption rate in PBMCs or muscle biopsy)
- Increase in endogenous mitochondrial peptide levels or improved MDP-to-reserve ratio

Later Phase (Weeks 24–52):

- Reversal or remission of metabolic syndrome criteria (e.g., normalization of fasting glucose or BP)
- Regression of hepatic steatosis or NASH (if present)
- Improvement in endothelial function, arterial stiffness, microalbuminuria
- Reduction in cardiovascular risk (e.g., improvements in carotid intima-media thickness, flow-mediated dilation)
- Maintenance or even increase of lean muscle mass
- Possible longevity or aging signal improvements (e.g., telomere length, senescence markers)

Of paramount importance is that peptide interventions are adjunctive rather than replacement for lifestyle interventions. The most durable benefit is likely when peptides facilitate improved metabolic plasticity that synergizes with diet and exercise.

It is important to remember that all peptide therapies carry potential risks some known, many unknown in humans alongside drug-level safety considerations. Key safety strategies include:

- Careful dose-escalation with DSMB oversight in early-phase trials;
- Frequent monitoring of liver and kidney function, electrolytes, complete blood count;
- Close observation of injection site reactions (erythema, swelling, pain);
- Monitoring for immunologic reactions or antibody formation;
- Vigilance for hypoglycemia, especially when combining insulin sensitizers or antidiabetic drugs;
- Monitoring off-target pathways (e.g., mTOR/IGF axis, proliferative signaling, cancer risk markers);
- Long-term observation for neoplastic, autoimmune, or organ toxicity;

- A washout period included between peptide cycles to reduce receptor desensitization risks;
- Predetermined stopping rules if serious adverse events occur.

Particular caution should apply when combining multiple peptides that may have overlapping intracellular pathways (e.g. AMPK activation, mTOR modulation). Synergistic or overactivation could conceivably provoke metabolic overshoots, catabolism, or unintended pro-apoptotic signaling. Given the limited human safety database, early trials should include extended follow-up (6–24 months) for late-onset effects. Biomarkers of DNA damage, senescence, telomere attrition, and proliferation may offer early detection of adverse long-term effects.

Conclusion

Metabolic syndrome arises from a breakdown of homeostatic circuits bridging the gut, adipose tissue, vasculature, and importantly, the mitochondria. Peptides serve as the language of inter-organ communication, stress adaptation, and metabolic coordination. While traditional peptide regulators such as GLP-1 and adipokines remain essential, the discovery of mitochondrial-derived peptides (MOTS-c, humanin, SHLPs) and the conceptual innovation of nanomized organ-specific peptides (NOPs) and Mito Organelles expand the therapeutic horizon. Klotho peptide fragments offer another axis linking metabolism and aging. Carefully engineered peptide combinations may one day permit restoration of metabolic resilience, reversing the spiral of mitochondrial dysfunction, insulin resistance, inflammation, and organ damage.

Yet, translation remains in early stages: pharmacokinetics, delivery, targeting, immune compatibility, and long-term safety demand rigorous exploration. The coming decade promises to test whether peptide therapy can evolve from promising molecular concept to clinical reality.

The concept of mitochondria-organellar peptides (MOs), bolstered by organ-specific micropeptides (OSPs/NOPs) and integrated with neuromuscular stimulation, offers a compelling, systems-level therapeutic paradigm for metabolic syndrome. By addressing both the mitochondrial engine and local tissue microenvironments, this dual-tiered strategy aspires to restore metabolic homeostasis more deeply than single-axis interventions.

Although much of the clinical roadmap remains speculative, the mechanistic foundation is increasingly robust, and the translational blueprint set forth here offers a starting template for first-in-human explorations. With careful design, biomarker-guided escalation, rigorous safety oversight, and iterative learning, the vision of peptide-driven metabolic repair may evolve from narrative paradigm to clinical reality in a daily practice of regenerative medicine physician.

CHAPTER 6

Peptide Therapeutics for Retina and Optic Nerve—Modulating Immunity, Regeneration & Neuroprotection

The retina and optic nerve are among the most demanding tissues in the the body, because of their high metabolic burden, structural complexity, and restricted regenerative capacity. Diseases such as retinitis pigmentosa (RP), glaucoma, and optic neuropathies converge on pathways of apoptosis, oxidative stress, glial activation, inflammation, and axonal loss. In recent years, the peptide class of therapeutics has emerged as an elegant and semi–modular toolset to influence these pathways: to modulate immune responses, protect neuronal and glial elements, and support regeneration. This chapter explores the mechanistic rationale, experimental evidence, delivery challenges, and future directions for peptides acting in the retina and optic pathway.

Pathobiology of Retinal Degeneration and Optic Neuropathy—the Rationale for Peptide Interventions

Inherited retinal degenerations, exemplified by RP, are genetically heterogeneous but share common downstream stress pathways. Photoreceptor degeneration triggers oxidative damage, mitochondrial dysfunction, microglial activation, breakdown of blood-retina barriers, and glial remodeling. These inflammatory and immune sequelae not only worsen ongoing cell loss but may also disrupt viable neighboring neurons. The degenerative milieu is thus self-amplifying: dying cells release danger signals (DAMPs), further activating innate immune receptors (e.g., Toll-like receptors, NLRP3 inflammasome) and recruiting maladaptive T cell responses. In RP, chronic microglial activation and elevated cytokines (e.g., IL-1β, TNF-α, IL-6) are commonly observed in both animal models and postmortem human tissue [157].

Meanwhile, in glaucoma and other optic neuropathies, retinal ganglion cells (RGCs) face insult via elevated intraocular pressure, ischemia, axonal transport disruption, and glial stress. Secondary inflammation, complement activation, and glial scar formation further impede neuronal survival and axonal regrowth. Stem cell-based strategies have been under exploration for glaucomatous nerve repair, but peptides offer a complementary or adjunctive dimension: small, tunable molecules with the capacity to cross barriers, modulate immunity, and deliver trophic signaling [158].

Because peptides can act on multiple nodes of the degenerative cascade, from mitochondrial stabilization to immunoregulation to glial reprogramming they are uniquely suited to intervene in tissues as delicate and complex as retina and optic nerve.

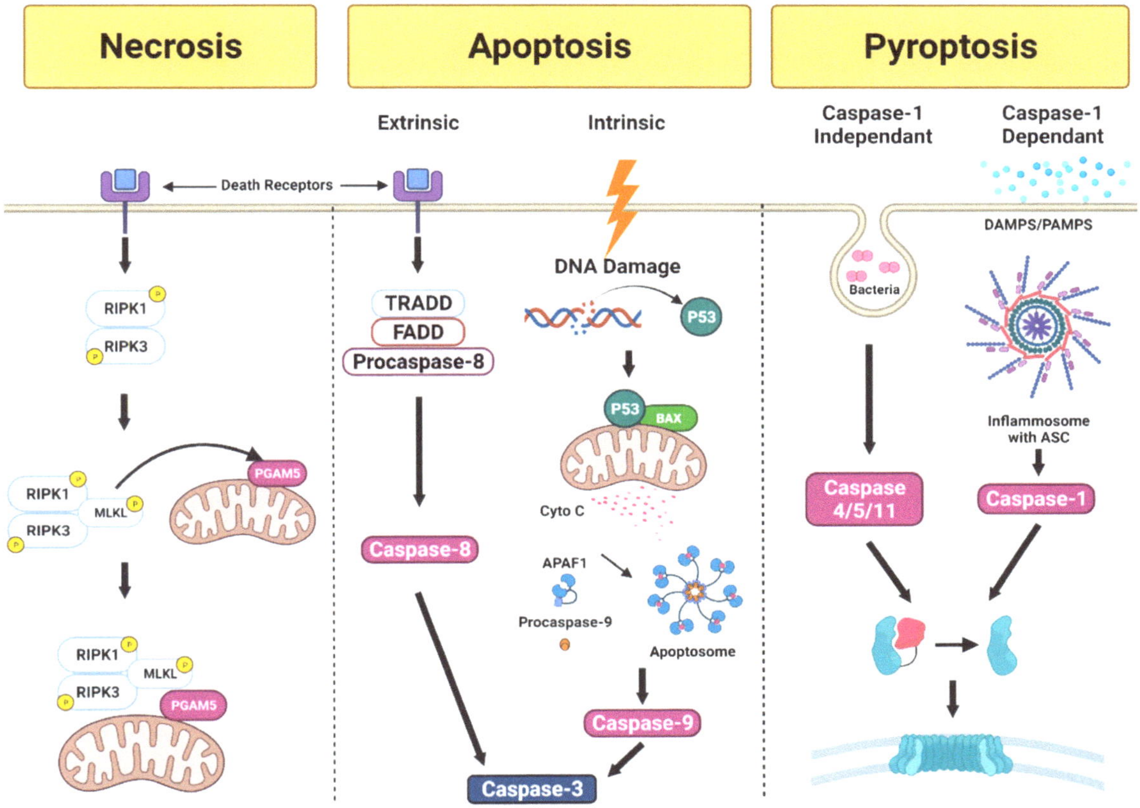

Fig 6.1. *Overview of necrosis, apoptosis, and pyroptosis pathways involved in retinal pigment epithelium (RPE) cell death in age-related macular degeneration. In necrosis, the necrosome forms complex proteins that attach to the mitochondrial membrane, triggering cell death. Apoptosis can be activated through the intrinsic or extrinsic pathways, which eventually result in the activation of caspase 3 and then cell death. Pyroptosis can occur through caspase 1-dependent or independent pathways, which lead to the generation of an N-terminal fragment that induces cell death (source: Kim, J., Lee, Y. J., & Won, J. Y. (2021). Molecular Mechanisms of Retinal Pigment Epithelium Dysfunction in Age-Related Macular Degeneration. International Journal of Molecular Sciences, 22(22), 12298).*

Bioactive Peptides in the Retina—Mechanisms of Action

Within retinal degeneration research, several classes of peptides have shown promise. Let's discuss the most promising options.

Melanocortin-derived peptides (α-MSH, KPV, analogs). The melanocortin peptides exert potent anti-inflammatory and immunoregulatory effects. They modulate microglial polarization, inhibit NF-κB activation, and reduce cytokine release. In retinal models, α-MSH analogs have been reported to suppress microglial activation and preserve photoreceptors [159]. The tripeptide fragment KPV (Lys–Pro–Val), derived from α-MSH, can likewise protect the blood-retinal barrier, regulate inflammatory mediators, and stabilize tight junctions in diabetic retinopathy models.

Mitochondria-targeted peptides are among the most advanced in translation is the tetrapeptide SS-31 (elamipretide), which localizes to the inner mitochondrial membrane, binds cardiolipin, maintains mitochondrial membrane potential, and reduces oxidative stress and apoptotic signaling. In canine RP models, daily SS-31 preserved outer retinal structure and slowed functional decline. Its ability to mitigate metabolic stress at the core of degenerative cascades makes it especially compelling [160].

Thymic peptides, including MO *Thymus* and Thymosin β4 (Tβ4) and regenerative peptides are the small actin-binding peptides known for cytoprotective, anti-fibrotic, and pro-repair properties. In light-injury retinal models, Tβ4 reduces gliosis, supports Müller glia responses, and helps maintain the integrity of the neurovascular interface. It may help preserve the blood-retina barrier and mitigate reactive glial remodeling [161].

Chaperone-derived mini-peptides, including the Nano organ Peptides from retina are the misfolded proteins and aggregation stress are features of retinal degeneration. Mini-peptides derived from α-crystallin (a small heat-shock protein) can stabilize misfolded proteins, inhibit caspase activation, and reduce photoreceptor apoptosis. The neuroprotective peptide NAP (NAPVSIPQ) derived from activity-dependent neuroprotective protein (ADNP) is another example: it exerts microtubule stabilization and neuroprotection in retinal injury models [162][163].

Antigen-specific tolerogenic peptides / antigen-adaptive selective immunotherapy, including the Autologous Specific Immunotherapy (AASI) are the more ambitious direction is the use of retina-derived antigen peptides (e.g., recoverin, arrestin, interphotoreceptor retinoid-binding protein [IRBP]) in tolerogenic formulations. The goal is to re-educate pathogenic T cell responses, expand regulatory T cells, and restore immunological tolerance without general immunosuppression. In experimental autoimmune uveitis and animal models of immune-mediated retinal damage, peptide-loaded tolerogenic dendritic cells or nanoparticle carriers have induced protective Treg responses and reduced effector T cell infiltration. Although no AASI trials exist yet in RP, the paradigm holds potential to stabilize inflammatory subtypes of retinal disease and complement regenerative strategies [164].

While much of the retinal peptide work has centered on photoreceptor and RPE support, the optic pathway offers parallel opportunities. Peptides capable of modulating glial scarring, promoting axonal growth, suppressing inflammation, or delivering neurotrophic support may play a role in glaucoma and optic neuropathies. One could envisage melanocortin peptides, mitochondrial stabilizers, or tolerogenic peptides applied to the optic nerve microenvironment to ameliorate RGC degeneration or support regenerative grafts. Although the specific literature on optic nerve peptide therapeutics is currently sparser, the conceptual framework is strongly analogous to retinal approaches, and cross-fertilization is promising [165][166].

In my decades of work spanning hundreds of clinics across the globe, I have witnessed firsthand the transformative potential of Mito Organelles peptides, particularly the formulations *Retina* and *Optic Nerve*, in restoring sight and redefining what was once considered irreversible vision loss. These peptides, meticulously derived from retinal and optic nerve mitochondria, act as masterful conductors within the eye, orchestrating repair at the most fundamental cellular level. Mito Organelles *Retina* revitalizes photoreceptors and retinal pigment epithelium, enhancing mitochondrial bioenergetics, quelling oxidative stress, and awakening dormant retinal progenitor cells to rebuild the architecture of vision itself. Simultaneously, Mito Organelles *Optic Nerve* repairs ganglion cells and regenerates axons, remyelinating and reconnecting them with the brain's visual centers, restoring the very highways through which light becomes perception.

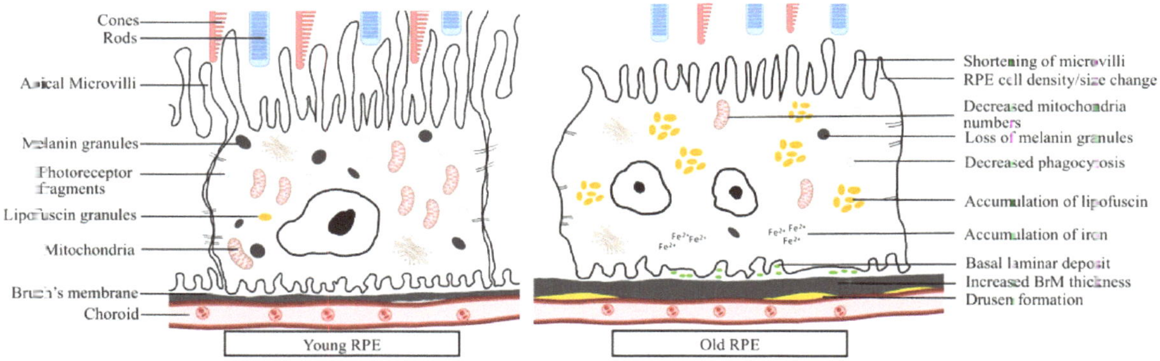

Fig 6.2. *Role of Mitochondria in Retinal Pigment Epithelial Aging and Degeneration (source: Front. Aging, 2022. Sec. Aging, Metabolism and Redox Biology)*

To achieve maximal impact, I administer these peptides via a triple-route strategy that reflects both precision and elegance: intramuscular injections, ocular drops, and sphenopalatine ganglion (SPG) blocks. Specifically, intramuscular administration is performed 2–3 times per week on alternate days for 15–20 weeks, allowing systemic mitochondrial support to reach retinal and optic nerve cells. The NOP *Retina* formulation is applied as daily eye drops, twice a day, providing targeted nourishment directly to the retinal layers. Finally, SPG blocks are delivered weekly or once every 10–14 days, facilitating direct neural access to the optic nerve and optimizing regeneration along central visual pathways.

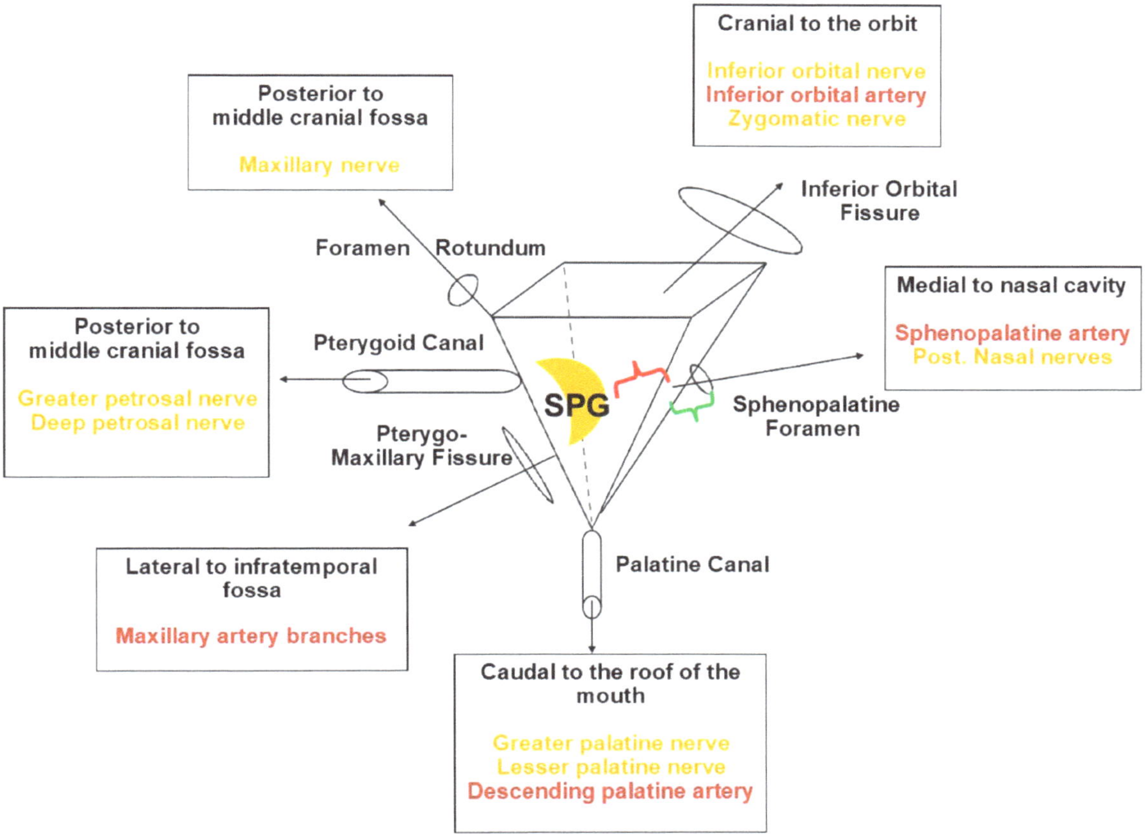

Fig 6.3. *Sphenopalatine ganglion and neural pathways it is involved in (source: Regional Anesthesia & Pain Medicine, 2020).*

The clinical outcomes observed in patients with diabetic retinopathy, glaucoma, ischemic retinal injury, and optic nerve atrophy have been remarkable: improved visual acuity, enhanced retinal thickness, and restored nerve conduction, often surpassing expectations in cases long deemed untreatable. What distinguishes these therapies is not merely their potency, but their synergy with the body's own biology. Unlike conventional interventions, which often treat symptoms or attempt to overpower the system, Mito Organelles peptides guide the eye back to its natural state of balance and function. In my personal experience, these molecules do not merely preserve vision, instead they essentially restore it, returning patients to a world they feared lost. In the realm of ophthalmic regeneration, *Retina* and

Optic Nerve are not just treatments, they are instruments of renaissance, elegant in design, profound in effect, and unmatched in their ability to awaken the dormant potential of the human eye.

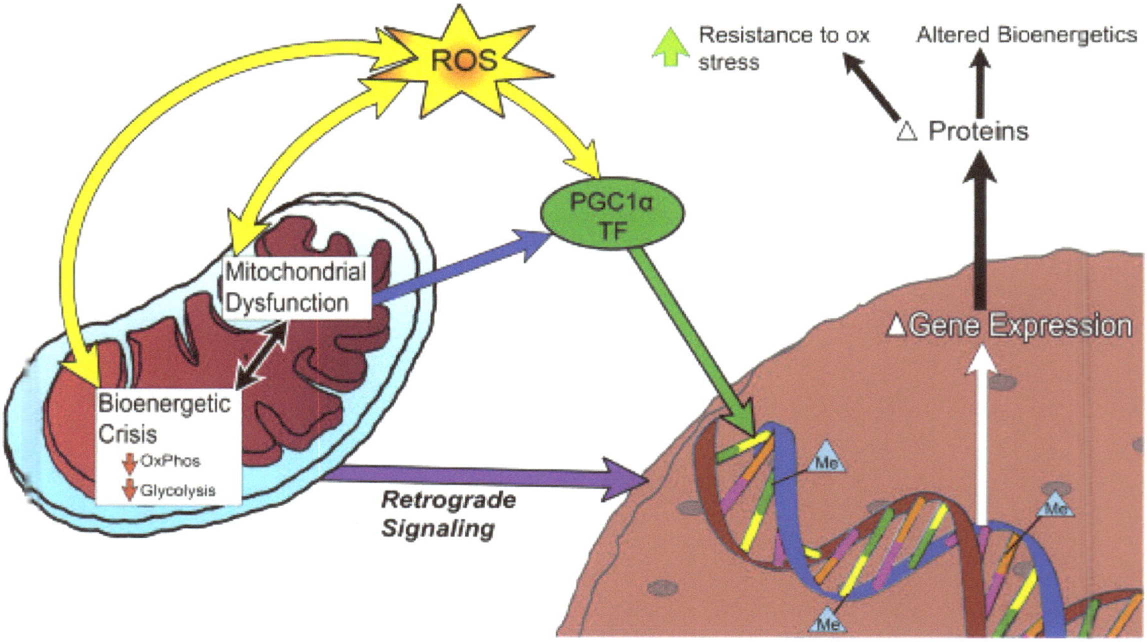

Fig 6.4. *AMD is associated with mitochondrial dysfunction and a bioenergetic crisis, documented by decreased OxPhos and glycolysis. Through restored mitochondrial retrograde signaling, these pathways restore gene expression and protein content of the cell (Source: Redox Biology, 2017).*

Integration with Stem/Progenitor Cell Therapies in Glaucoma

Stem cell–based approaches in glaucoma often focus on RGC replacement, neurotrophic support, or modulation of intraocular pressure–induced damage. The review on progenitor/precursor stem cells in glaucoma outlines the current status and challenges in translating these cellular therapies [158]. One critical barrier is the hostile microenvironment: inflammation, reactive glia, oxidative stress, and immunologic rejection impair graft survival and integration.

Here, peptides may serve as co-therapies. Administering a peptide that calms inflammation, fosters glial permissiveness, or sustains transplanted progenitor cells could significantly boost the success of stem cell grafts. For instance, a peptide that stabilizes mitochondrial health in transplanted RGC precursors may improve their survival under stress. Alternatively, a tolerogenic peptide approach may reduce immune rejection of allogeneic or iPSC-derived grafts by locally modulating host T cell responses. Thus, peptide–cell therapy synergy could be especially impactful in the optic nerve domain [167].

Delivering peptides into retinal and optic compartments is inherently challenging. The ocular barriers—cornea, sclera, vitreous, internal limiting membrane (ILM), and blood-retina barrier, limit simple diffusion of peptides. Moreover, systemic administration often results in enzymatic degradation, off-target dilution, and limited penetration [168].

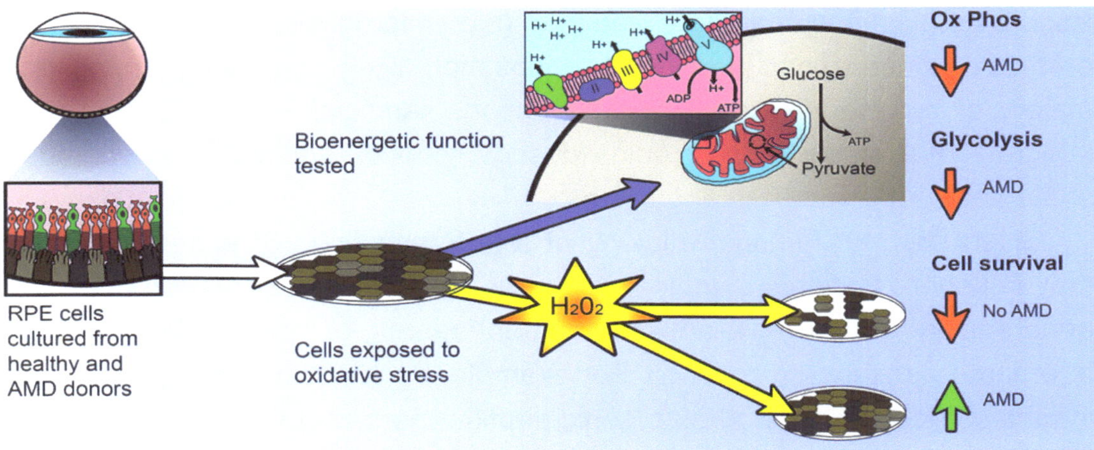

Fig 6.5. *Enhanced resistance to oxidative stress in retinal progenitor pigment epithelial cells from donors with age-related macular degeneration (Source: Redox Biology, 2017).*

To overcome these hurdles, several strategies are under investigation. Cyclization and PEGylation of peptides can extend half-lives and resist proteolysis. Nanoparticle encapsulation, liposomes, and exosome-based carriers can ferry peptides across ocular barriers and target them to the subretinal or perivascular space. Retinal homing peptides that bind selectively to degenerating photoreceptors or RPE surfaces may further concentrate payloads. In addition, combining peptide delivery with minimally invasive routes (intravitreal, subretinal, suprachoroidal) may optimize access [169].

For antigen-specific tolerogenic peptides, nanoparticle or microparticle platforms delivering antigenic peptides in tolerogenic form may support uptake by tolerogenic antigen-presenting cells in ocular tissues, promoting Treg induction and immune reprogramming [170].

Despite encouraging preclinical data, translation of peptide therapies in retina and optic nerve faces several hurdles. Manufacturing consistency, regulatory pathways, long-term safety, and patient stratification remain significant obstacles. Clinical endpoints in retinal degeneration are evolving beyond simple visual acuity to include field sensitivity, microperimetry, imaging biomarkers, and patient-reported outcomes.

Precision stratification will be vital. Multi-omic profiling (genetics, transcriptomics, proteomics) and imaging biomarkers (e.g., microglial activation maps, autofluorescence kinetics) can identify subgroups more likely to benefit from immunoregulatory or regenerative peptide interventions. Artificial intelligence models may integrate multimodal data to guide dosage, peptide selection, and combination strategies.

Given the multifactorial etiology of retinal and optic diseases, monotherapy may fall short. Rational combination therapies consisting of pairing peptides with gene editing, cell therapy, anti-complement agents, or small molecules are likely to emerge as standard practice. For example, transient immunosuppression during the induction phase of tolerogenic peptide therapy could reduce inflammation and allow better immune re-education. Similarly, peptides may be timed to support graft integration or to recalibrate glial responses post-cell transplantation.

One of the most exciting frontiers is designing multifunctional peptides: molecules engineered to combine mitochondrial targeting, immunomodulation, and trophic signaling in one scaffold. Coupled with smart delivery systems and patient-specific biomarker-informed design, peptides may bridge the gap between symptomatic management and true regeneration.

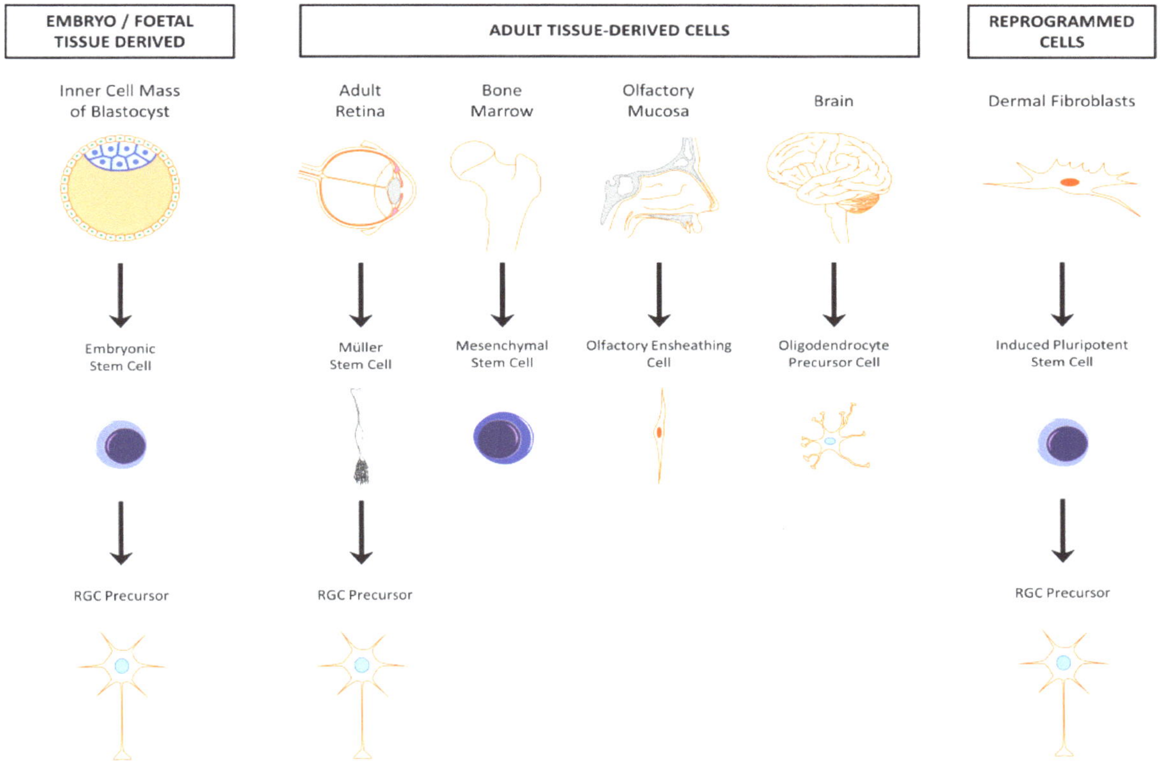

Fig 6.6. *Stem cell based therapies for glaucoma (source: The Mystery of Glaucoma, 2011).*

In conclusion, I want to mention that peptides are emerging as a sophisticated, tunable, and clinically translatable class of biologics for retinal and optic nerve disease. Their capacity to modulate immunity, support metabolism, and foster repair makes them well suited for the delicate and complex ocular environment. Though many challenges remain, particularly in delivery, stability, clinical translation, and regulatory acceptance, the conceptual and experimental foundation is strong. In the coming era of regenerative ophthalmology, peptides may well become indispensable adjuncts or even principal agents in treating retinal degenerations and optic neuropathies.

CHAPTER 7

Peptides in Neurodegenerative Disorders—Regeneration, Plasticity, and Disease Modification

Neurodegenerative diseases, including but not limited to Alzheimer's disease, Parkinson's disease, amyotrophic lateral sclerosis, Huntington's disease, and related disorders that pose one of the greatest challenges in modern medicine. Their progressive courses, lack of curative therapies, and the complexity of underlying pathophysiology demand novel approaches that go beyond symptomatic relief. Over the past decade, peptides have emerged as versatile therapeutic candidates, capable of modulating neuroinflammation, oxidative stress, protein misfolding, synaptic repair, and regenerative signaling. In this chapter, we examine how peptide therapeutics may shift the paradigm from neurodegeneration to neuroregeneration, how they might support neuroplasticity, and what translational obstacles must be overcome.

The Landscape of Neurodegeneration: Common Pathways and Therapeutic Niches

Although each neurodegenerative disease manifests distinct features, many share converging pathological hallmarks: accumulation of misfolded proteins (amyloid-β, tau, α-synuclein, TDP-43, huntingtin), mitochondrial dysfunction and oxidative stress, chronic neuroinflammation, synaptic loss, impaired proteostasis, disordered metal homeostasis, and failure of endogenous repair systems (neurogenesis, plasticity) [171].

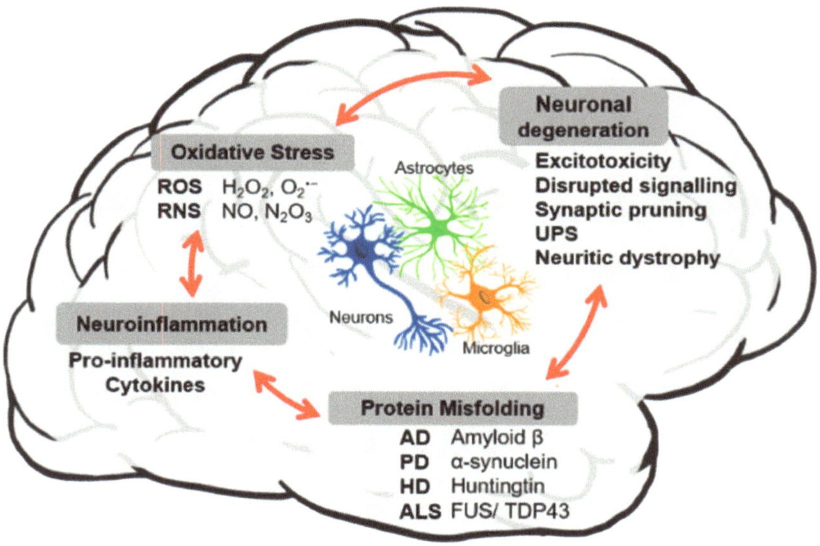

Fig 7.1. *Main hallmarks of neurodegeneration and neurodegenerative diseases–protein misfolding, neuroinflammation, neuronal degeneration and oxidative stress–shared between the major cellular types present in the brain such as neurons, astrocytes and microglia. UPS: ubiquitin–proteosome system, ROS: reactive oxygen species, RNS: reactive nitrogen system, AD: Alzheimer's disease, PD: Parkinson's disease, HD: Huntington's disease, ALS: amyotrophic lateral sclerosis. (Source: Carregosa, Diogo & Mota, Sara & Ferreira, Sofia & Alves-Dias, Beatriz & Loncarevic-Vasiljkovic, Natasa & Crespo, Carolina & Menezes, Regina & Teodoro, Rita & Santos, Cláudia. (2021). Overview of Beneficial Effects of (Poly)phenol Metabolites in the Context of Neurodegenerative Diseases on Model Organisms. Nutrients. 10.3390/nu13092940.)*

Traditional therapies have mostly focused on symptomatic relief but they fail to increase the brainspan. Such include the cholinesterase inhibitors and NMDA antagonists in Alzheimer's, dopamine replacement in Parkinson's, spasticity or supportive measures in ALS, but none fundamentally alter disease trajectory. This gap invites modalities that intervene at upstream or midstream nodes in degeneration, ideally promoting regeneration or resiliency. Bioactive peptides, by virtue of their high specificity, modifiability, and lower off-target toxicity, are promising candidates for this role [172].

Peptides can be designed to bind and inhibit aggregation of pathogenic proteins, modulate receptor signaling to favor trophic and anti-apoptotic pathways, deliver or mimic neurotrophic factors, regulate metal dyshomeostasis, and attenuate neuroinflammation. In Alzheimer's disease (AD), for example, peptide inhibitors of amyloid-β aggregation and tau phosphorylation are under active study. Peptide therapies may also facilitate endogenous neurogenesis and synaptic repair, shifting the balance from neuronal loss toward regeneration. Several recent reviews underscore the potential of bioactive peptides in neurodegenerative disease, highlighting both their promise and their challenges (e.g. low half-life, blood–brain barrier (BBB) penetration) [173][174].

In Alzheimer's disease, the amyloid cascade (aggregation of amyloid-β from APP cleavage) and tau hyperphosphorylation have dominated therapeutic strategies. However, the complexity of downstream neurodegeneration suggests a multipronged approach. Peptide-based inhibitors targeting amyloid-β assembly, modulators of tau pathology, and peptide mimetics of neurotrophic factors have been under development [175].

Peptides that interfere with amyloid-β oligomerization and fibril formation show promise. Peptide fragments, conformationally constrained ligands, or chaperone-mimicking peptides can bind Aβ species and block their aggregation or disassemble existing fibrils. Nanoparticle-assisted peptide delivery is a growing field: peptide inhibitors conjugated to nanoparticles can improve stability and crossing of the BBB, thereby enhancing their therapeutic index [176]. Some peptides are also being designed to chelate metal ions (e.g., Cu, Zn) involved in amyloid aggregation, offering a hybrid function of aggregation inhibition plus metal homeostasis.

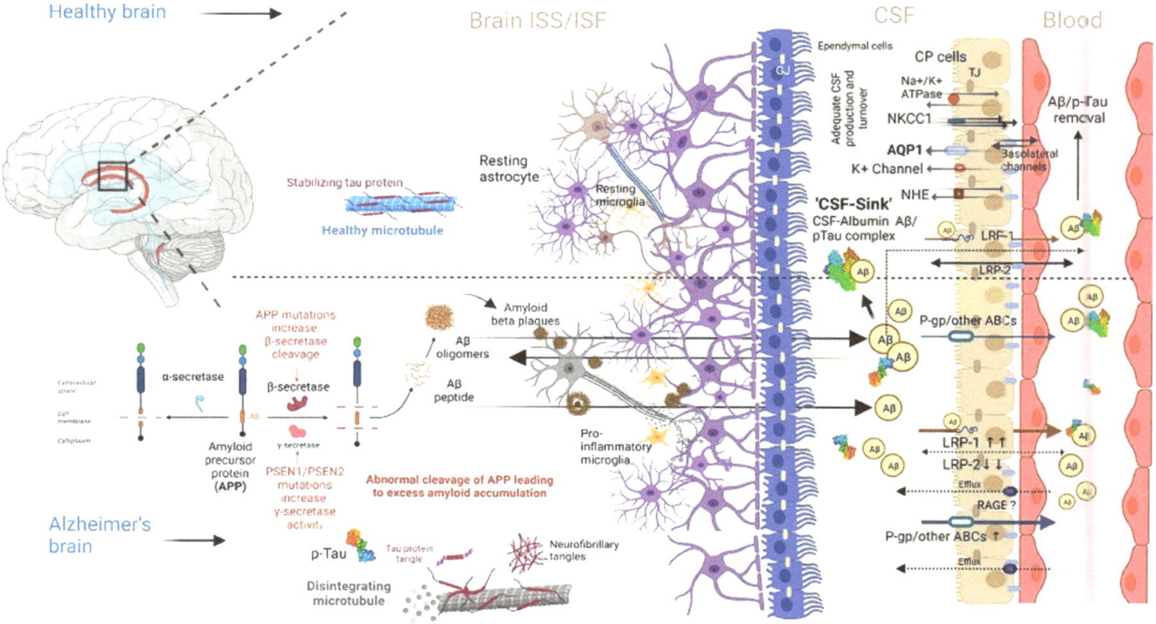

Fig 7.2. *Transportation dynamics of Aβ across the blood–brain barrier (BBB) into plasma in healthy and Alzheimer's brains demonstrating the 'plasma-Aβ sink' (source: Mondal R et al. Neurologia, 2025).*

Another promising approach is the use of small peptide mimetics of neurotrophic factors. Because recombinant neurotrophic proteins (like BDNF, NGF, CNTF) suffer from poor pharmacokinetics and limited brain penetration, small peptides that mimic key binding epitopes or downstream signaling motifs are attractive. One example is *P021*, a peptide mimetic of CNTF, which enhances hippocampal neurogenesis and BDNF expression, while suppressing tau hyperphosphorylation via inhibition of GSK-3β. P021 has favorable properties, including BBB permeability and oral bioavailability, and has demonstrated beneficial effects in animal models of AD [177][178]. The concept is that such peptide mimetics can shift the molecular balance toward synaptic repair, neuronal survival, and plasticity, hence increasing the brainspan in a big way.

Beyond aggregation and trophism, peptides may target other pathogenic axes in AD. For instance, the *J bs-5YP* peptide was recently shown, in senescent mice, to ameliorate cognitive deficits by modulating iron export. This peptide enhances transcription of the *Slc40a1* gene, which encodes ferroportin, thereby promoting iron efflux. In treated animals, brain iron load and free radical levels decreased, neuronal integrity improved, and behavioral measures of dementia were partially reversed. This is a striking demonstration of how a designed peptide can intercept a non-canonical axis of neurodegeneration (iron toxicity) and produce functional benefit. *J bs-5YP* crosses the BBB when administered orally, further underscoring its translational potential [179].

Diet-derived or plant/food-source peptides also hold potential. A black soybean-derived peptide (BSP1) has been shown in hippocampal neuronal cultures to modulate the AMPK/SIRT1 pathway, reducing BACE1 expression, APP processing, tau phosphorylation, and neuroinflammation (via NF-κB suppression) in models of lead-induced AD phenotypes. This suggests that naturally derived peptides may serve as adjuncts or leads in drug development efforts [180].

Taken together, the Alzheimer's peptide therapeutics pipeline is evolving toward integrative strategies: combining aggregation inhibitors, neurotrophic mimetics, metal modulators, and anti-inflammatory peptides into multi-target regimens. The goal is not simply to curb pathology but to redirect brain physiology toward regeneration, resilience, and functionally meaningful recovery. This conceptual shift from purely suppressing degeneration to actively rebuilding structure is gaining momentum in Alzheimer's pharmacology [181][182].

Parkinson's and Synucleinopathies: Targeting α-Synuclein with Peptides

Parkinson's disease (PD) is characterized by misfolded α-synuclein aggregation, mitochondrial dysfunction, oxidative stress, and neuroinflammation. Peptides designed to bind α-synuclein oligomers or fibrils can prevent further aggregation or enhance clearance by chaperone or proteasomal systems. In this space, the *aSynPEP-DB* database provides a useful resource: using computational screening across human neuropeptides, antimicrobial peptides, and diet-derived peptides, researchers have identified over 100 candidate peptides predicted to inhibit α-synuclein aggregation via selective binding to toxic species. For example, the endogenous human peptide *LL-37* emerged as a high-affinity binder to α-syn aggregates, suggesting a potentially endogenous regulatory role and serving as a scaffold for engineering improved derivatives [183][184].

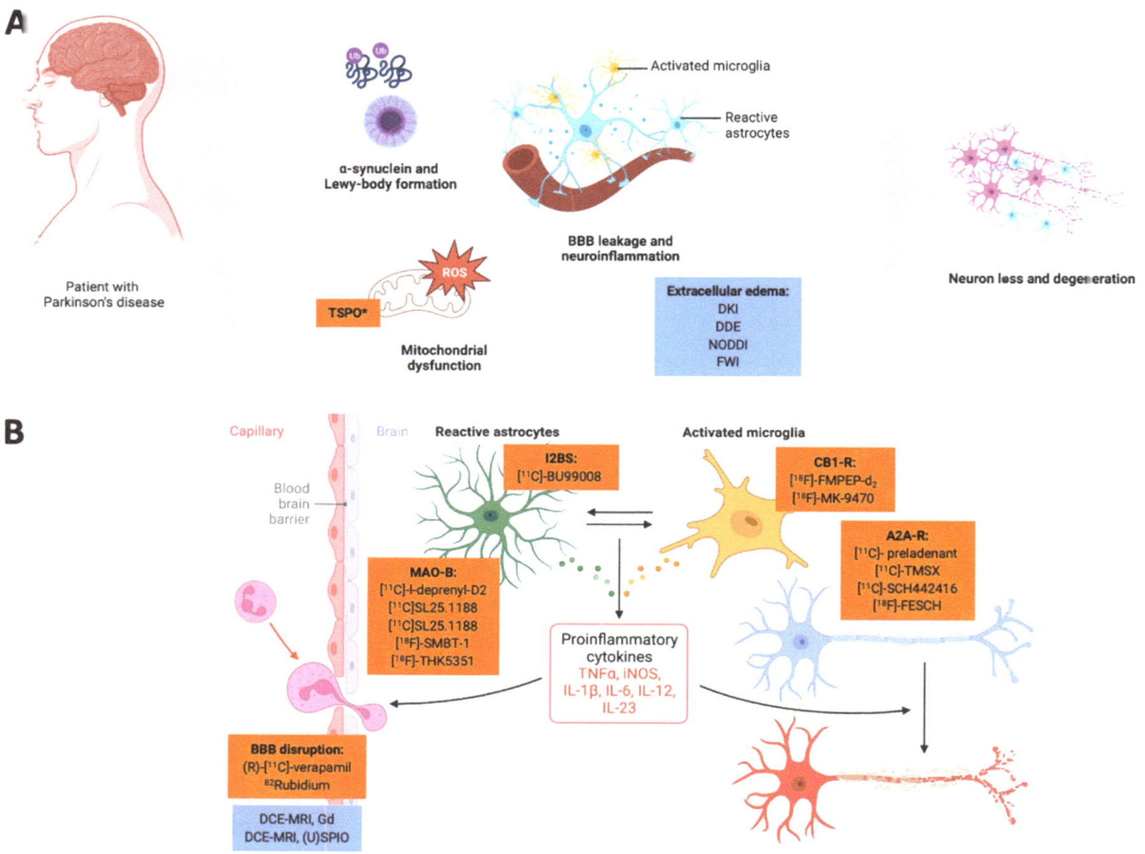

Fig 7.3. *The interconnected nature of neuroinflammation and mitochondrial dysfunction and how pathophysiology-orientated neuroimaging can be applied to study these disease mechanisms. In Panel (A), we demonstrate how a-synuclein deposition, mitochondrial dysfunction, and the tissue/cellular aspects of neuroinflammation act together in a vicious cycle to promote neurodegeneration. Radiotracers are highlighted in orange, and MRI-based neuroimaging approaches are highlighted in blue. Here, TSPO can also be considered an unspecific marker of the mitochondria. BBB leakage and the extracellular edema component of neuroinflammation are usually investigated by (advanced) diffusion-weighted MRI methods. In Panel (B), we illustrate how (pre-)clinical radiotracers can address the cellular and humoral neuroinflammatory responses. The closeup on the BBB also highlights novel*

MRI-based approaches to assess BBB integrity (source: Pizarro-Galleguillos, B. M., Kunert, L., Brüggemann, N., & Prasuhn, J. (2023). Neuroinflammation and Mitochondrial Dysfunction in Parkinson's Disease: Connecting Neuroimaging with Pathophysiology. Antioxidants, 12(7), 1411. https://doi.org/10.3390/antiox12071411).

In the past over 45 years I come to realize that the main point here is that Mito Organelles and NOP peptides can act as molecular "chaperones" or modulators of aggregation homeostasis limiting toxic species while sparing monomeric function. Because α-syn aggregation is central to PD pathology, these peptide strategies hold real promise if delivered with sufficient organ specificity and stability to ensure precision in bioregeneration [185].

While much peptide work has concentrated on AD and PD, the principles generalize to other neurodegenerative disorders. In amyotrophic lateral sclerosis (ALS), aggregation of TDP-43 or SOD1, excitotoxicity, and glial inflammation are key targets. Peptides capable of modulating glutamate receptor signaling, suppressing excitotoxic pathways, or enhancing motor neuron trophic support may be therapeutic. In Huntington's disease, peptide inhibitors of mutant *huntingtin* aggregation or modulators of downstream apoptotic signaling could slow disease progression [186][187].

Review literature underscores that peptides such as vasoactive intestinal peptide (VIP), glucagon-like peptides (GLP-1 analogs), neurotensin, and cholecystokinin may have neuroprotective roles in multiple neurodegenerative contexts. These peptides may mitigate oxidative stress, improve mitochondrial function, regulate calcium signaling, or dampen neuroinflammation [188][173]. The challenge is to adapt or re-engineer them for delivery into the central nervous system, enhance their stability, and minimize degradation.

One of the most compelling frontiers is the deployment of peptides not only to slow degeneration, but to reinvigorate plasticity and regeneration. In Alzheimer's, for instance, enhancing adult hippocampal neurogenesis or promoting synaptic rewiring may help restore cognitive reserve. The pathology of AD includes a marked impairment of endogenous neurogenesis, possibly mediated by toxic milieu, inflammation, and niche exhaustion. Strategies to rescue or amplify neural stem cell (NSC) niches will be critical. The role of peptides here is multifold: (1) direct stimulation of NSC proliferation or differentiation via mimicry of growth factors or extracellular niche cues; (2) modulation of glial or vascular niche factors to restore a permissive environment; (3) suppression of inflammatory or oxidative stress that would otherwise impair plasticity. Reviews argue that facilitating endogenous neurogenesis, in conjunction with degeneration-modifying strategies, is a promising path forward in AD therapy [189][181].

Peptide mimetics of neurotrophins (e.g., BDNF, NGF) can support synaptic repair, dendritic growth, and circuit remodeling. Endogenous peptides such as irisin and melatonin, or peptides derived from metabolic or circadian signaling hubs, have been considered for their pleiotropic effects on neuronal resilience and plasticity in Alzheimer's models [190]. By linking metabolic or systemic signals to neural repair, these peptides may help realign brain-wide health with local regeneration.

A central obstacle for peptide therapies in neurodegeneration is the blood–brain barrier, enzymatic degradation, and short systemic half-life. Brain targeting requires either inherent BBB permeation (via favorable structure or transporter binding) or active delivery systems. Cell-penetrating peptides (CPPs) are often employed as carriers or fusion partners to facilitate BBB crossing and intracellular uptake. Nanoparticle conjugation, exosome-loaded peptides, or liposomal vehicles can protect peptides from proteolysis and target them to specific brain regions or cell types. In the context of Alzheimer's, peptide inhibitors conjugated to nanoparticles show improved brain delivery and reduced off-target exposure [176]. In more advanced applications, "*nano-organo peptides*" tailored to target deep brain nuclei (e.g., thalamic relay regions) are being proposed, as in the context of Alzheimer's network dysfunction [191].

Structural modification of peptides (cyclization, D-amino acids, PEGylation, backbone stabilization) can enhance proteolytic resistance. Rational design to minimize immunogenic epitopes and optimize receptor affinity is also crucial. Monitoring pharmacokinetics, brain distribution, off-target uptake, and potential immunogenicity will be key in translating promising peptide leads into therapeutic candidates.

Despite the conceptual promise, peptide therapeutics in neurodegenerative disease remain largely at the preclinical stage. Several challenges must be addressed. First, optimizing BBB permeability without losing target specificity or exposing peripheral toxicity is nontrivial [192]. Second, the complex and multifactorial nature of neurodegeneration suggests that monotherapy peptides may not suffice; rational combination strategies may be needed, but that increases complexity, regulatory burden, and risk of interactions [193]. Third, long-term safety and immunogenicity of peptide therapies, particularly in aged or immunosenescent populations, must be carefully evaluated. Fourth, robust biomarkers and trial designs are needed to detect early regenerative effects, plasticity changes, or disease modification (rather than just symptomatic improvement). Finally, cost, manufacturing scalability, and delivery logistics (especially for repeated dosing) weigh heavily in translation [95].

Promising approaches may include coupling peptides with gene therapy or viral vectors (to express peptide derivatives in situ), using inducible release systems, or combining peptides with cell- or exosome-based therapies. Rational patient stratification using genetics, imaging, fluid biomarkers, and network models will be essential to match peptide candidates to responsive subpopulations [194].

The evolving vision for peptide therapeutics in neurodegenerative disease is bold: not merely to stanch decline, but to restore connectivity, promote renewal, and rebuild neural resilience. This will require integration of peptide-based aggregation modulators, neurotrophic mimetics, anti-inflammatory and metabolic stabilizers, and plasticity-enhancing agents, all delivered via advanced targeting platforms. As the boundary between neuroprotection and neuroregeneration blurs, peptides may become indispensable tools in a new class of regenerative neuromedicine.

Emerging clinical trends in Alzheimer's therapeutics emphasize this transition from single-pathway small molecules to biologics, combinatorial regimens, and regenerative strategies [195][196]. The time is ripe for peptides to step into that space, bridging molecular precision with regenerative ambition.

Peptide-Based Treatment Protocols: Clinical Approaches with Mito Organelles and Regenerative Peptides

While much of the scientific literature on peptides for neurodegeneration remains preclinical or investigational, certain peptide-based protocols have already entered clinical use within the context of integrative and regenerative medicine. One of the most clinically relevant peptide classes in this domain is the Mito Organelles *CNS*, a bioregulatory peptide complex derived from mitochondrial fractions of porcine or ovine origin, designed to target cellular energy metabolism, reduce neuroinflammation, and support neuroplastic repair.

Mito Organelles *CNS* peptides are administered intramuscularly, typically two to three times per week on alternate days, in treatment cycles lasting 12 to 15 weeks, followed by a rest period of several weeks before the cycle is repeated. This pulsed protocol allows for biological integration, adaptation, and avoidance of immune tolerance or receptor downregulation. The cumulative therapeutic effect of Mito Organelles is observed across repeated cycles, as mitochondrial biogenesis, oxidative balance, and neuroprotective signaling progressively improve with consistent stimulation.

The rationale for mitochondrial-targeted peptide therapy in neurodegenerative conditions stems from the central role of mitochondrial dysfunction in neuronal degeneration. Mitochondria in aging neurons are subject to fragmentation, depolarization, and bioenergetic decline. They produce excess reactive oxygen species (ROS), activate inflammasome complexes (e.g., NLRP3), and release cytochrome c and other apoptotic signals [197]. Mito Organelles peptides aim to stabilize mitochondrial membrane integrity, normalize ATP production, and reduce oxidative stress, thereby shifting the cell away from a pro-apoptotic state toward survival and plasticity.

Studies and clinical observations indicate that Mito Organelles peptides enhance the expression of mitochondrial superoxide dismutase (MnSOD), upregulate PGC-1α (peroxisome proliferator-activated receptor gamma coactivator 1-alpha), and promote mitochondrial DNA repair and replication. These processes collectively support mitochondrial biogenesis, restore calcium buffering, and reduce the release of DAMPs (damage-associated molecular patterns), which are major triggers of neuroinflammation [198].

By mitigating mitochondrial dysfunction, Mito Organelles *CNS* peptides indirectly modulate microglial activation. In neurodegenerative diseases, chronic microglial activation leads to a sustained release of inflammatory cytokines such as IL-1β, TNF-α, and IL-6. These not only harm neurons but impair neurogenesis and synaptic integrity. Regular intramuscular administration of mitochondrial peptides has been shown to downregulate NF-κB signaling, reduce glial reactivity, and protect against myelin and synapse degradation [199].

Clinically, patients undergoing Mito Organelles *CNS* peptide therapy report improvements in cognitive clarity, emotional stability, sensory integration, motor coordination, and sleep regulation. These effects are particularly notable in patients with early-stage Alzheimer's disease, Parkinson's disease, multiple sclerosis, and even neurodevelopmental conditions such as autism spectrum disorder (ASD). The benefits tend to accumulate gradually over each 12–15-week cycle, with many practitioners observing enhanced responses in second and third cycles compared to the first. This suggests a progressive remodeling effect at the level of mitochondrial–neuronal networks.

I come to realize that in integrative clinical practice, Mito Organelles *CNS* peptides are often used synergistically with other neuroregenerative modalities such as neural progenitor cells, exosome therapy, transcranial photobiomodulation, and cerebrolysin. For example, Mito Organelles administered prior to neural stem cell transplantation may help "precondition" the neuroenvironment by reducing inflammation, stabilizing mitochondrial membranes, and enhancing redox potential, thus improving graft survival and integration. The Mito Organelles *CNS* formulation is designed to enhance the functional longevity of neural cells what we describe as the cellspan of the brain, thereby supporting an expanded and more resilient brainspan. Given that cognitive vitality is the very foundation of how we perceive, interpret, and savor existence, sustaining the brain's performance is not merely desirable; it is essential to the experience of a life well-lived.

Protocols also incorporate adjunctive peptides to support neuroendocrine modulation, gut-brain axis integrity, and detoxification. Peptides such as Thymosin β4, *Pineal peptides*, and *Cortex* peptides are sometimes layered into protocols in a phased or rotation-based manner. The approach emphasizes biological synergy supporting not just neurons but also glial cells, immune cells, endothelial function, and systemic metabolic health.

Treatment personalization is central to these protocols. Patients are typically stratified based on metabolic state, neuroimaging patterns, cognitive profiling, and inflammatory biomarkers. This allows clinicians to tailor the dose and frequency of Mito Organelles and supporting peptides to achieve optimal neuroplastic and anti-inflammatory responses.

In Alzheimer's disease and mild cognitive impairment (MCI), Mito Organelles *CNS* therapy has been associated with delayed progression, improved verbal fluency, better executive function, and more stable sleep-wake cycles, which is a likely result of improved mitochondrial support in the suprachiasmatic nucleus and pineal-cortical axis. In Parkinson's disease, reductions in tremor amplitude, gait stabilization, and emotional regulation have been noted, particularly when peptides are combined with nutritional mitochondrial cofactors (e.g., CoQ10, NAD+ precursors).

In autism spectrum disorder (ASD), where mitochondrial dysfunction is frequently observed, Mito Organelles *CNS* have shown clinical benefit in reducing sensory hypersensitivity, motor dyspraxia, and emotional dysregulation. These outcomes are believed to stem from enhanced neuronal energy buffering, improved detoxification pathways, and stabilization of neural network oscillations.

I come to realize that Mito Organelles therapy is safe and well-tolerated as I have never seen any problem after injecting it, with no known long-term adverse effects in standard clinical dosing ranges. Its low immunogenicity and physiological origin make it suitable for chronic cyclic administration, an essential feature in lifelong neurodegenerative and neurodevelopmental conditions.

The incorporation of peptide protocols such as Mito Organelles *CNS* into neurodegenerative disease management reflects a growing shift from symptomatic control to biologically integrative repair. Rather than merely suppressing one pathological node, mitochondrial peptides target fundamental subcellular processes, i.e. energy generation, ROS balance, and apoptotic resistance that underpin neuronal health and resilience.

Combined with disease-modifying agents, cognitive rehabilitation, neuromodulation, and lifestyle interventions, peptide therapy has the potential to reshape the clinical trajectory of neurodegenerative disorders. More rigorous randomized trials are needed to validate long-term efficacy, refine dosing strategies, and explore optimal combinations. Nonetheless, the evolving real-world data points to a future in which peptides form a cornerstone of precision neuroregeneration.

Application of Mito Organelles Peptide Therapy in Stroke Recovery

While the pathophysiology of stroke differs mechanistically from chronic neurodegenerative diseases, the aftermath of ischemic or hemorrhagic cerebrovascular events often triggers similar secondary processes: mitochondrial failure, oxidative stress, inflammation, neuronal apoptosis, and glial scarring. In my personal clinical practice, I come to realize that these shared mechanisms create a compelling rationale for applying mitochondria-targeted peptides, particularly Mito Organelles *CNS*, in early post-stroke neurorestorative care.

Following the acute management phase of ischemic stroke, including thrombolysis or mechanical thrombectomy there is a critical window during which cellular salvage, synaptic recovery, and network reorganization can be actively supported. This neuroreparative phase spans days to weeks and is highly responsive to interventions that stabilize cellular metabolism, mitigate inflammation, and enhance neuroplasticity. It is within this context that Mito Organelles peptide protocols have shown clinical promise.

The Mito Organelles *CNS* stroke protocol involves daily intramuscular injections for 40 consecutive days, starting as early as possible, ideally within the first 3–5 days after stroke onset, once the patient is medically stabilized. This intensive administration schedule is designed to provide continuous support to the metabolically stressed and damaged neurons and glia during the vulnerable subacute phase, when secondary injury cascades are still active and neuroinflammatory responses are peaking.

Following the initial 40-day course, patients typically transition to a maintenance protocol (e.g., 2–3 times per week for an additional 8–12 weeks) depending on clinical response and rehabilitation progress. If needed, further cycles are repeated after a short rest period of 3–4 weeks. It is always a good idea to add Mito Organelles *Placenta* as well to use concurrently for 12-15 weeks protocol 2-3 times per week for better results.

In the acute-to-subacute phase after stroke, neurons within the ischemic penumbra, which is the metabolically compromised but potentially salvageable region surrounding the infarct core that exhibit mitochondrial depolarization, ATP depletion, calcium dysregulation, and oxidative stress. These processes lead to excitotoxicity, caspase activation, and programmed cell death if not reversed. Simultaneously, glial activation, BBB compromise, and infiltration of peripheral immune cells contribute to neuroinflammation and secondary injury.

Mito Organelles peptides, through their bioregulatory action on mitochondrial membrane potential, electron transport chain function, and oxidative phosphorylation, support the reactivation of cellular energy production. This preserves neuronal viability, reduces excitotoxic damage, and improves the survival of astrocytes and oligodendrocytes, which are essential for maintaining structural and functional brain connectivity.

Furthermore, Mito Organelles peptides have been observed to inhibit excessive ROS production, stabilize the mitochondrial permeability transition pore (mPTP), and upregulate protective pathways involving NRF2, PGC-1α, and SIRT3, all of which are key regulators of mitochondrial integrity and stress resistance. The resulting reduction in oxidative damage and inflammation supports neurogenesis, angiogenesis, and remyelination—the processes vital for stroke recovery.

Patients undergoing post-stroke Mito Organelles *CNS* therapy frequently demonstrate accelerated recovery of motor and cognitive functions, improved speech and coordination, and greater responsiveness to physiotherapy and occupational rehabilitation. These effects appear to be most pronounced when therapy is initiated early and maintained consistently throughout the neurorecovery phase.

Clinicians have reported improved muscle tone normalization, gait retraining, and fine motor coordination, as well as restoration of autonomic balance and reduced central fatigue. In patients with post-stroke aphasia or cognitive slowing, enhanced alertness, focus, and speech fluency are often observed within weeks of initiating therapy. These outcomes are believed to result not only from neuroprotection but from enhanced synaptic plasticity and improved connectome reorganization driven by more efficient neuronal metabolism.

Additionally, the modulation of glial responses, especially the reduction of reactive astrocytosis and microglial priming it appears to contribute to better outcomes in terms of infarct resolution, white matter repair, and long-term cognitive preservation. The cumulative effect is a neurorestorative trajectory that diverges from the typical post-stroke decline or plateau, enabling patients to achieve more complete functional recovery.

The 40-day intensive Mito Organelles protocol is especially effective when integrated with structured neurorehabilitation programs, including physical, occupational, and cognitive therapies. Mitochondrial support enhances neuronal plasticity, thereby increasing the efficacy of rehabilitative training and helping to consolidate new motor and cognitive patterns.

Some clinicians combine Mito Organelles with *Cortex peptides*, Neuroglia peptides, Cerebrolysin, or exosome therapies to further augment neuroplastic repair. The goal is to create a biological environment conducive to regeneration, in which damaged circuits can be reorganized and functional networks reestablished with minimal scarring and maximal synaptic fidelity.

The growing body of clinical experience with Mito Organelles therapy in stroke suggests that mitochondrial peptides may emerge as first-line neurorepair agents in the subacute care of cerebrovascular disease. By intervening at a critical juncture of the post-injury timeline, when neurons are on the precipice between survival and death, these peptides can decisively shift the cellular fate toward recovery.

As stroke care evolves to incorporate regenerative principles alongside acute intervention, mitochondrial peptide therapy offers a safe, scalable, and biologically rational strategy to maximize long-term functional outcomes. Future directions may include use in stroke prevention (in high-risk individuals with mitochondrial dysfunction), chronic stroke rehabilitation, and adjunctive neurocognitive support in vascular dementia.

As I am coming to the closure of this chapter I come to realize that in the long arc of human history, few frontiers are as consequential as the one we now face: the fate of the human mind as the body grows old. For millennia, longevity was a privilege of the fortunate; today, it is increasingly a predictable outcome of modern medicine. And yet, a question haunts these gains: what is the point of reaching 100 or even 120 if you are bedridden, confused, or incapacitated at 75?

As researchers, clinicians, and storytellers of biology, we are slowly learning that years added to life are hollow unless life is added to those years. Longevity means nothing without healthspan, and healthspan, in turn, depends profoundly on what we might call brainspan, the durability of the neural networks that shape memory, identity, creativity, and connection. Ultimately, these are anchored in what could be described as cellspan: the vitality of the cells that allow the brain to remain itself. At birth, the human body, an exquisitely synchronized consortium of approximately 37.2 trillion cells, possesses one of its greatest biological endowments: a remarkably high density of stem cells. Estimates suggest that in early life, roughly 1 in every 10,000 cells carries true stem-like potential, giving the newborn organism its unparalleled capacity to grow, repair, and regenerate. Yet this reservoir begins to decline almost from the moment development is complete. By the age of 25, when the body contains roughly 30–35 trillion cells after natural tissue remodeling, the stem-cell density has diminished to approximately 1 in 100,000 cells. By the age of sixty, with the organism comprising a similar order of magnitude leaving approximately 30 trillion cells, the pool contracts even further, falling to an estimated 1 stem cell per million cells.

And although the body never reaches a literal count of zero, the functional availability of stem cells in the final years of life becomes so diminished, so biologically silent, that the regenerative machinery approaches a practical standstill. In this sense, the drama of human aging can be measured not merely in years but in the gradual depletion of this once-plentiful cellular aristocracy—the slow fading of the very cells that orchestrate repair, restore resilience, and sustain the vitality of the human form.

Peptides, the small, ancient messengers have emerged at this intersection. They stand at the crossroads between what evolution wrote into our biology billions of years ago and what biotechnology now dares to rewrite. Through their ability to modulate repair pathways, synaptic resilience, inflammation, and cellular signaling, they offer a blueprint, perhaps still early, still incomplete, of how we might preserve cognition as we preserve life.

For decades, the idea of biological age reversal belonged to myth or metaphor. Now it has migrated into the domain of measurable possibility. Research teams around the world have reported early signs that biological age may be shifted, sometimes by several years, through targeted interventions that influence cellular repair and epigenetic regulation. In exploratory self-tracking studies, even individuals have observed shifts that resemble a biological "rewinding." In my own case, preliminary biomarker tests conducted under research conditions suggested a movement from a chronological age of 64 toward a biological profile closer to 46.

These results do not claim certainty; they claim potential, a signal rising above the noise that deserves deeper investigation.

What matters is not the specific number, nor the vanity of youth recaptured, but the direction of the evidence: our biology may be more malleable than we once believed.

If the 20th century taught us how to prevent early death, the 21st may teach us how to prevent early decline.

The breakthrough we now glimpse, though still nascent, still demanding rigorous trials, however is the possibility of increasing longevity through healthspan and brainspan via cellspan. This is not a promise of immortality, but an invitation to pursue a future where growing older does not mean fading away. A future where a vibrant mind can inhabit a long-lived body. A future in which neurodegeneration is not an inevitability but a solvable puzzle.

And perhaps most importantly: A future where the last decades of life are not merely endured, but lived—awake, connected, purposeful.

The story of peptides in neurodegeneration is still being written. But for the first time, it feels less like a story about slowing decline and more like one about reclaiming possibility.

CHAPTER 8

Peptides as Therapeutic Modalities in Gastrointestinal Disorders

In recent decades, gastrointestinal health has become a critical frontier not only because of recognized diseases such as Crohn's disease and ulcerative colitis, but also because of the alarming rise in disorders of gut barrier dysfunction ("leaky gut"), food intolerances, and subclinical inflammation in populations eating highly processed and nutritionally imbalanced diets. In this environment, peptides (short chains of amino acids that are larger than small molecules yet more manageable than full-length proteins) have captured scientific and clinical interest as biologically precise modulators of barrier function, immune signaling, and mucosal repair.

Modern nutrition plays a central role in the growing burden of gut disorders. Highly processed foods dominate many diets, bringing with them excess refined sugars, unhealthy fats, additives, emulsifiers, and low fiber; nutrient densities are often skewed, and essential micronutrients (zinc, selenium, vitamin D, omega-3) may be deficient. These dietary patterns can disrupt the normal homeostasis of the gut barrier: tight junctions become compromised, gut permeability increases, microbial diversity declines, and low-grade, chronic inflammation ensues. Processed food additives (such as certain emulsifiers and artificial sweeteners) have been shown in animal and mechanistic studies to degrade the mucous layer, destabilize gut microbiota, and induce mucosal immune responses. These risk factors are not theoretical, instead they map onto epidemiologic trends, with increasing incidence and earlier onset of inflammatory bowel disease, rising prevalence of gastrointestinal functional disorders, and emergence of non-communicable diseases linked to low-grade systemic inflammation.

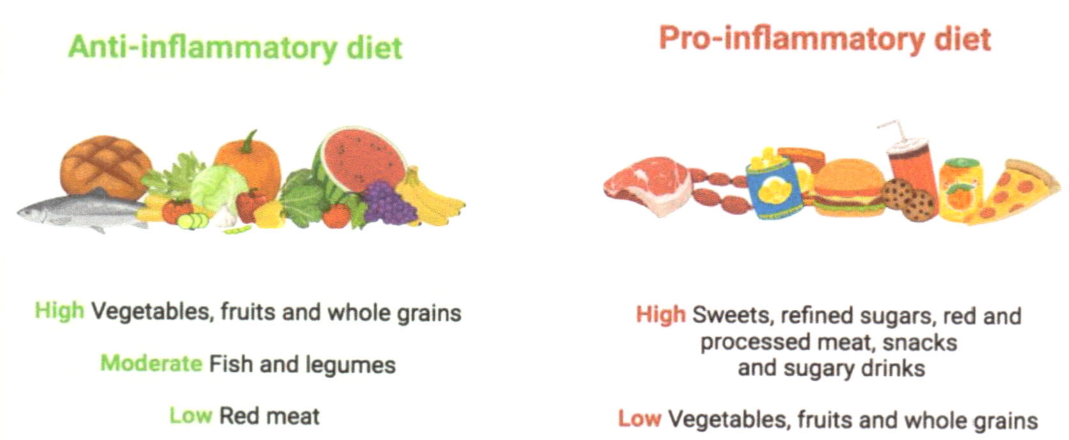

Fig 8.1. *Low-Grade Inflammation and Ultra-Processed Foods*

Against this backdrop, peptides represent an especially promising therapeutic modality. Their intermediate molecular weight positions them in a "sweet spot" of biological activity: they are large enough to interact with specific molecular targets (receptors, signaling cascades, cell-adhesion proteins), yet small enough potentially to penetrate tissues or mucosal layers if delivered appropriately. In disorders of gut barrier dysfunction and chronic inflammation, such as those increasingly seen in modern nutritional contexts, peptides have the capacity to restore tight junction integrity, modulate deleterious immune activation, and stimulate mucosal healing.

However, despite their promise, peptides encounter significant challenges. Enzymatic degradation in the gastrointestinal tract, rapid clearance, poor bioavailability (especially via the oral route), susceptibility to acidic pH and proteases, and difficulty achieving targeted delivery are all substantial obstacles. Formulation strategies, such as enteric coatings, encapsulation in nanoparticles or hydrogels, mucoadhesive delivery systems, or molecular engineering to resist degradation are essential to realize their therapeutic potential.

In modern era where diet is often less a source of nourishment and more a source of potential insult, the study of peptides as therapeutic agents in gastrointestinal medicine is not only scientifically compelling but socially and clinically urgent. As processed food consumption continues to rise globally, the imbalance in modern nutrition magnifies the need for interventions that go beyond symptom control, aiming to repair, restore, and maintain the gut's barrier defenses. Peptides thus hold potential as next-generation therapeutics, not merely supplementing but intervening at the root level of disease processes that are increasingly being driven by dietary and environmental factors.

Pathophysiology: Leaky Gut, Crohn's Disease, and Colitis

The conceptual anchor for peptide-based therapy in gastrointestinal disease is the integrity of the epithelial barrier. The term "leaky gut syndrome" refers to a state of pathological permeability of the intestinal barrier, where tight junction disruptions permit luminal antigens, microbial products, or other noxious molecules to infiltrate the lamina propria and trigger immune activation. Although "leaky gut syndrome" remains a controversial clinical diagnosis, the underlying phenomenon of increased intestinal permeability is well documented in inflammatory bowel disease (IBD), metabolic conditions, and other systemic disorders.

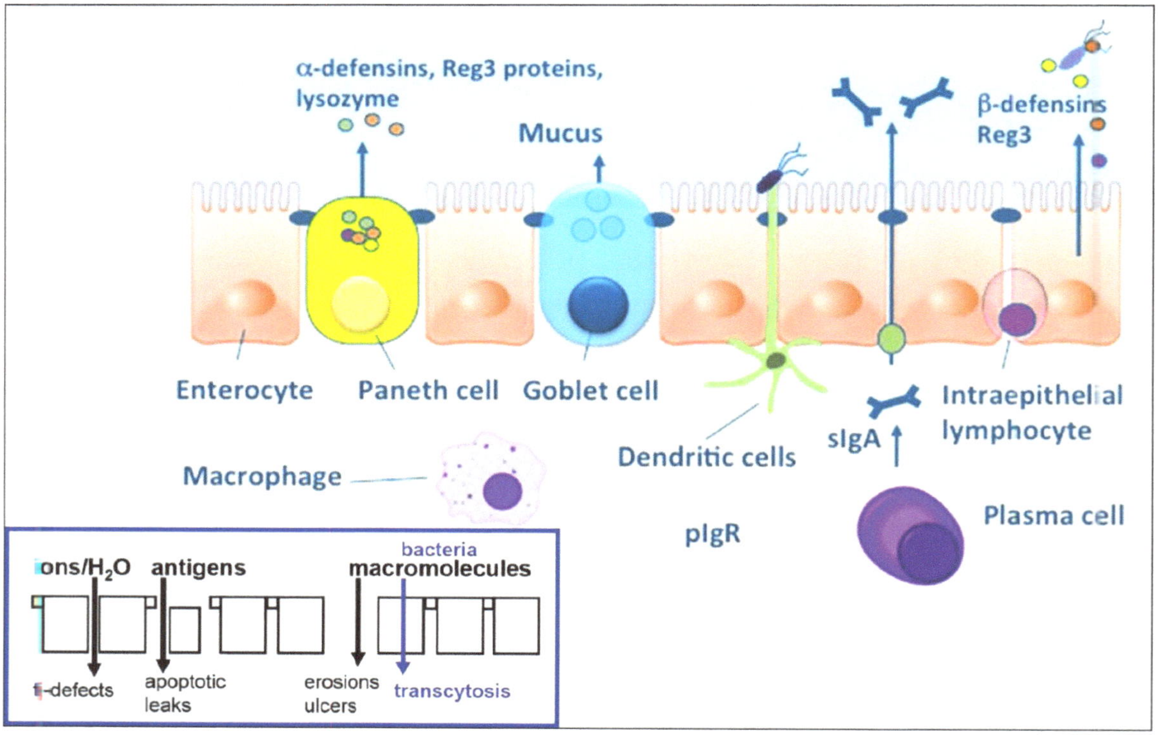

Fig 8.2. *Leaky gut: mechanisms, measurement and clinical implications (source: Camilleri M. Leaky gut: mechanisms, measurement and clinical implications in humans Gut 2019;68:1516-1526.)*

In Crohn's disease (CD) and ulcerative colitis (UC), the interplay of barrier dysfunction, dysregulated mucosal immunity, and microbial dysbiosis constitutes a vicious cycle. In Crohn's disease, Paneth cell dysfunction and reduced *defensin* production (especially in ileal disease) may reduce antimicrobial peptide defenses [200]. In colonic Crohn's disease, there is evidence of reduced induction of β-defensins, elafin, and cathelicidin LL-37, alongside impaired mucosal antiproteases [200]. Meanwhile, ulcerative colitis features extensive mucosal damage with crypt loss, goblet cell depletion, and direct injury to the colonic epithelium. Both pathologies may share barrier breakdown, translocation of bacterial products such as lipopolysaccharide (LPS), and amplification of proinflammatory cytokine cascades (IL-1β, TNF, IL-6) that perpetuate tissue injury and chronicity.

In the context of immune responses to the intestinal microbiota, several coordinated mechanisms play crucial roles in maintaining intestinal homeostasis. Goblet cells contribute by secreting mucin glycoproteins that form a protective mucus layer, while plasma cells produce immunoglobulin A (IgA), which helps neutralize pathogens and prevent microbial translocation. Intestinal epithelial cells detect microbial components via pattern recognition receptors such as Toll-like receptors (TLRs) and NOD2 (nucleotide-binding oligomerization domain-containing protein 2), triggering the release of antimicrobial peptides that help regulate microbial populations. Dendritic cells (DCs) also play a central role by capturing microbial antigens and migrating to Peyer's patches and mesenteric lymph nodes, where they initiate the differentiation of B cells into IgA-secreting plasma cells. Additionally, dendritic cell sampling of polysaccharide A (PSA) from *Bacteroides fragilis* promotes the induction of regulatory T cells (Tregs), which produce interleukin-10 (IL-10), a key anti-inflammatory cytokine that contributes to immune tolerance and mucosal homeostasis. Host-derived antimicrobial proteins, such as REG3γ (Regenerating islet-derived protein 3 gamma), not only offer direct protection against pathogenic bacteria but also shape the composition of the gut microbiota. These complex interactions between epithelial cells, immune cells, and commensal microbes ensure a balanced immune response, preventing both excessive inflammation and microbial overgrowth. Key molecules involved in these processes include IL-10, MYD88 (myeloid differentiation primary-response protein 88), and M cells (microfold cells), all of which contribute to the dynamic regulation of mucosal immunity [201].

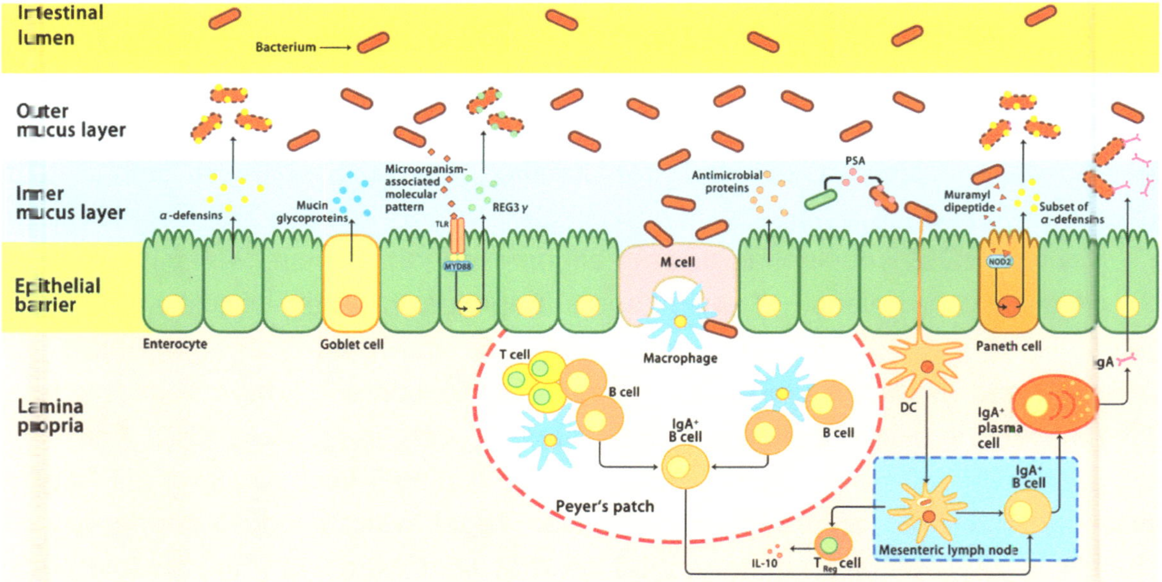

Fig 8.3. *Host immune responses to intestinal microbiota (source: Zhang, Front. Immunol., 2017).*

It is within this context that therapeutic peptides are being explored: Can a peptide restore tight junction integrity, modulate immune responses, or promote mucosal healing without systemic immunosuppression?

Peptides in GI therapy fall broadly into several mechanistic classes: tight junction modulators, anti-inflammatory/regulatory peptides, reparative or trophic peptides, and peptide-based biologics (e.g., antibody fragments or receptor antagonists). A useful recent review ("Peptide-based therapeutic and delivery strategies for inflammatory bowel disease") outlines these categories and the design challenges (stability, delivery, targeting) that must be overcome [202].

One especially compelling mechanistic axis is the regulation of tight junctions. A peptide that can reverse "leakiness" in the gut may reduce antigenic provocation and break the feed-forward loop of inflammation. *Larazotide acetate* (also known as AT-1001) is a prototypical example: an octapeptide that antagonizes zonulin signaling, a key mediator of tight junction disassembly. In vitro, larazotide promotes assembly of tight junction proteins (ZO-1, occludin, claudins), fosters actin rearrangement, and resists disassembly induced by gliadin fragments or cytokines [203][204]. In ex vivo intestinal injury models in pigs, larazotide enhances transepithelial electrical resistance (TEER), reduces serosal-to-mucosal LPS flux, and improves claudin-4 localization in repairing epithelium [205]. Clinically, larazotide has been tested in celiac disease patients to reduce gluten-induced permeability and symptom activation [206][204]. Although primarily evaluated in celiac disease, the barrier-restorative mechanism makes it of interest for IBD and leaky gut syndrome more broadly.

Beyond barrier modulation, anti-inflammatory peptides constitute a rich vein of innovation. The 2023 systematic review "Anti-Inflammatory Peptides as Promising Therapeutics Agent Against Inflammatory Bowel Diseases" identified several candidates that act via suppression of TNF cytotoxicity, stabilization of junctional proteins, modulation of microbiota, or rebalancing cytokine networks [207]. Among these, *H-SN1* (a snake-venom–derived peptide) and *GLP-2 dimer (GLP-2②)* emerged as effective in preclinical IBD models, reducing TNF levels, MPO activity, and histologic damage [207]. Additional peptides such as *Ac2-26* (an annexin A1 mimic) and *αs2-casein–derived peptides* (together with synbiotics) have shown capacity to restore microbiotal balance and mitigate inflammation [207]. Peptides such as *AMP-18 (Gastrokine-1)* and *MBCP* (derived from buffalo milk) function to stabilize tight junctions and reinforce barrier integrity [202].

An interesting frontier is *NIPEP-IBD*, a synthetic peptide targeting integrin β1. In murine IBD models, NIPEP-IBD localized selectively to impaired colonic epithelium, reduced immune cell infiltration, decreased proinflammatory cytokines, and preserved epithelial structure [208]. The emphasis here is not only dampening inflammation but promoting mucosal restitution.

A further class of peptides includes hybrid designs: one recent study engineered eight hybrid peptides combining antimicrobial motifs (e.g., LL-37, YW12D, cathelicidin fragments) with thymic regulatory peptides (e.g., thymopentin, thymosin α1) to balance antibacterial and immunomodulatory effects in intestinal inflammation [209]. Other peptides with immunoregulatory or helminth-derived origins, such as *SJMHE1* (a helminth-derived peptide), have been tested in DSS-induced colitis models, where they reduce disease activity, modulate Th1/Th17 biases, and promote regulatory T cell profiles [210].

Yet another avenue is bioactive peptides in dietary sources. For instance, wheat peptides (a complex mixture containing >300 peptide species) were shown to mitigate DSS-induced colitis in mice, in part by activating the Keap1-Nrf2 antioxidant axis and preserving barrier integrity [211]. Similarly, hydrolyzed salmon peptides reduced histopathological inflammation and cytokine signatures in IBD models compared with fish oil [212]. Sea conch peptide hydrolysates also ameliorated colitis and restored microbiota balance in murine models [213]. These "nutraceutical peptides" may serve as adjuncts to more targeted peptide therapeutics.

The value of such peptides lies in their capacity to modulate barrier and immune function with (potentially) fewer systemic side effects compared to broad immunosuppressants. Yet challenges remain oral bioavailability is poor due to proteolysis; site-specific delivery is difficult; and pharmacokinetics are typically short-lived. Peptide-based strategies thus often incorporate formulation technologies, such as PEGylation, nanoparticle encapsulation, hydrogels, mucoadhesive carriers, colon-release systems aiming to protect against enzymatic degradation and achieve mucosal targeting [202].

Recent research has delved deeply into the mechanistic and experimental foundations of peptide-based therapies for gastrointestinal diseases, highlighting their multifaceted roles in modulating gut immunity, restoring barrier integrity, and promoting mucosal healing [209]. One area of innovation lies in the development of hybrid peptides, which are engineered by combining antimicrobial sequences with immunoregulatory domains. These constructs are designed to simultaneously target dysbiosis and immune dysregulation, the two central features of conditions such as Crohn's disease and ulcerative colitis. By integrating these dual functions, hybrid peptides can suppress pathogenic microbial overgrowth while also tempering proinflammatory signaling pathways, offering a more comprehensive therapeutic effect [214].

In parallel, advances in peptide formulation have addressed longstanding challenges related to stability and targeted delivery. The gastrointestinal tract is a highly proteolytic environment, where unmodified peptides are rapidly degraded by enzymes and rendered therapeutically inactive. This has spurred the use of chemical modifications, such as cyclization, terminal capping, or substitution with D-amino acids, as well as the development of specialized delivery platforms, including nanoparticles, hydrogels, and enteric-coated capsules. These innovations help to protect peptides from premature breakdown, enhance mucosal adhesion, and enable site-specific release within inflamed or damaged regions of the gut [215].

Experimental models of colitis and Crohn's-like inflammation have provided compelling preclinical evidence for the efficacy of these peptide-based interventions. Peptides administered either systemically or locally have demonstrated the capacity to reduce inflammatory biomarkers, such as TNF-α, IL-1β, and IL-6, while concurrently promoting epithelial regeneration and tight junction reassembly. These effects translate to measurable improvements in histological architecture, reduced disease activity scores, and restoration of intestinal barrier function. Such findings underscore the therapeutic potential of peptides not merely as symptom modulators, but as agents capable of intervening at the root of gastrointestinal pathology [216].

Mito Organelles *Intestinal Mucosa* is a specialized biologic preparation derived from purified cell extracts of intestinal endothelial tissue obtained from SPF (specific-pathogen-free) rabbits. These cell fractions are rich in mitochondrial components and biomolecular signals specific to gut mucosal regeneration [217]. By harnessing the natural bioactivity of mitochondrial elements, such as signaling peptides, metabolic cofactors, and micro-vesicular components, Mito Organelles *Intestinal Mucosa* supports the repair and regeneration of damaged intestinal epithelium, increasing its cellspan. Through the increased cellspan of the intestinal mucosa the gutspan increment is achieved. This therapy is particularly effective in cases of chronic mucosal inflammation, epithelial barrier breakdown, and ulceration, often seen in patients with irritable bowel syndrome, ulcerative colitis, Crohn's disease, or gut dysbiosis associated with long-term dietary imbalances and toxic load [218]. In addition, the gut–brain axis is the two-way communication network that links gastrointestinal system and central nervous system. It involves neural pathways (especially the vagus nerve), hormones and immune system signals. The gut microbiome (the flora and fauna of the organism represented by the trillions of microbes inside the intestines) is a system system that allows gut to influence the brain function and the brain, in its turn, to influence the gut function, hence in a way gutspan can increase the brainspan.

The healing effects of Mito Organelles therapy are notably enhanced when used in a synergistic integrative protocol. This includes *HMD detoxification* (to reduce systemic heavy metal burden), hydrocolonic therapy (to cleanse the large intestine and reduce toxic reabsorption), and a proenzyme-symbiotic complex administered over 2–4 months. The proenzyme-symbiotic supports digestive enzyme balance and microbiota restoration, both essential for reducing endotoxemia and resetting mucosal immunity. Together, this multi-pronged approach reduces local and systemic inflammation, facilitates epithelial renewal, and restores the functional integrity of the gut lining [217].

The clinical protocol for Mito Organelles *Intestinal Mucosa* typically involves intramuscular injections of 2 to 3 vials per week over a 15-week course, with some protocols combining the therapy with MO *LPPSIMKE* and MO *Adrenal Cortex*, which may contain adrenochrome, a biologically active compound known for its vascular and cellular stabilizing effects. The inclusion of MO *LPPSIMKE* and MO *Adrenal Cortex* with adrenochrome may enhance mucosal microcirculation and reduce oxidative tissue damage in highly inflamed intestinal environments. Patients undergoing this protocol often report improvement in symptoms such as bloating, cramping, irregular bowel habits, and mucosal sensitivity within 6–8 weeks, with deeper regenerative effects becoming evident after the full 15-week regimen. When applied consistently and in combination with detoxification and microbiome support, Mito Organelles *Intestinal Mucosa*" presents a compelling therapeutic option for integrative gut healing and long-term mucosal resilience.

Proposed Peptide Protocols and Expected Outcomes

Because few peptide treatments are yet standard-of-care, the following protocols are essentially illustrative or adapted from preclinical and early-phase trial literature. They should be regarded as hypothetical frameworks rather than prescriptions.

Protocol A: Larazotide for Barrier Restoration in IBD (based on Pilot Human Study)

- Inclusion criteria: Patients with mild-to-moderate UC or Crohn's disease in remission but with documented increased intestinal permeability (e.g., lactulose-mannitol test or zonulin assays).

- Intervention: Larazotide acetate oral capsules, 0.5 mg to 1 mg three times daily before meals (this dosing mirrors off-label use in celiac studies) [206].
- Duration: 8—12 weeks.
- Outcomes: Primary—change in permeability metrics (e.g., urinary excretion ratios), biomarkers of barrier integrity (e.g., fecal zonulin, occludin/claudin expression in biopsy). Secondary—clinical symptom scores, fecal calprotectin, endoscopic mucosal healing, adverse events.
- Expected results: A moderate reduction in permeability, partial normalization of tight junction protein localization, and improved symptom scores in a subset. Given that larazotide has shown protective effects in vitro and ex vivo on tight junctions, these effects are biologically plausible [203].

Protocol B: H-SN1 Administration in DSS-Induced Colitis Model (Murine)

- Protocol: Treatment groups receive intraperitoneal or oral H-SN1 peptide (e.g., 1–5 mg/kg) daily from day 0 through day 10; control group receives vehicle.
- Readouts: Body weight loss, disease activity index (DAI: stool consistency, bleeding), colon length, histologic scoring, expression of proinflammatory cytokines (IL-1β, TNF, IL-6), myeloperoxidase (MPO) activity, tight junction protein expression, microbial community analysis.
- Expected outcomes: Compared to controls, H-SN1–treated mice should show attenuated weight loss, lower DAI, preserved colon length, reduced cytokine levels, lower MPO activity, and improved mucosal architecture. Indeed, prior studies have demonstrated that H-SN1 and GLP-2② reduce TNF cytotoxicity and histologic damage in IBD models [207].

Protocol C: NIPEP-IBD Colon-Targeted Delivery in IBD Mouse Model

- Design: Use a colon-targeting prodrug or polymeric capsule that yields NIPEP-IBD selectively in the colon (e.g., pH-triggered release).

Administer daily dosing (e.g., 10 mg/kg colon-delivered) for 14–21 days in a dextran sulfate sodium (DSS) or TNBS colitis model.

- Readouts: As above (DAI, histology, cytokines, infiltration). Additional imaging (e.g., fluorescence labeling) to confirm localization of NIPEP-IBD to damaged epithelium.
- Expected outcomes: Reduced epithelial injury, lower inflammatory infiltrate, restoration of tight junction protein expression, and maintenance of remission. In preliminary reports, NIPEP-IBD binds selectively to injured epithelium and reduces cytokine infiltration in colonic tissue [208].

Interpreting such experiments, one might expect moderate gains in barrier function and inflammation control, especially as adjuncts to conventional therapies. The true translational leap will be to replicate these in human subjects, ensure pharmacokinetics allow effective dosing, and confirm safety.

Despite the promise, peptide therapeutics in GI disease face substantial hurdles. Enzymatic degradation in the stomach and small intestine severely limits systemic absorption. Proteases, peptidases, and acidic pH quickly neutralize many peptides. As such, most current peptide GI therapies rely on local mucosal action rather than systemic exposure, and require protective delivery systems (e.g., enteric coatings, nanoparticle encapsulation, mucoadhesive polymers). Off-target effects and immunogenicity (antibody induction against the peptide) must be carefully evaluated, as well as toxicity at higher doses.

Another challenge is achieving selective targeting to diseased mucosa without affecting healthy tissue. Overly broad barrier tightening could impede nutrient absorption or interfere with normal epithelial renewal dynamics. Also, in active disease, heavy inflammation may render epithelial response to peptides blunted.

A promising direction is integrated peptide-biologic hybrids or engineered microbial delivery systems (e.g., probiotic strains genetically modified to express peptide on demand). The review by Ge et al. emphasizes biomaterial-assisted delivery, PEGylation to enhance half-life, and local hydrogel scaffolds to protect peptides until release at the mucosa. Combining peptide therapy with microbiome modulation (e.g., synbiotics) may also provide synergistic benefit, for instance, casein-derived peptides with synbiotics have been used in animal colitis models.

Finally, carefully designed human trials will be critical. Biomarker endpoints (permeability assays, tight junction gene expression, mucosal histology) may allow early signal detection before large-scale efficacy trials.

The topic of peptide therapy in gastrointestinal disease is one of cautious optimism. The theoretical rationale is compelling: a peptide that restores epithelial barrier integrity, modulates local immune responses, and fosters mucosal healing could break the cycle of antigen-driven inflammation at the gut interface. Early successes (e.g., larazotide in celiac settings, H-SN1 in murine colitis) support this vision, but translation into human IBD remains nascent. Well-designed protocols, advanced delivery strategies, and rigorous safety evaluation will be required to move from bench to bedside. As our understanding of gut barrier biology, peptide engineering, and mucosal immunology deepens, the peptide class may eventually take its place alongside biologics and small molecules in the armamentarium against Crohn's disease, ulcerative colitis, and "leaky gut"–associated disorders.

CHAPTER 9

Peptide-Based Strategies for Cartilage Regeneration in Osteoarthritis: Mitochondrial Therapeutics and Mito Organelles Integration

(with Prof. Jonathan R.T. Lakey, B.Sc., M.Sc., Ph.D)

Osteoarthritis (OA) is a chronic, progressive, and debilitating joint disorder that ranks among the most common musculoskeletal diseases globally. It is marked by the gradual degradation of articular cartilage, persistent low-grade synovial inflammation, and pathological remodeling of the subchondral bone. Clinically, OA manifests with joint pain, stiffness, reduced mobility, and eventually functional impairment, making it a leading cause of disability, especially among the aging population. Current estimates suggest that over 500 million people worldwide are affected by OA, with incidence rising sharply in relation to aging, obesity, sedentary lifestyles, and joint injury [219][220].

While once classified as a mechanical "wear-and-tear" condition, OA is now recognized as a complex, multifactorial disease that involves not only biomechanical overload but also chronic low-grade inflammation, altered cellular signaling, epigenetic changes, and importantly, mitochondrial dysfunction within joint tissues [221]. This paradigm shift has revealed OA to be a metabolically active disease of the whole joint, involving crosstalk between cartilage, subchondral bone, synovium, ligaments, and adipose tissue. Notably, the failure of chondrocytes, which are the key cells responsible for maintaining the cartilage extracellular matrix has been directly linked to impaired mitochondrial function, increased oxidative stress, and apoptosis, all of which contribute to progressive joint degradation.

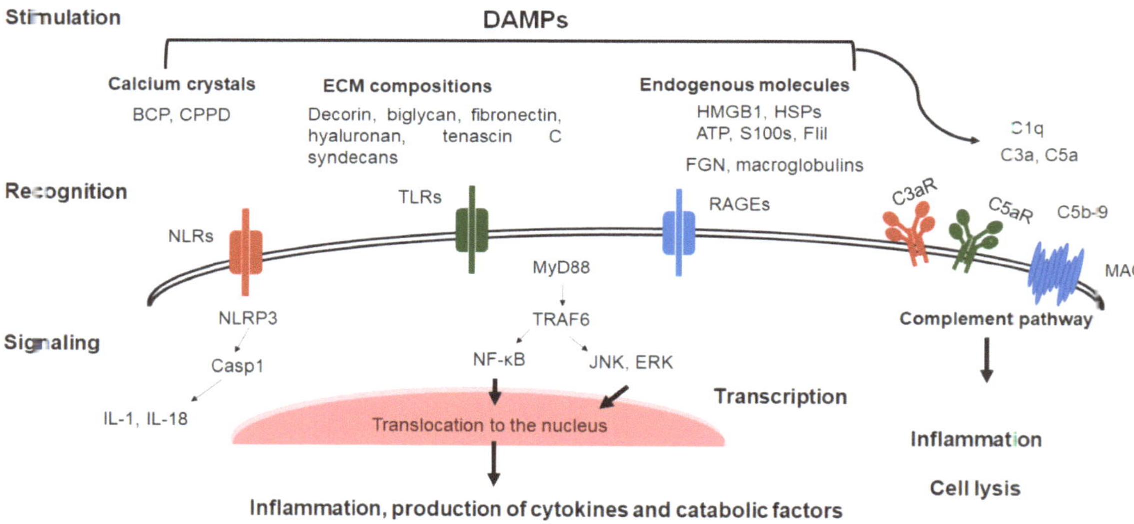

Fig 9.1. *The role of DAMPs in the initiation of LGI. DAMPs, including cartilage compositions, crystals, endogenous molecules, and plasma proteins, are recognized by PPRs, including NLRs, TLRs, and RAGEs resulting in the activation of several signaling pathways involved in the production of proinflammatory cytokines and proteolytic enzymes by macrophages and chondrocytes. The binding of DAMPs to complement molecules activate the complement pathway resulting in cell activation leading to inflammatory responses and cell lysis (source: Terkawi MA, Ebata T, Yokota S, Takahashi D, Endo T, Matsumae G, Shimizu T, Kadoya K,*

Iwasaki N. Low-Grade Inflammation in the Pathogenesis of Osteoarthritis: Cellular and Molecular Mechanisms and Strategies for Future Therapeutic Intervention. Biomedicines. 2022).

Despite the enormous burden posed by OA on public health systems, available therapies remain largely palliative, focusing on symptomatic relief rather than disease modification. Non-steroidal anti-inflammatory drugs (NSAIDs), intra-articular corticosteroids, analgesics, and physical therapy remain the mainstay of treatment but do little to halt or reverse the underlying cartilage degeneration. In advanced stages, surgical interventions such as joint replacement become the only recourse, though these carry significant costs, complications, and limitations [222].

This therapeutic stagnation has fueled growing interest in regenerative medicine approaches, which seek to restore joint homeostasis, repair cartilage, and modulate inflammatory and metabolic dysfunctions. Among the most promising strategies are peptide-based therapeutics, the small bioactive sequences capable of mimicking growth factors, signaling molecules, and repair mediators. When used in combination with mitochondrial biologics such as Mito Organelles (MO) *Cartilage* and MO *Placenta*, these therapies hold the potential to target both the energy deficits and anabolic insufficiency seen in OA. MO *Cartilage* provides mitochondrial support tailored to cartilage tissue, while MO *Placenta* contributes broader regenerative and immunomodulatory organelles that enhance systemic healing capacity. Together, they form a novel platform that integrates bioenergetic repair with structural regeneration, offering hope for truly modifying the course of osteoarthritis [223].

Mitochondrial Dysfunction in Cartilage Degeneration

Articular cartilage is a highly specialized, avascular connective tissue that lines the surfaces of synovial joints, enabling smooth articulation and efficient load distribution. It is composed predominantly of an intricate extracellular matrix (ECM), which provides the biomechanical properties necessary for joint function, including tensile strength and resistance to compressive forces. Embedded within this dense ECM is a sparse population of metabolically active yet non-proliferative cells known as chondrocytes, which are solely responsible for the synthesis, maintenance, and turnover of the cartilage matrix.

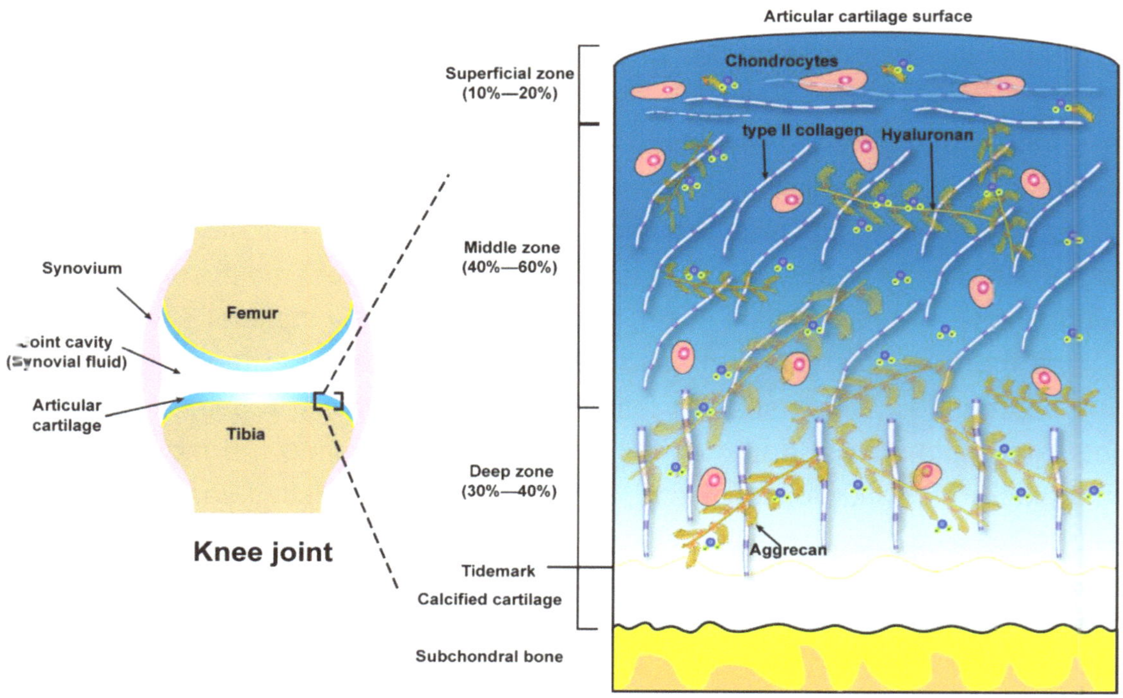

Fig 9.2. *Schematic illustration of the knee joint and the structure, compositions of articular cartilage from the surface to subchondral bone (source: Li, Y., Yuan, Z., Yang, H., Zhong, H., Peng, W., & Xie, R. (2021). Recent Advances in Understanding the Role of Cartilage Lubrication in Osteoarthritis. Molecules).*

In healthy adult cartilage, chondrocytes maintain a finely balanced anabolic–catabolic equilibrium, characterized by the production of matrix components such as type II collagen, the primary structural protein of hyaline cartilage, and aggrecan, a large proteoglycan essential for water retention and load-bearing capacity. At the same time, these cells exert tight regulatory control over matrix-degrading enzymes, including matrix metalloproteinases (MMPs) such as MMP-1 and MMP-13, and a disintegrin and metalloproteinase with thrombospondin motifs (ADAMTS), notably ADAMTS-4 and ADAMTS-5, which are primarily responsible for aggrecan degradation. This dynamic yet balanced process allows cartilage to respond adaptively to physiological mechanical loads while preserving tissue integrity.

However, in the context of OA, this homeostatic balance becomes progressively disrupted. Chondrocytes undergo phenotypic shifts toward a hypertrophic or inflammatory state, marked by the downregulation of anabolic genes and a concomitant upregulation of catabolic and pro-inflammatory mediators. One of the central molecular disruptions in this transition is mitochondrial dysfunction, which plays a critical role in driving both chondrocyte senescence and ECM degradation.

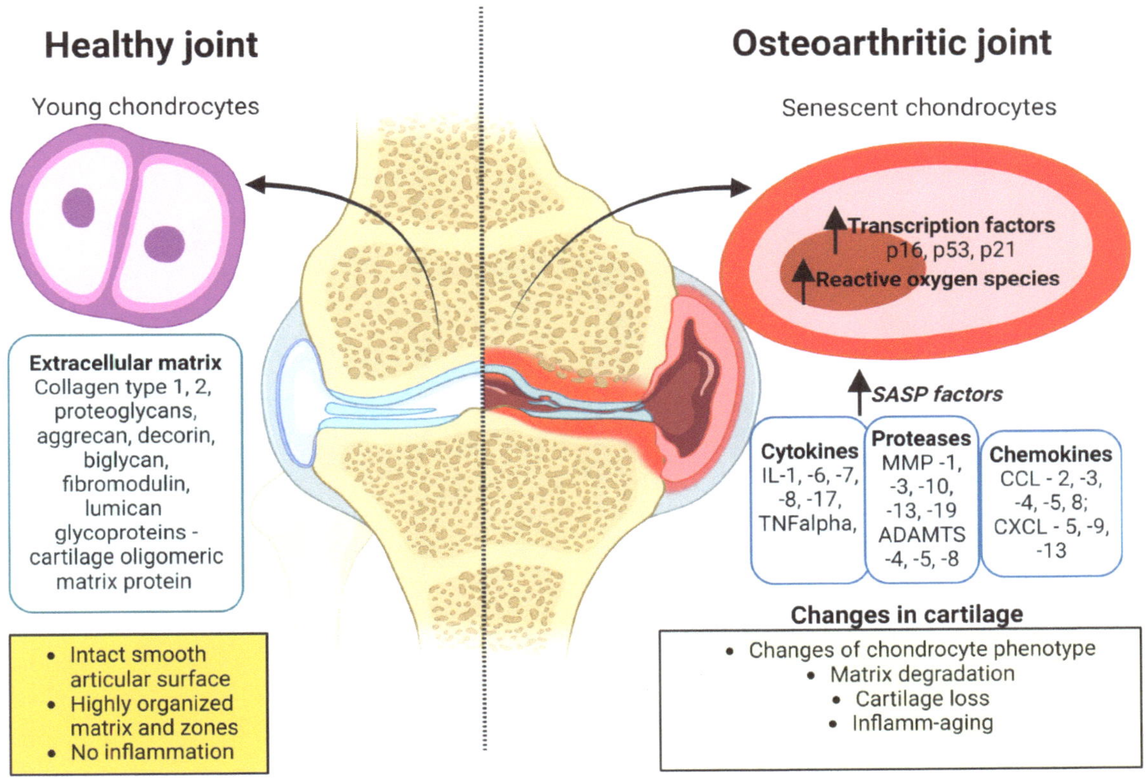

Fig 9.3. *Differences between a healthy joint and an osteoarthritic joint (source: Atasoy-Zeybek, A., Showel, K.K., Nagelli, C.V. et al. The intersection of aging and estrogen in osteoarthritis. npj Womens Health 3, 15 (2025)).*

In OA cartilage, mitochondria, which is essential for ATP production, redox signaling, and apoptotic regulation exhibit structural and functional impairments, including swelling, loss of cristae architecture, decreased oxidative phosphorylation capacity, and increased production of reactive oxygen species (ROS). These changes result in oxidative stress, which further amplifies the expression of catabolic enzymes through the activation of signaling cascades such as NF-κB, MAPKs, and AP-1, contributing to ECM breakdown. Additionally, oxidative damage to mitochondrial DNA (mtDNA) and a reduction in mitochondrial biogenesis impair the chondrocytes' ability to recover from stress, leading to a vicious cycle of matrix degradation and cellular senescence.

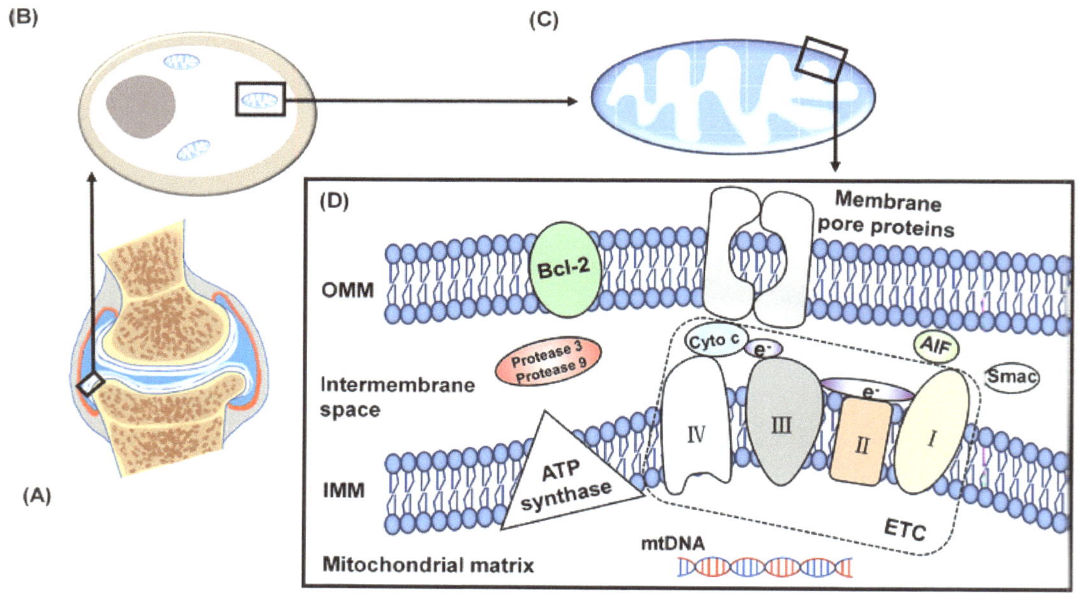

Fig 9.4. *Mitochondrial structure in chondrocytes. (A) The schematic diagram of the articular cartilage structure. Cartilage is composed of dense ECM and chondrocytes. ECM mainly contains aggrecan and type II collagen. (B) Mitochondria are randomly distributed in the cytoplasm of chondrocytes under physiological conditions. The distribution of mitochondria in chondrocytes is related to the demand of ATP. (C) The general morphology of mitochondrion. Mitochondrion is a kind of double-membrane organelle. Mitochondrial inner membrane folds to form cristae. (D) Mitochondrial double-membrane structure. The OMM contains membrane pore proteins and Bcl-2 family proteins. The IMM mainly contains complexes I, II, III, and IV of ETC and ATP synthase. Functional proteins in the intermembrane space between*

OMM and IMM include but are not limited to Cyto c, AIF, Smac, and proteases 3 and 9. The mitochondrial matrix contains mtDNA and proteins related to energy metabolism. ECM = extracellular matrix; ATP = adenosine triphosphate; OMM = outer mitochondrial membrane; Bcl-2 = B-cell leukemia/lymphoma-2; IMM = inner mitochondrial membrane; ETC = electron transport chain; Cyto c = cytochrome c; AIF = apoptosis-inducing factor; Smac = second mitochondrial-derived activator of caspases; mtDNA = mitochondrial deoxyribonucleic acid (source: Kan, Shiyi & Mengmeng, Duan & Liu, Yang & Wang, Chunli & Xie, Jing. (2021). Role of Mitochondria in Physiology of Chondrocytes and Diseases of Osteoarthritis and Rheumatoid Arthritis. CARTILAGE. 13. 194760352110638. 10.1177/19476035211063858.).

Emerging evidence also suggests that dysfunctional mitochondria promote the release of damage-associated molecular patterns (DAMPs), which engage pattern recognition receptors (e.g., TLRs and NLRs) on chondrocytes and synoviocytes, initiating sterile inflammation within the joint. This inflammatory microenvironment perpetuates catabolic signaling and suppresses cartilage repair mechanisms, accelerating the progression of OA [224].

Mitochondria in chondrocytes are essential not only for ATP production but also for managing redox signaling, calcium homeostasis, and apoptosis regulation [225]. In OA, chondrocyte mitochondria exhibit reduced membrane potential, diminished biogenesis, and excessive production of ROS, all of which accelerate ECM breakdown and cell death [226]. Damaged mitochondria also activate pro-inflammatory pathways, including NF-κB and NLRP3 inflammasomes, thereby amplifying joint inflammation and matrix catabolism [227]. Moreover, mitochondrial DNA (mtDNA) released from apoptotic chondrocytes may act as damage-associated molecular patterns (DAMPs), perpetuating immune responses in the synovium [228][229].

Given this centrality of mitochondrial dysfunction, therapeutic interventions aimed at restoring mitochondrial health hold significant promise for halting or reversing cartilage degeneration. Recent studies have demonstrated that mitochondrial transplantation from mesenchymal stem cells to recipient chondrocytes can reduce oxidative stress and improve cartilage integrity in OA models [230]. These findings underpin the rationale for using mitochondrial-rich extracts, such as Mito Organelles derived from placental and cartilage tissues, in regenerative OA protocols.

Mito Organelles Cartilage and Placenta: A Novel Bioactive Paradigm

Mito Organelles (MO) are biologically active organelle extracts obtained from specific tissues of healthy, specific-pathogen-free (SPF) animal sources. These extracts are enriched in mitochondrial proteins, enzymes, bioenergetic cofactors, and signaling peptides. MO Cartilage is specifically derived from joint cartilage tissue, whereas MO Placenta is harvested from placental tissue, known for its regenerative and immunomodulatory properties [231].

In osteoarthritic contexts, the hypothesis is that MO injections, which are administered intramuscularly, serve as systemic trophic support, restoring chondrocyte mitochondrial efficiency, improving redox balance, and enhancing the cellular responsiveness to anabolic signaling. MO therapies are believed to act at multiple levels: improving ATP production, upregulating antioxidant enzymes like superoxide dismutase (SOD), stabilizing mitochondrial membrane potential, and modulating gene expression related to ECM synthesis and inflammation [231].

Clinical protocols involving MO *Cartilage* and MO *Placenta* often recommend intramuscular administration of 2 to 3 vials per week over a 12- to 15-week course. In more advanced or refractory OA cases, a higher frequency of 3 vials per week has been used, sometimes in combination with other peptides such as NOP *Synovia*, a compound proposed to improve microvascular integrity and oxygen delivery. The use of these therapies is typically integrated into broader regenerative strategies, including physical rehabilitation, dietary optimization, and concurrent peptide administration.

Other Peptide Therapeutics in Cartilage Restoration

Peptides offer a unique therapeutic window for cartilage repair due to their ability to modulate signaling pathways, promote anabolic gene expression, and reduce catabolic mediators without the long-term risks associated with systemic immunosuppression or steroids. Among the most investigated peptide strategies are those based on human growth hormone (HGH) and its secretagogues, BPC-157, and cartilage-targeting biopeptides such as the PEDF 29-mer [232][233].

Human growth hormone, and more frequently its secretagogues (such as

GHRP-2, GHRP-6, and ipamorelin), stimulate the endogenous release of growth hormone, which in turn elevates insulin-like growth factor 1 (IGF-1)—a potent anabolic signal in chondrocytes. IGF-1 has been shown to enhance type II collagen and aggrecan synthesis, suppress MMP-13 and ADAMTS5, and protect against chondrocyte apoptosis [234]. Clinical and experimental data support that GH/IGF-1 therapies improve joint function and pain scores, especially when combined with biomechanical support.

The BPC-157 is the 15-amino-acid peptide is derived from a gastric protein and has been studied for its roles in angiogenesis, tendon healing, and gastrointestinal repair. In joint contexts, BPC-157 has demonstrated effects on vascularization, nitric oxide modulation, and tissue remodeling (Sikiric et al., 2018). While data on cartilage-specific outcomes remain limited, animal studies suggest it supports joint capsule healing and reduces joint pain. Its subcutaneous administration (200–500 mcg/day) is commonly reported in integrative protocols [235].

PEDF 29-mer Peptide is one of the most promising intraarticular peptides. It is the 29-amino-acid fragment of pigment epithelium-derived factor (PEDF) has demonstrated chondroregenerative effects in rodent models of OA. Delivered in hyaluronic acid (HA), PEDF 29-mer promotes chondrocyte proliferation, increases matrix deposition, and reduces synovitis via STAT3 signaling [236]. When combined with systemic peptide support and mitochondrial therapy, PEDF 29-mer may act synergistically to rebuild cartilage matrix [236].

Advances in phage display and molecular engineering have produced peptides that home to damaged cartilage, improving drug delivery and retention. These include sequences that bind collagen type II, aggrecan, or fibronectin domains, and when linked to therapeutic agents, allow localized, sustained regenerative effects [237]. These targeted systems may be particularly valuable in conjunction with Mito Organelles, where bioavailability to cartilage is otherwise a limitation.

In practical clinical settings, the integration of Mito Organelles (MO) with peptide-based therapeutics has evolved into comprehensive, multi-phase regenerative protocols tailored to the severity and anatomical complexity of OA. This integrated approach aims to address not only the symptomatic burden of OA but also its underlying cellular, mitochondrial, and extracellular matrix pathologies. The therapeutic synergy lies in concurrently supporting mitochondrial function, stimulating anabolic peptide signaling, and mitigating chronic inflammation.

A typical protocol begins with a priming phase that employs Mito Organelles *Cartilage* or MO *Placenta*, administered intramuscularly at a frequency of 2–3 vials per week over a period of 6 to 8 weeks. MO *Cartilage* provides mitochondrial and extracellular vesicle support derived from healthy cartilage tissue, enhancing energy metabolism within recipient chondrocytes, upregulating antioxidant enzymes (e.g., SOD2, catalase), and restoring mitochondrial membrane potential. This primes the chondrocyte microenvironment by reducing oxidative stress, downregulating catabolic mediators such as matrix metalloproteinase-13 (MMP-13), and promoting a phenotypic shift from a senescent to a reparative state. MO *Placenta*, rich in trophic factors and immunomodulatory organelles, augments systemic repair responses and is particularly valuable in patients with inflammatory or autoimmune components of OA.

Following mitochondrial priming, the tissue regeneration phase is initiated by introducing anabolic peptides, including growth hormone secretagogues (e.g., ipamorelin, GHRP-2, or CJC-1295) and BPC-157. These are administered subcutaneously once or twice daily, depending on the compound and patient-specific parameters. Growth hormone secretagogues stimulate pulsatile release of endogenous GH, thereby increasing circulating insulin-like growth factor-1 (IGF-1) levels. IGF-1 acts on chondrocytes to enhance type II collagen synthesis, promote proteoglycan deposition, and inhibit apoptosis via the PI3K/Akt signaling pathway. BPC-157, a 15-amino acid stable gastric peptide, supports angiogenesis, fibroblast activity, and modulates nitric oxide pathways, which in turn enhances synovial perfusion and tissue remodeling. Its efficacy in promoting tendon and ligament repair suggests similar reparative roles in joint capsule and periarticular structures.

In advanced or focal joint degeneration, particularly involving localized cartilage defects or post-traumatic osteoarthritis, intraarticular delivery of the PEDF 29-mer peptide formulated in hyaluronic acid (HA) for sustained joint residence is employed. This 29-amino acid fragment derived from pigment epithelium-derived factor (PEDF) promotes chondrocyte proliferation, inhibits synovial angiogenesis, and downregulates pro-inflammatory cytokines via STAT3 signaling activation.

Typically administered once every two weeks for a total of 3–5 injections, PEDF 29-mer serves as a potent stimulus for local cartilage regeneration and synovial quiescence.

Throughout the treatment course, mechanical load modulation and physical therapy are indispensable. Controlled movement and joint loading guided by physiotherapists are used to direct collagen alignment, prevent fibrosis, and promote mechanotransduction signaling in regenerating cartilage. These biomechanical cues are crucial for integrating newly synthesized extracellular matrix and stabilizing joint function.

Adjunctive therapies are often tailored based on the OA phenotype. Inflammatory OA variants may benefit from ozone therapy, which exerts oxidative preconditioning effects, increases local oxygenation, and modulates Nrf2-mediated antioxidant defenses. For biologic augmentation, platelet-rich plasma (PRP) or mesenchymal stem cell (MSC) therapies may be incorporated to provide growth factors (e.g., TGF-β, VEGF) and progenitor support. PRP injections are generally administered intraarticularly at 2–3-week intervals, while MSCs may be delivered via intraarticular or intravenous routes, depending on protocol and patient profile.

Expected clinical outcomes typically begin to emerge within 6 to 8 weeks, with full effect often observed by 12 weeks post-initiation. Patients frequently report reductions in joint pain and stiffness, along with improvements in range of motion, gait stability, and daily functional capacity. Objective improvements are documented through both biochemical markers, including decreased serum and synovial fluid levels of MMP-13, cartilage oligomeric matrix protein (COMP), and C-terminal telopeptide of type II collagen (CTX-II) and radiologic evidence of cartilage stabilization or thickening via MRI or ultrasound.

Patient-reported outcomes are quantified using standardized tools such as the Western Ontario and McMaster Universities Arthritis Index (WOMAC) or the Knee Injury and Osteoarthritis Outcome Score (KOOS). Improvements in these scores often reflect enhanced pain control, reduced functional limitation, and better joint quality of life. In select patients with early to moderate OA, these integrated peptide-mitochondrial protocols have demonstrated not only symptom control but also potential disease-modifying effects, delaying or eliminating the need for joint replacement surgery.

In summary, the integration of Mito Organelles therapy with regenerative peptides and biomechanical rehabilitation offers a novel, multi-dimensional strategy for managing osteoarthritis. By addressing the energetic, biochemical, and structural deficits of degenerative joint disease, these protocols represent a paradigm shift from symptomatic management to targeted regeneration.

Osteoarthritis remains one of the most therapeutically underserved chronic diseases. However, the integration of peptide therapeutics with mitochondrial support via Mito Organelles *Cartilage, Placenta as well as NOPs Synovia* represents a novel and biologically grounded strategy to restore joint integrity. These therapies address the disease at its metabolic core: reversing mitochondrial dysfunction, reactivating chondrocyte anabolism, and modulating inflammation. As further clinical trials and translational research emerge, these protocols may become a cornerstone of regenerative rheumatology.

CHAPTER 10

Thymic Peptides and Thymus Extracts in Regenerative and Peptide-Based Medicine

(with Prof. Thomas Skutella, MD, PostDoc)

Historical Foundations and Scientific Rationale

The thymus gland, once thought to be vestigial, has emerged as a central organ in the regulation of adaptive immunity, particularly T-lymphocyte development and homeostasis. Its involution beginning in early adulthood coincides with a progressive decline in immune function, often described under the umbrella term "immunosenescence." This physiological regression is characterized by reduced output of naïve T cells, a skewed T-cell receptor (TCR) repertoire, and diminished immunosurveillance. Such changes contribute to increased susceptibility to infections, malignancy, chronic inflammation, and impaired tissue regeneration in the elderly.

Interest in thymic peptides and extracts for therapeutic use emerged in the mid-20th century, spurred by observations that crude thymus tissue preparations from calves or pigs conferred immune-enhancing effects in both animals and humans. These observations led to the isolation and characterization of biologically active thymic peptides such as thymosin α1, thymopoietin, thymulin, thymosin β4, and the clinically investigated thymostimulin. Synthetic analogs were subsequently developed to ensure greater consistency, purity, and safety in administration.

The therapeutic potential of these molecules spans oncology, infectious disease, and increasingly, the field of regenerative and anti-aging medicine. Their proposed benefits derive from the capacity to reconstitute or mimic thymic function, enhance T-cell mediated immunity, modulate inflammatory responses, and support recovery from immunosuppressive therapies such as chemotherapy or radiation.

Mechanisms of Action and Immunological Implications

The biologic activity of thymic peptides operates through intricate immunomodulatory pathways. These peptides act both within the thymus to support T-cell differentiation and in the periphery to modulate immune function [238]. Thymosin α1 for instance, enhances the differentiation and function of CD4+ and CD8+ T cells, increases natural killer (NK) cell cytotoxicity, and promotes the maturation of dendritic cells. It also exerts influence on the cytokine milieu, favoring a shift toward a more robust Th1-mediated immune response through upregulation of interleukin-2 (IL-2), interferon-gamma (IFN-γ), and tumor necrosis factor-alpha (TNF-α) [239].

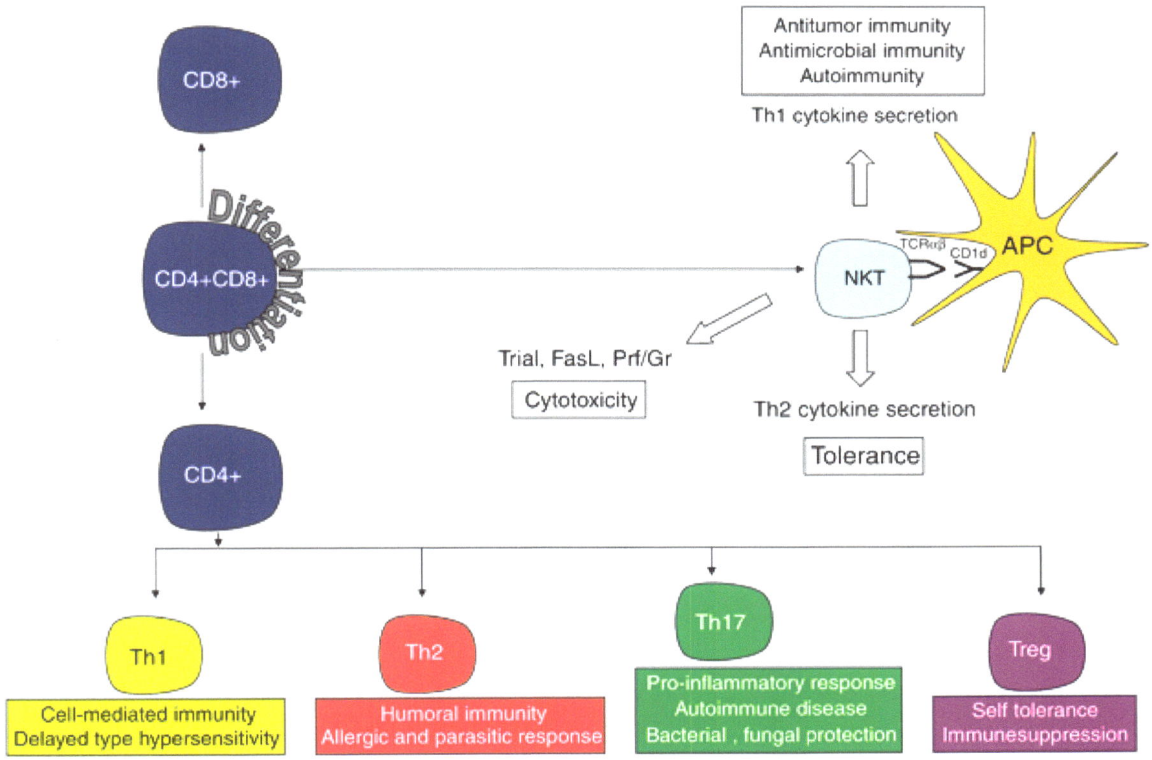

Fig 10.1. *Differentiation of CD4+CD8+ T cells and activation of NKT cells. CD4+CD8+ T cells can differentiate in CD4+, CD8+, and NKT cells (that can be double negative for CD4/CD8 or may be single positive for CD4 or CD8). CD4+ T cells differentiate in Th1, Th2, Th17, and Treg. (Source: Balato, Anna & Unutmaz, Derya & Gaspari, Anthony. (2009). Natural Killer T Cells: An Unconventional T-Cell Subset with Diverse Effector and Regulatory Functions. The Journal of investigative dermatology. 129. 1628-42. 10.1038/jid.2009.30.)*

Similarly, thymopoietin and thymulin influence the maturation and function of T-cell subsets, including regulatory T cells (Tregs), and may play a role in maintaining peripheral tolerance. Emerging data suggests that thymosin β4 has a role beyond immunomodulation, including promotion of angiogenesis, wound healing, and inhibition of fibrosis, further aligning it with regenerative processes [240].

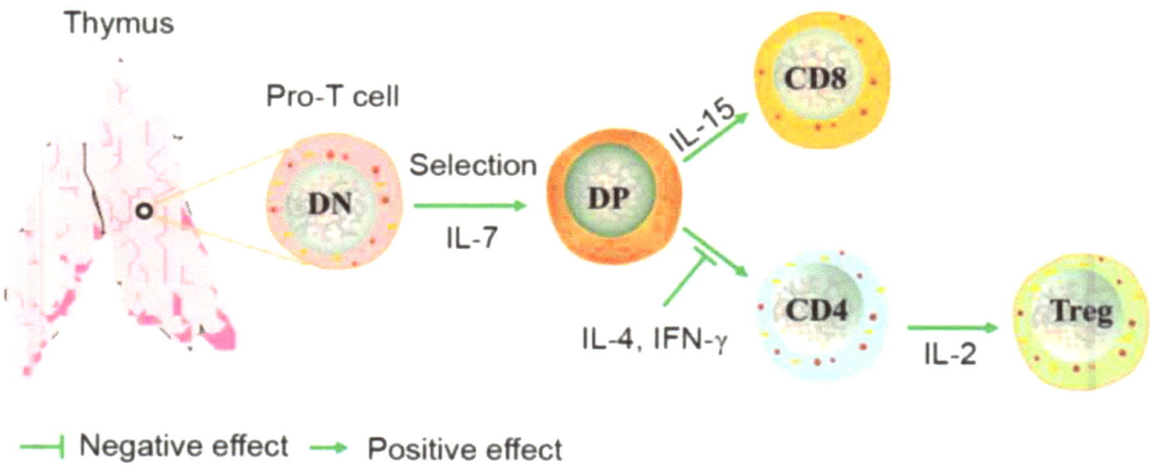

Fig 10.2. *Role of cytokines in T cell development. CD, cluster of differentiation; DN, double negative; DP, double positive; IL, interleukin; Treg, regulatory T cell (source: Yan, F., Mo, X., Liu, J., Ye, S., Zeng, X., & Chen, D. (2017). Thymic function in the regulation of T cells, and molecular mechanisms underlying the modulation of cytokines and stress signaling (Review). Molecular Medicine Reports, 16, 7175-7184. https://doi.org/10.3892/mmr.2017.7525)*

At the molecular level, thymic peptides have been shown to upregulate transcription factors critical to thymopoiesis, such as FoxN1, and stimulate thymic epithelial cell (TEC) proliferation. One recent preclinical model demonstrated that peptide-rich fish collagen induced TEC regeneration and gene expression associated with thymic architecture restoration via NF-κB signaling. These findings provide mechanistic support for therapeutic strategies aimed at reversing thymic involution through exogenous peptide administration [241].

The thymus gland plays a pivotal role in the development and maintenance of the adaptive immune system. Beyond T-cell education, the thymic microenvironment includes a range of non-lymphoid cell types, i.e. thymic epithelial cells (TECs), fibroblasts, macrophages that maintain complex inter-organelle networks. These networks give rise to a diverse molecular repertoire within the thymus, including peptides derived from mitochondria, nuclear matrix, endoplasmic reticulum, and lysosomes.

Cellular extract preparations, particularly those derived from embryonic or neonatal thymic tissue, often contain partially purified subcellular fractions or nanostructures including mitochondria-rich fragments. These formulations may be further enriched via ultracentrifugation or nanofiltration, yielding organelle-specific peptide complexes (e.g., "*nano-organo peptides*") capable of interfacing with recipient cells via endocytosis or receptor-mediated uptake [242].

The most robust clinical evidence supporting the use of thymic peptides originates from studies in oncology. In a Cochrane systematic review conducted by Wolf et al. (2011), data from 26 randomized controlled trials (RCTs) involving over 2,700 patients with solid tumors or hematological malignancies were analyzed to assess the efficacy of thymic peptides as adjuncts to conventional chemotherapy and radiotherapy. The analysis found that while overall survival (OS) and tumor response rates were not significantly altered by thymic peptide administration, there was a statistically significant reduction in treatment-related infectious complications. Specifically, patients receiving thymic peptides experienced lower rates of severe infections and, in some trials, less pronounced chemotherapy-induced neutropenia [243].

Thymostimulin, a partially purified thymic extract containing a mixture of peptides, has been the subject of clinical interest. In small-cell lung cancer, head and neck tumors, and gastrointestinal malignancies, several clinical trials have reported reduced infection rates, improved tolerance to chemotherapy, and, in some cases, prolonged survival compared to control groups. However, limitations in trial design, including lack of blinding, small sample sizes, and variable extract composition, have precluded broad consensus regarding its efficacy in tumor control [243].

Thymosin α1 has garnered regulatory approval in several countries, particularly for use in viral infections and as an adjuvant in hepatitis B and C therapy. Its application in oncology has been more cautious, though preliminary studies suggest possible synergy with checkpoint inhibitors and cancer vaccines. Given its defined molecular structure and favorable safety profile, thymosin α1 remains among the most promising thymic peptides for further clinical development.

Mitochondrial Thymic Peptides: Origin and Function

Mitochondrial peptides, whether encoded in the mitochondrial genome (e.g., humanin, MOTS-c) or derived from mitochondrial proteins (e.g., cytochrome c fragments, TFAM-derived peptides), are emerging as systemic regulators of aging and cell resilience. In thymic tissues, where mitochondrial turnover is rapid during T-cell development, these peptides are abundant and biologically active [242].

Mitochondrial-derived peptides (MDPs), particularly those found in thymic organelle and nano-organelle extracts, exert a multifaceted influence on cellular homeostasis through both intracellular and systemic signaling pathways. Their therapeutic relevance in regenerative and anti-aging medicine is anchored in their ability to modulate mitochondrial dynamics, redox status, metabolic flexibility, and cell survival mechanisms. These actions are mediated by distinct, yet interrelated, molecular pathways that contribute to improved cellular resilience, enhanced immune function, and attenuation of senescence-related dysfunctions.

One of the principal actions of mitochondrial peptides involves the activation of peroxisome proliferator-activated receptor gamma coactivator 1-alpha (PGC-1α), a transcriptional coactivator that orchestrates the expression of genes involved in mitochondrial replication, oxidative phosphorylation, and antioxidant defense. Through coactivation of nuclear respiratory factors (NRF1 and NRF2), PGC-1α enhances transcription of mitochondrial DNA (mtDNA)-encoded genes and promotes replication of mitochondrial genomes, thereby expanding the mitochondrial network within metabolically active tissues [244].

NRF2 serves as a critical redox-sensitive transcription factor that enhances the expression of genes encoding antioxidant enzymes such as heme oxygenase-1 (HO-1), glutathione peroxidase, and superoxide dismutase (SOD). Activation of the PGC-1α/NRF2 axis by MDPs restores mitochondrial abundance and functionality, particularly in tissues compromised by age, oxidative damage, or metabolic stress [245].

A hallmark of mitochondrial aging is the accumulation of ROS, which causes oxidative damage to mitochondrial membranes, proteins, and DNA. Mito Organelles *Thymus* have demonstrated robust antioxidant properties, not by direct free radical scavenging, but through the upregulation of endogenous antioxidant systems and the reduction of mitochondrial proton leak. These peptides help preserve the *mitochondrial membrane potential (ΔΨm)*, a key bioenergetic parameter essential for ATP synthesis via oxidative phosphorylation.

Stabilization of the mitochondrial membrane also inhibits the release of cytochrome c and other pro-apoptotic factors into the cytosol, thereby reducing the initiation of the intrinsic apoptotic cascade. By protecting mitochondrial integrity, MDPs maintain cellular viability under metabolic and inflammatory stress conditions.

Mitophagy, the selective autophagic clearance of damaged or depolarized mitochondria, is a key component of mitochondrial quality control. MDPs have been shown to facilitate mitophagic flux by activating key signaling mediators such as *PINK1 (PTEN-induced kinase 1)* and *Parkin*, which tag damaged mitochondria for lysosomal degradation. This process is essential for preventing the accumulation of dysfunctional organelles that contribute to oxidative stress, inflammation, and cellular senescence.

By promoting mitophagy, mitochondrial peptides support mitochondrial turnover and renewal, ensuring that only functional mitochondria are retained within the cell. This effect is particularly relevant in long-lived cells such as neurons, immune cells, and stem cells, where mitochondrial integrity is essential for sustained function [246].

Mitochondrial peptides exert systemic metabolic effects by modulating energy-sensing pathways, most notably through activation of AMP-activated protein kinase (AMPK). AMPK serves as a master regulator of cellular energy homeostasis and is activated under conditions of ATP depletion or mitochondrial stress. By enhancing AMPK activity, MDPs improve glucose uptake, increase fatty acid oxidation, and promote mitochondrial biogenesis, the mechanisms that contribute to enhanced insulin sensitivity and metabolic flexibility.

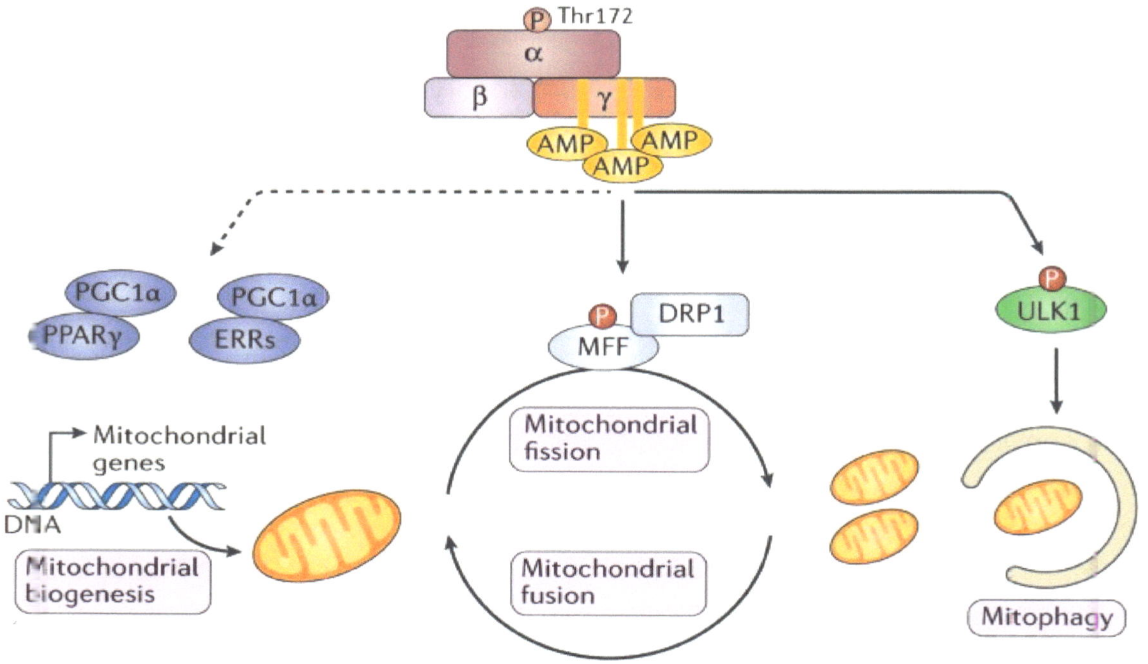

Fig 10.3. *AMPK: guardian of metabolism and mitochondrial homeostasis (source: Nature reviews, Molecular biology).*

Mito Organelles *Thymus* has been shown to translocate to the nucleus under stress conditions and regulate nuclear gene expression involved in metabolism, inflammation, and stress resistance. These mitokines thereby bridge mitochondrial function with endocrine-like systemic effects, influencing whole-body glucose homeostasis and insulin signaling pathways. Such actions have clear implications for the treatment of metabolic syndrome, type 2 diabetes, and age-associated insulin resistance [242].

Beyond their metabolic roles, Mito Organelles *Thymus* provide robust anti-apoptotic protection, especially in immune and barrier-forming tissues. Humanin, for example, has been shown to inhibit Bax translocation to mitochondria and block activation of caspase-dependent apoptotic pathways. These effects are crucial for the preservation of T-cell populations in the context of thymic involution and immune exhaustion, as well as for the maintenance of epithelial integrity in organs vulnerable to aging or injury (e.g., gut, skin, lungs) [242].

Furthermore, these peptides modulate intracellular calcium signaling and ER stress responses, reducing susceptibility to apoptosis in response to cytokine exposure, oxidative insult, or nutrient deprivation.

Other mitochondrial peptides, like Humanin and MOTS-c are now recognized not only as mitochondrial by-products but as *mitokines*—the signaling molecules of mitochondrial origin that exert systemic, hormone-like effects. Unlike traditional cell-autonomous mitochondrial regulators, mitokines are released into the extracellular space and bloodstream, where they act on distant tissues to regulate stress adaptation, metabolism, and inflammation [247].

Preclinical studies in murine models have demonstrated that exogenous administration of Humanin or MOTS-c extends lifespan, improves physical endurance, enhances cognitive performance, and mitigates age-related pathologies [15]. These findings support the hypothesis that mitochondrial peptides function as intercellular communicators of mitochondrial status, potentially coordinating organism-wide responses to energetic and oxidative stress.

When incorporated into Thymic Mito Organelles or Nano-Organo Peptide extracts, these peptides may act synergistically with thymic-derived hormones such as thymosin α1, thymulin, and thymopoietin. This combination supports both immunological regeneration by enhancing thymopoiesis and restoring T-cell diversity and metabolic resilience, by revitalizing mitochondrial function in immune and stromal cells.

The synergistic action of thymic cytokines and mitochondrial peptides has the potential to:

- Reprogram senescent immune cells
- Improve stem cell viability and engraftment
- Reverse inflammaging phenotypes
- Reinvigorate thymic epithelial cell (TEC) function via mitochondrial repair.

By targeting both the immune and metabolic dimensions of aging, these complex peptide therapies offer a comprehensive approach to systemic rejuvenation.

"*Nano-organo Peptides*," or *ultrafiltrates* of subcellular components smaller than whole organelles but larger than simple peptides, are increasingly studied for their ability to modulate cellular behavior through inter-organellar cross talk. These may include vesicular particles, microRNA-containing exosomes, and nanoscale remnants of peroxisomes or lysosomes, all carrying functional peptides, nucleotides, and lipids.

In thymic nano-organelle extracts, functional bioactive fractions have been shown to:

- Induce epigenetic remodeling via histone deacetylase inhibition;
- Enhance proteostasis and autophagic flux in senescent cells;
- Modulate telomerase activity in progenitor T cells;
- Normalize nuclear-mitochondrial interactions, promoting cell survival;
- Regulate inflammation, particularly via NF-κB and inflammasome attenuation.

Such extracts can be delivered parenterally (commonly intramuscularly or subcutaneously), and their nanoscopic size allows tissue penetration and cellular internalization without eliciting antigenic responses [231].

Mitochondrial-derived peptides, particularly when delivered in the context of thymic nano-organelle extracts, represent a promising class of bioactive molecules in regenerative and anti-aging medicine. Their capacity to enhance mitochondrial biogenesis, suppress oxidative stress, activate autophagic pathways, and exert endocrine-like effects across multiple tissues underscores their potential to restore cellular homeostasis and delay aging-related decline. When integrated into thymic peptide therapy protocols, these Mitochondrial peptides may provide a mechanistically robust intervention to enhance immune competence, metabolic balance, and organismal resilience.

Regenerative and Anti-Aging Medicine: Immunosenescence and Thymic Rejuvenation

In the field of regenerative and anti-aging medicine, thymic peptides are being investigated for their ability to counteract the age-related decline in immune competence. Clinical observations reported by Chan et al. (2023) describe the use of thymus extracts and synthetic peptides in aging patients experiencing recurrent infections, delayed wound healing, and general immunologic decline. Patients receiving multi-week courses of thymic peptides demonstrated improvements in immunologic markers, including increased CD4+/CD8+ ratios, enhanced NK cell activity, and normalized immunoglobulin levels [248].

Although most such studies are open-label or observational, the results suggest a role for thymic peptides in rejuvenating immunologic function. The effect may be particularly significant when used in conjunction with hormonal modulation (such as growth hormone or IGF-1 therapy), micronutrient optimization, and regenerative protocols involving stem cells. In a case series involving thymus extract therapy combined with mesenchymal stem cell infusions, patients showed not only immunologic restoration but also improvements in subjective markers of vitality, skin tone, and cognitive clarity.

These findings echo earlier pilot studies, including the 1999 Foundation for Immunology and Nutrition review, which documented normalized delayed-type hypersensitivity (DTH) responses, improved immune profiles, and even potential antitumor effects in selected patient cohorts [Trial J. Cooperation between early acting delayed-type hypersensitivity T-cells and cultured effector cells in tumor rejection. Cancer Res. 1988 Nov 1;48(21):5922-6. PMID: 3262417.].

Table 10.1. Protocols for thymic peptides / thymus extracts in immunomodulation and anti-aging

Clinical Setting	Agent(s)	Dose / Route / Duration	Outcomes Tracked / Monitoring
Cancer patients undergoing chemotherapy/ radiotherapy (adjunctive therapy)	Purified thymus extracts (e.g., thymostimulin, thymus fraction V) or synthetic peptides (e.g., thymosin α1, thymopentin)	Administer pTE or sTP in addition to standard therapies; in trials, frequency varied (e.g., twice weekly or per cycle), routes often intramuscular; duration corresponds with chemo cycles; many studies ~4-8 weeks or per cycle of treatment	Monitor infectious complications (rate/severity), neutropenia, white cell counts, tumor response, overall survival; equitable safety follow-up including side effects, tolerability
Post-immuno-suppression / aging / immune recovery	Thymus extract or thymic peptides, possibly with stem cell support	Longer courses (several weeks to months); possibly cycles (3-6 months), sometimes repeated; routes: injectable or oral (depending on preparation)	Endpoints: naive T cell count, T cell receptor diversity, immune function (e.g., vaccine response, DTH), rate of infections, possibly general health metrics in aging (skin, wound healing)

Clinical Setting	Agent(s)	Dose / Route / Duration	Outcomes Tracked / Monitoring
Anti-aging / immunosenescence in elderly / middle age	Thymic peptides or extracts, possibly combined with lifestyle, nutritional, and hormonal support	Lower intensity, longer durations, e.g., daily or several times per week injections / dosing; cycles of several weeks to months; possibly repeated every few months	Monitor immune-phenotyping (CD4/CD8, NK, regulatory T cells), inflammatory markers, infection rates, quality of life, safety (autoimmunity, malignancy risk)

Clinical Protocols in Thymic Peptide Therapy

Protocols for thymic peptide administration vary considerably depending on clinical context, patient age, immune status, and therapeutic goals. In oncology settings, thymic peptides are commonly administered as adjunctive agents during or between chemotherapy cycles. For example, thymosin α1 may be given subcutaneously at a dose of 1.6 mg twice weekly over a 4–12-week period. Thymostimulin has been administered intramuscularly at 100 mg three times weekly in patients undergoing radiochemotherapy [249].

In anti-aging and immune rejuvenation applications, protocols tend to be longer in duration and are often delivered in cycles. A commonly described regimen involves 1.6 mg of thymosin α1 administered twice weekly for 8 to 12 weeks, repeated every six months based on response and tolerability. Some protocols include concurrent supplementation with zinc and selenium to support thymic hormone activity. Clinical monitoring typically includes lymphocyte subset analysis (CD3, CD4, CD8, NK cells), inflammatory markers (CRP, IL-6), and periodic evaluation of infection frequency and vaccine responsiveness [250].

In experimental regenerative settings involving stem cell co-therapy, thymic peptides are used to prepare or support the thymic niche, aiming to facilitate engraftment or differentiation of progenitor cells into functional T-lymphocytes [251]. These combined protocols remain investigational but may represent the future of multi-modal immune rejuvenation.

Based on existing evidence and analogous protocols, the following could be considered as a blueprint for thyme peptide applications:

- *Patient Selection:* Middle-aged or older adult (e.g., ≥ 50 years) with signs of immune decline (frequent infections, slow wound healing, low T cell counts or naive/memory T cell imbalance), with no active malignancy, acceptable baseline health, no major autoimmunity.
- *Baseline Assessment:* Full immune panel (CBC with differential, CD4/CD8/naive/memory subsets, NK cells, regulatory T cell proportion), functional immune tests (vaccine challenge or recall antigen), inflammatory markers (CRP, IL-6 etc.), metabolic profile.
- *Agent:* Choose a well characterized thymic peptide (e.g., synthetic thymosin α1) or standardized thymus extract with known potency. If using extract, verify purity.
- *Route / Dose / Schedule*: For example, synthetic thymosin α1 at e.g., 1.6 mg subcutaneously twice per week for 8-12 weeks; or thymus extract intramuscularly twice weekly for several weeks, possibly repeating cycles every 3-6 months. Adjust dose by body weight or immune parameter response.
- *Adjuncts:* Combine with nutritional optimization, moderate resistance exercise, adequate sleep, control of inflammation, possibly hormone optimization (e.g., correcting vitamin D deficiency, modulating sex steroids if applicable).
- *Monitoring During Therapy:* Every 4-8 weeks: immune cell subsets, infection rate, adverse events; every 3 months: functional immune tests, general wellness, autoimmunity markers; consider periodic imaging or screening if cancer risk is elevated.

- *Duration and follow-up*: Initial course of 8-12 weeks, assess response (immune parameters, infections). If favorable, consider further cycles (e.g., 3-6 months apart). Follow up for at least 1 year for safety.

Standard Thymosin α1 protocol:

- Standard: 1.6 mg SC twice weekly
- High-dose protocols: 3.2 mg daily for sepsis (though TESTS trial showed no benefit)
- Duration: 4-12 weeks, repeated every 3-6 months
- Route comparison: SC preferred (half-life ~2 hours); IV continuous infusion studied for maintaining therapeutic levels
- PEGylation to extend half-life mentioned in patents but not clinically available

Standard Thymostimulin protocol:

- 100 mg IM 3x weekly during chemotherapy cycles
- Variable extract composition limits reproducibility

Standard Thymosin β4 protocol:

- Topical application for wounds: effective at nanogram concentrations
- Systemic: 5-30 mg/kg in animal studies; human dose ~5 mg intradermal 2x weekly

Standard Thymalin protocol:

- 10 mg IM/SC daily for 5-10 consecutive days
- 1-4 cycles per year for immune support and anti-aging

Standard Epitalon protocol:

- 5-10 mg daily for 10-20 days, repeated 2-4 times per year
- Sublingual, SC, or IM administration

Thymic peptides have generally demonstrated a favorable safety profile in clinical trials and real-world applications. Adverse effects, when reported, are usually limited to local injection site reactions, transient flu-like symptoms, or mild gastrointestinal disturbances. There is minimal evidence suggesting a significant risk of autoimmune activation or neoplastic progression when used appropriately and in controlled doses [252][253][254].

Nevertheless, several limitations must be acknowledged. First, the heterogeneity of thymic extract preparations, particularly those derived from animal sources, introduces variability in peptide composition and bioactivity. Synthetic peptides offer greater standardization but may not capture the full spectrum of biologically active components present in whole gland extracts. Second, much of the clinical literature is based on studies conducted prior to modern trial design standards, with limited placebo control or long-term follow-up. Third, regulatory challenges persist, with many thymic peptides categorized as experimental or off-label therapies in most jurisdictions.

Ongoing research is aimed at clarifying the role of thymic peptides in comprehensive regenerative strategies. Studies are investigating their combination with IL-7, GH/IGF-1 axis modulation, and immune checkpoint therapies. Parallel work is exploring the potential of lab-grown thymic epithelial cells or induced thymopoietic stem cells, potentially supported by thymic peptides, to reconstitute thymic function in aging or immunodeficient individuals [255].

The transcription factor FOXN1 is the master regulator of thymic epithelial cell (TEC) differentiation and function, governing the structural and molecular programs necessary for thymopoiesis. In a landmark study, Bredenkamp et al. (2014) demonstrated that forced FOXN1 expression in aged murine models was sufficient to completely regenerate thymic architecture, cellularity, and functional output, effectively restoring thymopoietic capacity to levels comparable with young adult mice. The rejuvenated thymus displayed reestablished cortical and medullary organization, increased naïve T-cell export, and enhanced T-cell receptor (TCR) diversity.

These findings position FOXN1 upregulation as arguably the most promising single-target intervention for thymic rejuvenation. Given FOXN1's upstream role in regulating TEC differentiation, its modulation could serve as a unifying mechanism to reverse multiple aging-associated defects. Ongoing research focuses on gene therapy vectors, small-molecule activators, and epigenetic reprogramming strategies capable of safely enhancing FOXN1 activity in situ. Comprehensive exploration of FOXN1-based therapies is therefore essential to understanding and potentially translating thymic regeneration into clinical practice.

Keratinocyte Growth Factor (KGF; FGF7) acts through the FGFR2IIIb receptor, which is expressed on thymic epithelial cells, to promote proliferation, survival, and structural maintenance. Multiple preclinical and clinical studies have demonstrated that KGF preserves thymopoiesis during graft-versus-host disease (GVHD), protects TECs from cytotoxic injury, and accelerates thymic recovery following irradiation or chemotherapy. In murine models, KGF administration enhances thymic size, increases thymocyte counts, and restores T-cell reconstitution after bone marrow transplantation. Several clinical trials (e.g., NCT00748582, NCT00314297) have evaluated KGF in the context of hematopoietic stem cell transplantation, with encouraging results regarding immune reconstitution and mucosal protection. Despite this evidence base, KGF is often underrepresented in discussions of thymic regeneration. Its inclusion is critical, as it represents one of the few clinically tested TEC-protective agents with demonstrated translational potential.

IL-7 is indispensable for thymocyte survival, proliferation, and T-cell homeostasis. Therapeutic IL-7 administration has been shown, in both preclinical models and early-phase human trials, to significantly enhance thymopoiesis, expand peripheral naïve T-cell pools, and increase TCR repertoire diversity following hematopoietic stem cell transplantation or lymphodepletion. Recombinant human IL-7 (rhIL-7) has advanced through several clinical studies demonstrating favorable safety and biologic activity, making it one of the most clinically actionable immunorestorative cytokines. IL-7's dual role in promoting thymic-dependent and thymic-independent T-cell recovery makes it a versatile candidate for both aging and post-treatment immune reconstitution strategies. Prominent inclusion of IL-7 therapy in discussions of thymic rejuvenation is therefore warranted, as it bridges mechanistic understanding with real-world clinical applicability.

IL-22, a member of the IL-10 cytokine family, has emerged as a key mediator of epithelial regeneration across multiple tissues, including the thymus. Preclinical studies have demonstrated that IL-22 directly stimulates TEC proliferation and repair following injury, acting via STAT3-dependent transcriptional programs to restore thymic microarchitecture. In models of radiation-induced or inflammatory thymic damage, IL-22 administration facilitated recovery of thymic cellularity and accelerated immune reconstitution. These findings suggest that IL-22 functions as a pro-regenerative cytokine within the thymic niche and may represent a complementary therapeutic avenue alongside KGF and FOXN1-based strategies.

Recent 2024 research employing single-cell transcriptomics has identified distinct populations of age-associated thymic epithelial cells (aaTECs) that accumulate progressively with age. These aberrant TEC subsets exhibit altered gene expression profiles, reduced FOXN1 activity, and heightened expression of senescence-associated and inflammatory markers. Functionally, aaTECs appear to act as "molecular sinks" for growth factors, including KGF and IL-7, thereby sequestering regenerative signals and impairing thymic restoration. Targeting aaTECs—through selective depletion, reprogramming, or modulation of their secretory phenotype—represents an entirely new therapeutic frontier. Understanding the biology of aaTECs may be essential for overcoming intrinsic barriers to thymic regeneration in aged individuals.

The most recent trial—the TESTS trial (The Efficacy and Safety of Thymosin α1 for Sepsis) reported in 2025, is to date the largest randomized controlled trial evaluating the immunomodulatory peptide Thymosin α1 in sepsis [302]. Conducted across 22 centres in China between September 2016 and December 2020, the study enrolled 1,106 adults aged 18-85 diagnosed with sepsis according to Sepsis-3 criteria, randomised 1:1 to receive thymosin α1 (552) or placebo (554). Participants received subcutaneous injections every 12 hours for 7 days unless discontinued. The primary endpoint was 28-day all-cause mortality: 23.4% in the thymosin α1 group versus 24.1% in the placebo arm (hazard ratio 0.99; 95% CI 0.77-1.27; P = 0.93), indicating no statistically significant mortality reduction in the overall cohort. Notably, pre-specified subgroup analyses suggested potential benefit in older patients (≥60 years) and in those with diabetes (HR 0.58; 95% CI 0.35-0.99; P for interaction 0.04), although these findings require cautious interpretation and validation. Safety profiles were similar between groups, with no unexpected adverse events attributed to thymosin α1. Overall, while the TESTS trial importantly establishes the feasibility and safety of large-scale thymosin α1 use in sepsis, it stops short of confirming a clear survival benefit in an unselected sepsis population, pointing to the need for more targeted studies.

Integration of thymic peptide therapy into broader frameworks of regenerative medicine may involve sequential or concurrent use with senolytics, stem cells, epigenetic modulators, or lifestyle-based interventions. Thymic peptides represent a versatile and evolving class of agents in regenerative and peptide medicine. Their ability to modulate immune function, restore T-cell homeostasis, and potentially reverse aspects of biological aging offers a compelling rationale for their integration into both clinical and preventive medicine. As the field advances, high-quality trials and precision medicine frameworks will be essential to fully unlock their therapeutic potential.

CHAPTER 11

Peptides in Aesthetic Dermatology

In my forty over years in the industry in Europe and Germany with Switzerland and China and even Middle East the field of dermatology and particularly aesthetic dermatology has witnessed a significant paradigm shift in the use of bioactive peptides. Originally explored in topical cosmeceutical formulations, peptides have now emerged as central agents in a new generation of therapeutic strategies aimed at promoting skin health, rejuvenation, and structural repair. This transition from surface-level applications to more advanced injectable modalities reflect a broader understanding of skin biology and molecular dermatology, as well as a growing demand for non-surgical interventions that yield clinically meaningful results with minimal downtime.

Peptides, defined as short chains of amino acids, function as key regulatory molecules within the skin's extracellular matrix (ECM). Their ability to act as cell-signaling agents allows them to influence a wide array of biological processes, including fibroblast proliferation, collagen and elastin synthesis, angiogenesis, and inflammatory modulation. These mechanisms form the foundation of their therapeutic potential in cutaneous rejuvenation. As our understanding of peptide structure–function relationships have matured, so too has the capacity to engineer specific peptide sequences that mimic natural matrikines or growth factors, offering a targeted and biocompatible approach to skin regeneration.

The evolution of peptide use in aesthetic dermatology has been driven not only by advances in molecular pharmacology and delivery systems but also by a growing body of clinical evidence supporting their efficacy. Initially confined to skincare formulations, peptides have become a central component of injectable therapies, particularly within the scope of mesotherapy. This minimally invasive technique, involving the intradermal injection of peptide-based cocktails, aims to deliver active compounds directly into the dermis, circumventing the limitations of topical penetration and enabling more precise targeting of cellular processes within the dermal matrix.

Today, injectable peptides are employed to address multiple aspects of cutaneous aging, including the loss of elasticity, increased surface roughness, fine lines, wrinkles, and textural irregularities. Their use is often integrated into comprehensive treatment protocols alongside other modalities such as microneedling, laser therapies, and energy-based devices, thereby enhancing the overall regenerative response.

This chapter provides a comprehensive exploration of peptide therapy in dermatology, with a particular emphasis on its applications in aesthetic medicine. It begins by reviewing the biological roles of peptides in skin physiology and the mechanistic pathways through which they exert reparative and regenerative effects. It then explores the classification of therapeutic peptides, focusing on signal peptides, carrier peptides, enzyme-inhibiting peptides, and neurotransmitter-inhibiting peptides, each with distinct dermatologic implications.

Furthermore, the chapter critically examines the clinical utility of injectable peptide therapies, highlighting their advantages, limitations, and areas of ongoing investigation. A detailed analysis is presented of a recent comparative case study involving two distinct peptide formulations such as F1, composed of low molecular weight peptides (1–10 kDa), and F2, a combination of both low (1–10 kDa) and medium–high molecular weight peptides (45–65 kDa). This study, conducted over a six-week period with consistent injection protocols, provides quantifiable data on improvements in skin texture, wrinkle reduction, collagen and elastin biosynthesis, and patient satisfaction outcomes. By contextualizing this experimental data within the broader landscape of peptide-based treatments, the chapter aims to elucidate both the current state of clinical evidence and the potential for future developments in the field.

In doing so, this chapter not only serves as a scientific primer on peptide-based dermatologic therapy but also as a clinical guide for practitioners seeking to incorporate evidence-based peptide strategies into their aesthetic practice. Through a synthesis of molecular insights, clinical data, and therapeutic considerations, it lays the groundwork for informed decision-making and individualized treatment planning in the rapidly advancing domain of peptide therapeutics.

Skin aging, dermal matrix degradation and the theoretical basis for peptides

With advancing chronological age and cumulative photodamage, the skin undergoes structural alterations that underpin the clinical features of laxity, sagging, rough texture and wrinkles. Microscopically, these changes include fragmentation and reduced synthesis of type I and type III collagen fibrils, alterations in type VII collagen at the dermal–epidermal junction, degeneration of elastic fibres, and a decline in tropoelastin and total dermal elastin content [256][257]. The mechanical consequences of these microstructural changes encompass diminished resilience, reduced firmness and increased skin laxity.

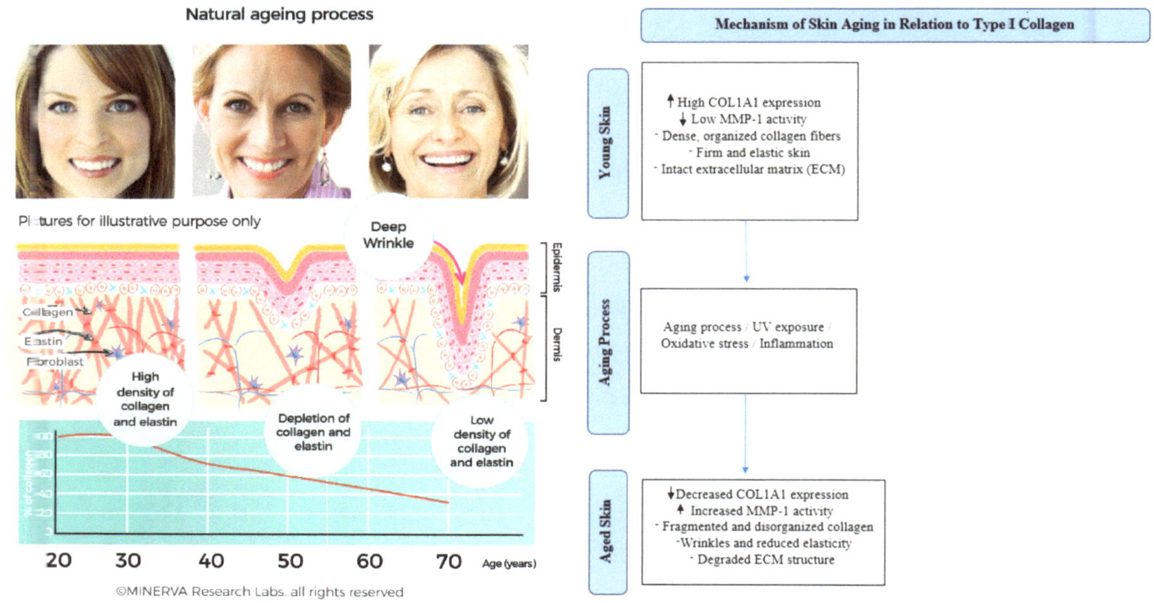

Fig 11.1. *Collagen content of skin is maximal between the 2nd and 3rd decade, after which there is a slow depletion and loss of collagen (and associated ECM components such as elastin and GAGs). The loss of collagen is clearly correlated with changes to appearance attributes which are typically referred to as fines lines and wrinkles (source: MINERVA Research Labs Ltd, London).*

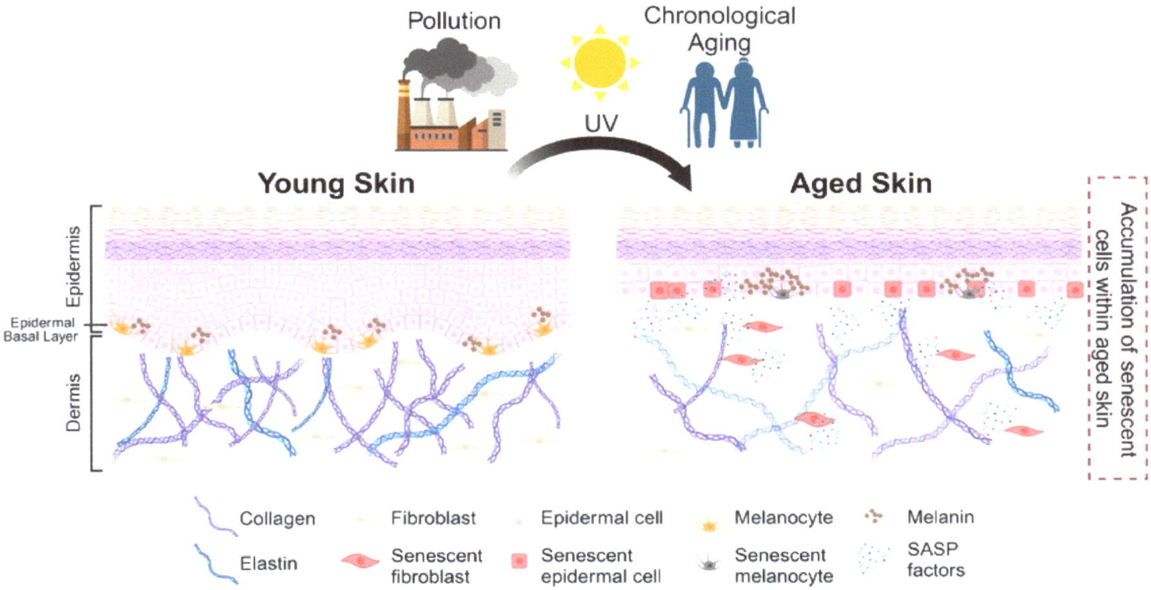

Fig 11.2. *Schematic representation of skin aging. Intrinsic and extrinsic factors (e.g., chronological aging, pollution, UV exposure) result in the accumulation of senescent cells in aged skin. In the aged skin, physiological changes occur–such as thinning of epidermis, flattening of dermal-epidermal junction (DEJ), hyperpigmentation, loss of melanocytes and degradation of collagen and elastin as indicated–that result in the manifestation of various aging phenotypes (source: Chin T., Front Physiol, 2022).*

Peptides operate in this environment by acting as signaling molecules or "messengers" to dermal fibroblasts and other matrix-producing cells. The term peptide in this context refers to short chains of amino acids derived from endogenous proteins (matrikines) or synthetically engineered analogues. As described in the literature, peptides transmit biochemical messages: for example, fragments of degraded collagen can themselves stimulate fibroblasts to synthesize new collagen in response to the perceived "damage" signal [257]. Topical and injectable peptides therefore aim to replicate or augment these signaling functions: by stimulating collagen and elastin synthesis, improving hydration via enhanced glycosaminoglycan production, strengthening the skin barrier, and reducing inflammation or oxidative stress [258].

Mechanistically, several categories of peptides have been defined: signal peptides (which stimulate matrix synthesis), carrier peptides (which facilitate nutrient or trace metal transport), neurotransmitter-inhibiting peptides (which reduce muscle contraction and thereby dynamic wrinkle formation) and enzyme-inhibiting peptides (which may inhibit matrix metalloproteinases) [259]. In aesthetic dermatology, emphasis has often fallen on signal peptides (e.g., palmitoyl pentapeptide-4) and neurotransmitter-inhibiting peptides (e.g., acetyl hexapeptide-8, also known as Argireline) given their anti-wrinkle and firming potential [260].

Nonetheless, it is important to emphasise the limitations: topical peptide formulations must contend with the 500 Dalton rule of skin penetration, the vehicle formulation, concentration, stability, and the fact that many clinical studies on topicals have been small or short-duration [261]. Additionally, while peptides are generally well tolerated, they are not a panacea and require realistic expectations: as one commentary noted, “peptides help with good-looking skin, but don’t expect ‘Botox in a bottle” [262].

Injectable peptide therapies and mesotherapy in aesthetic dermatology

In my forty-five years in aesthetic dermatology, the paradigm of simply applying peptides topically has given way to minimally invasive injection techniques, which are often loosely grouped under the umbrella of ‘*mesotherapy*’ or intradermal micro-injections of peptide-enriched cocktails, either alone or in combination with hyaluronic acid, vitamins, nucleotides or growth factors. The concept is to deliver the active substances directly into the dermis or dermal–epidermal junction thereby bypassing the skin barrier limitations of topical delivery [257]. The injections may also provoke a mild controlled injury response, thereby stimulating fibroblast activation via a wound-healing cascade, which may synergise with the peptide signals.

However, it should be emphasized that published, high-quality evidence for mesotherapy remains limited, variable and in many cases inconclusive. In my experience I come to realize that NOP and MO work better than anything else. A landmark study of six volunteers receiving mesotherapy injections for periorbital rejuvenation demonstrated no statistically significant changes in clinical outcomes or in immunohistochemically measured collagen (types I, III, VII), newly synthesized collagen, elastin or tropoelastin at end-treatment or three months later [263]. More recently, reviews emphasize that the variability of injected cocktails, lack of standardization of protocols, and absence of robust controlled trials limit the ability of mesotherapy to be universally recommended [264]. Nonetheless, the concept remains biologically plausible and is increasingly adopted in aesthetic practice, often in combination with lasers, microneedling or other adjunctive therapies [265].

In the context of aesthetic dermatology, injectable peptide treatments are typically directed toward improving skin tightness/firmer appearance, reducing fine lines and wrinkles, enhancing skin texture/roughness, improving dermal elasticity and hydration, and augmenting the results of other procedures with minimal downtime. Protocols vary, but many practitioners use multiple sessions spaced every 2–4 weeks, injecting small volumes over target areas such as periorbital, cheeks, forehead, neck or décolletage.

In a recent comparative case study (published via PrimeScholars) the efficacy of two injectable peptide formulas was evaluated in an aesthetic dermatology context. Formula 1 (F1) comprised peptides of molecular weight 1–10 kDa, which corresponds to the Nano Organo Peptides (NOP) range, whereas Formula 2 (F2) comprised a combination of peptides of 1–10 kDa plus higher molecular weight peptides of 45-65 kDa, which represents the Mito Orgenelles (MOs) range. Both groups comprised ten volunteers, with injections twice weekly for six weeks, delivering 2 mL into the upper face region. All 20 volunteers completed the protocol [266].

At the end of the six-week treatment period, skin tightening, and texture improvement were reported as 45–50 % for F1 (NOP) and 60–75 % for F2 (MO). At three months post-treatment the improvements were 35–45 % for F1 and 50–60 % for F2. Clinical improvement of wrinkles ranged from good to moderate in F1 and good in F2. Starting from week 3, average surface roughness decreased: for F1 a 14.1 % decrease was observed, reaching 19.7 % by end of treatment; for F2 the reductions were 27.6 % by end of treatment and 34.5 % at three months post. Total wrinkle height decrease was 23.4 % (F1 end) and 17.3 % (F1 at three months) versus 26.7 % (F2 end) and 25.0 % (F2 at three months). Immunohistochemically, collagen type I and type III expression increased to 68.6 % and 67.2 % (F1) and 69.0 % and 69.4 % (F2), respectively ($P < 0.05$). Newly synthesized collagen was quantified as 14.6 % before treatment, 17.5 % at end and 16.3 % at three months post for F1; for F2 they were 14.7 %, 18.0 % and 17.2 %. Type VII collagen changes were 10.2 % vs 10.6 % at baseline, 11.2 % vs 12.6 % at end and 10.9 % vs 11.9 % at three months post (F1 vs F2). Total dermal elastin and tropoelastin levels increased in F2 compared with F1: e.g., baseline 13.2 % vs 14.2 % (F1 vs F2), end of treatment 14.2 % vs 16.8 %, three months later 13.8 % vs 15.2 % ($P < 0.05$). Patient satisfaction measured by the GAIS (Global Aesthetic Improvement Scale) was high in both groups after four weeks. The authors concluded that minimally invasive mesotherapy with NOP and MO demonstrated effectiveness supported by both instrumental and clinical evaluations, with MO yielding statistically superior outcomes and a more prolonged effect than NOP. Clinically, MO appeared particularly effective in the periorbital area (numerous fine lines smoothing) whereas NOP showed a highly noticeable effect on the forehead region. The authors suggested future practice may consider combining both formulas in different target areas to achieve maximal results [267].

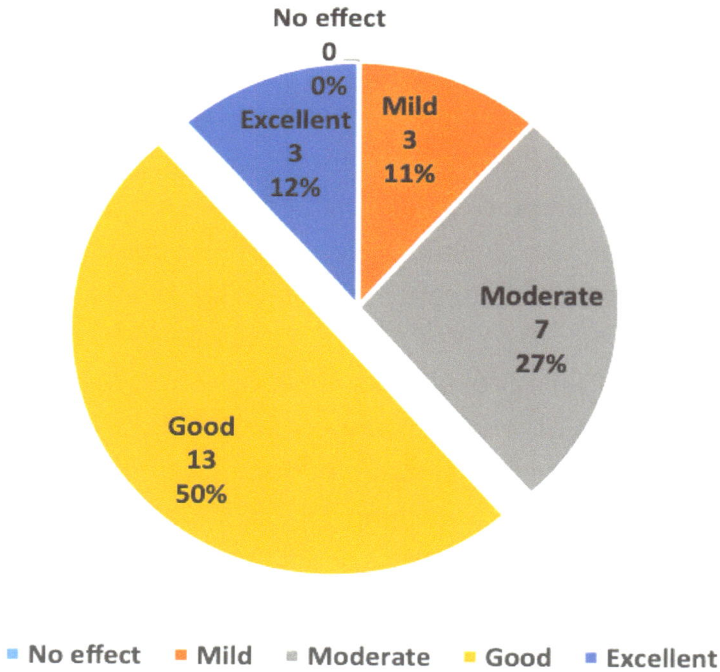

Fig 11.3. *Evaluation of outcomes of the mesotherapy based on the 5-point scale (3 months post-treatment) (source: Klokol D. et al., 2016).*

This case-study is particularly notable because it presents histological/immunohistochemical quantification of matrix components as well as objective roughness and wrinkle height metrics. Nevertheless, several caveats must apply: the study cohort is small (n = 10 per arm), the formulas are proprietary and their exact peptide sequences are not disclosed, placebo or control arms are not described in detail, and longer-term follow-up is limited. The results are encouraging but must be interpreted within the broader context of evidence.

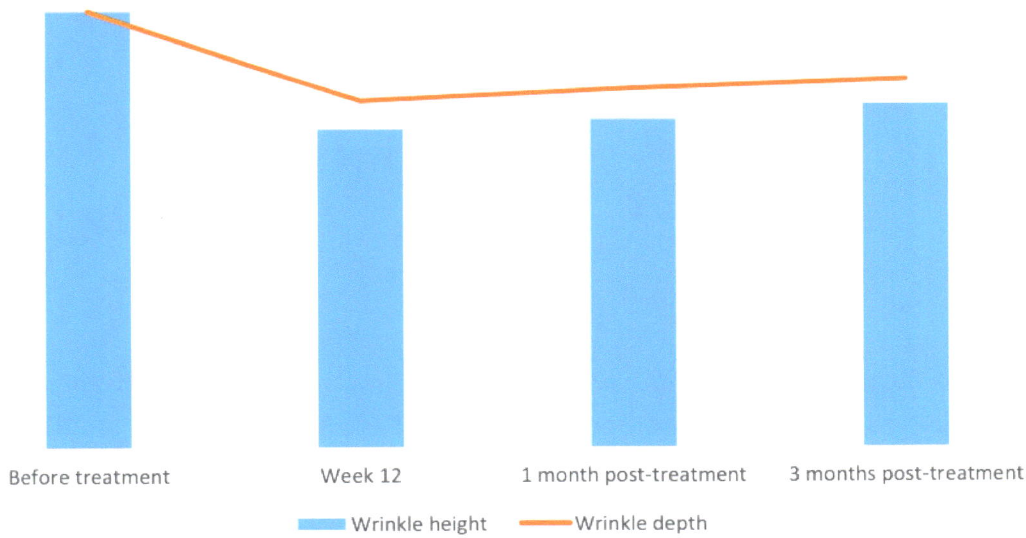

Fig 11.4. *Changes in total wrinkle height and depth before and after the treatment ("crow's feet") (source: Klokol D. et al., 2016).*

From a mechanistic perspective the finding that the inclusion of higher molecular weight peptides (45–65 kDa) improved outcomes suggests that larger peptides (or perhaps peptide complexes) may confer additional signaling or scaffold effects beyond the very low molecular weight peptides. This contrasts somewhat with the typical challenge of dermal delivery of large molecules, but when injected intradermally this limitation is circumvented. The comparison shows that not only the presence of peptides per se but the molecular-weight spectrum and formulation design may materially influence the clinical efficacy in aesthetic applications.

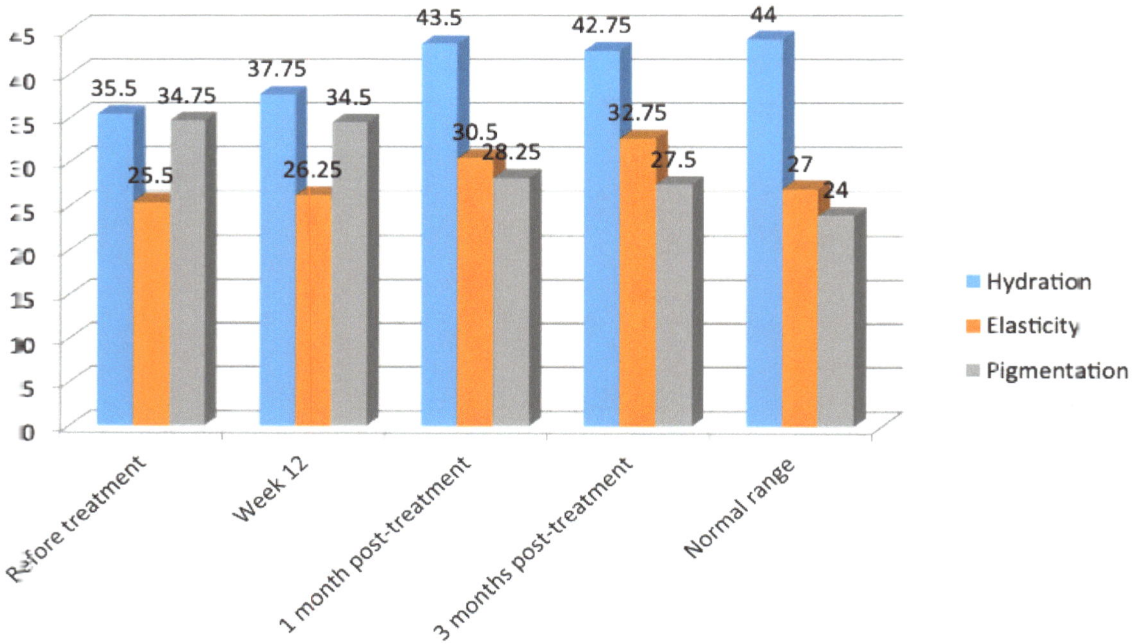

Fig 11.5. *Changes in skin hydration, elasticity and melanin levels in observed patients before, during and after the mesotherapy with SPMCE (source: Klokol D. et al., 2016).*

The application of peptides in aesthetic dermatology must be approached with both scientific rigor and realistic expectations. In practice:

1. Patient selection and indication: Ideal candidates are those with early to moderate skin laxity, textured skin, fine lines, or early signs of dermal matrix decline, but not advanced volume loss requiring deep lifting or surgical intervention. Peptide injections may serve as adjuncts to lasers, microneedling, energy-based devices, fillers or neuromodulators rather than stand-alone 'miracles'.
2. Formulation matters: The case study highlights that different peptide formulations (molecular weight, combination vs single, injection regimen)

yield different outcomes. Clinicians should scrutinize the composition, concentration, vehicle and compatibility of peptide injectables. The ability to reach the target dermal compartment and to deliver sufficient peptide bioactivity is key.

3. Injection protocol and technique: The protocol of twice weekly injections for six weeks (as used in the case study) is more intensive than many mesotherapy protocols (often every 2–4 weeks for 4–6 sessions). Therefore, expectations must be calibrated accordingly. Injection depth, volume (in the case study 2 mL upper face) and spacing must be standardized for reproducibility. Also, the possibility that the act of injection itself (micro-trauma) may contribute to fibroblast activation must be considered when assessing results.
4. Adjunctive therapies: Given that peptides work via signaling and matrix stimulation, their maximal effect may be realized in combination with other treatments. For example, microneedling or fractional lasers create dermal injury and upregulated repair pathways; delivering peptides in that post-injury window may enhance fibroblast response. Many clinics already combine mesotherapy peptide injections with laser or radiofrequency [257].
5. Safety and tolerability: Peptides are generally well tolerated, especially when compared to other injectables like neuromodulators or fillers. Topical peptide products have low irritation potential [268]. For intradermal injections, standard disclaimers of injection therapy (erythema, bruising, swelling) apply. The limited data on long-term safety of novel peptide cocktails mandates ongoing caution and informed consent.
6. Outcome measurement and maintenance: Objective metrics, such as skin roughness, wrinkle height, dermal matrix immunohistochemistry which are rarely accessible in routine practice, but clinicians should nevertheless monitor texture, firmness, patient-perceived improvement and photographic documentation. Maintenance protocols are likely required, as dermal remodeling is an ongoing process and the case study showed diminishing effect after cessation (e.g., NOP reduced from 45–50 %

improvement at end to 35–45 % at three months). Planning for booster sessions or combination therapies is prudent.

7. Cost-benefit and patient counseling: It is critical to manage patient expectations: whereas peptides can improve skin quality, they do not replace volume loss correction, surgical lifts or deep rhytid excision. As noted, the literature cautions that peptides are not "Botox in a bottle". Patients should be informed regarding the incremental nature of improvement, the need for compliance (multiple sessions) and the potential need for adjunctive treatments.

In the evolving landscape of aesthetic dermatology, the concept of xenogeneic organ-specific peptides and cell-derived extracts has emerged as a compelling frontier. Among these, formulations described as "*skin-placenta-mesenchyme*" (SPM) and the extended "*skin-placenta-mesenchyme-collagen-elastin*" (SPMCE) cocktails represent a novel class of mesotherapy agents whose theoretical and mechanistic bases warrant careful scientific scrutiny. These preparations are predicated on the premise that extracts derived from skin, placental and mesenchymal tissues further augmented with collagen and elastin proteins that may act as biologically active cocktails that stimulate dermal repair, enhance ECM synthesis, improve skin elasticity and hydration, and ultimately reduce the appearance of wrinkles and textural ageing.

At the molecular level, the dermal ageing process is characterized by a series of changes in the extracellular matrix: a reduction in collagen types I and III production, disruption of the organized fibrillar network, degradation and loss of elastin fibres, decreased tropoelastin synthesis, flattening of the dermal–epidermal junction, and diminished hydration and glycosaminoglycan content. These matrix alterations translate clinically into increased skin laxity, roughness, fine lines and wrinkle formation. Peptide-based interventions aim to reverse or attenuate these changes by signaling fibroblasts, modulating metalloproteinase activity, and promoting new ECM deposition. This mechanistic framework underpins the rationale for the use of complex organ-derived cocktails.

Formulations derived from skin, placenta and mesenchyme incorporate an array of bioactive molecules, the small peptides, growth factors, amino acids, trace elements, and ECM fragments. For example, placental extracts have been shown to contain a broad spectrum of amino acids (alanine, aspartic acid, arginine, histidine, leucine, lysine, phenylalanine, proline, tyrosine, tryptophan, valine) that have been implicated in fibroblast stimulation and collagen biosynthesis [269]. The "Mito Organelles™ *SPMCE*" formulation, described in the literature as containing skin-, placenta- and mesenchyme-derived peptides and proteins plus collagen and elastin, has been evaluated in mesotherapy for facial rejuvenation and has demonstrated improvements in skin hydration, reduction of skin roughness and promotion of new collagen and elastin fibres.

The underlying biological narrative is that when these organ-specific extracts are delivered intradermally via mesotherapy, they act in several complementary ways. First, the peptides and growth-factor–rich extracts engage dermal fibroblasts, encouraging proliferation, migration and synthesis of collagen and elastin. For instance, studies in vitro have shown that collagen peptides (0.3-8 kDa) significantly increased fibroblast elastin synthesis while inhibiting matrix metalloproteinase-1 (MMP-1) and MMP-3 release [270].

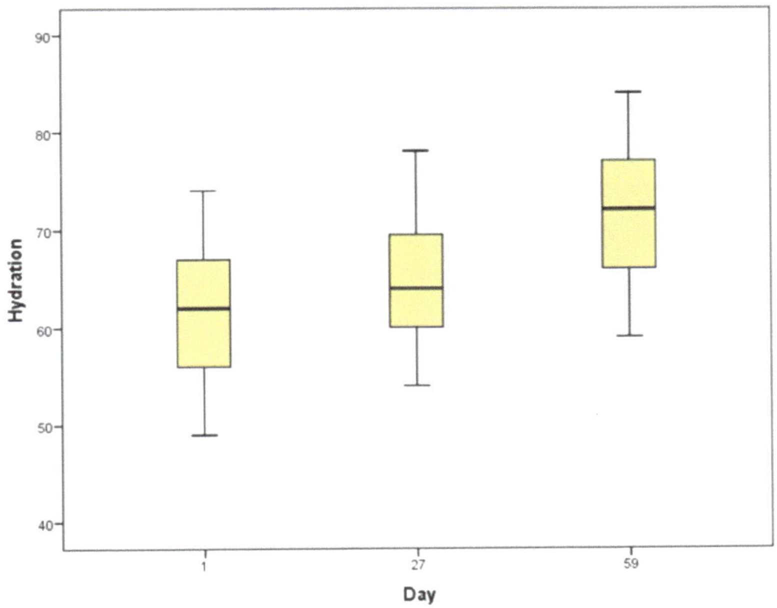

Fig 11.6. *Boxplots of Hydration measurement at Day-1, Day-27 and Day-59 of the treatment period (source: Chernykh V, 2020).*

This supports the concept that peptide signals may shift the fibroblastic environment towards matrix production rather than degradation. Second, the presence of amino acids and trace elements derived from placental or mesenchymal origin may serve as substrate or co-factors for matrix biosynthesis, and also exert antioxidant and anti- Third, the inclusion of pre-formed proteins such as collagen and elastin in the cocktail may provide a scaffold or template effect that assists newly synthesized matrix fibres to align and integrate, potentially accelerating structural remodeling. The study by Klokol et al. reported that mesotherapy with *skin-placenta-mesenchyme-collagen-elastin* extracts (SPMCE) in a cohort of 26 women improved hydration, reduced skin roughness, and increased biosynthesis of new collagen and elastic fibres, as evidenced by histochemical analysis [267].

As applied to aesthetic facial rejuvenation, the predicted and observed effects of these cocktails include enhancement of dermal collagen content, improved elastin fibre architecture, increased skin firmness and resilience, better hydration and water-binding capacity, and reduction in fine lines and wrinkles. By injecting these bioactive extracts into the upper reticular dermis and superficial papillary dermis, one aims to rekindle the dermal fibroblast and ECM network that has become quiescent or degraded due to aging, photo-damage or intrinsic factors. The improved collagen content restores dermal thickness and tensile strength, while enhanced elastin and tropoelastin production augment elastic recoil and reduce skin sagging. The cumulative effect is a smoother surface texture, fewer visible creases, firmer skin, and improved cutaneous “quality”, i.e., improved skin tone, luminosity, hydration and tactile softness.

It is also plausible that the mesenchyme-derived extracts bring mesenchymal stromal cell (MSC) factors or matrix-modulating peptides that influence fibroblast differentiation and matrix remodeling. While direct MSC transplantation is not performed in these cocktails, cell-derived extracts may contain paracrine signaling molecules that activate the resident dermal cells. In this way, the skin-placenta-mesenchyme cocktails serve as a hybrid between regenerative cell therapy and peptide-based dermal remodeling.

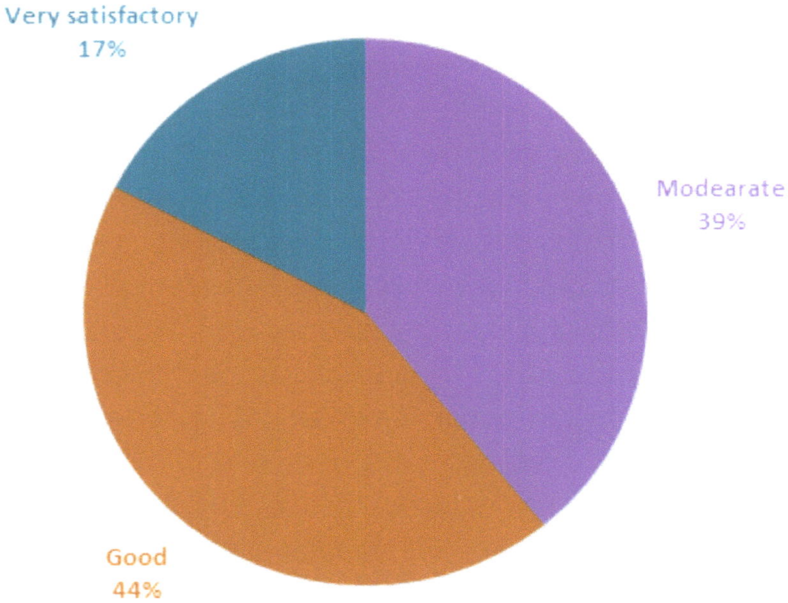

Fig 11.7. *Summary of the clinical outcomes (source: Chernykh V, 2020)*

Clinically, data support that the use of such cocktails via mesotherapy is safe, feasible and yields measurable improvements in skin structure and patient satisfaction. The aforementioned cohort study demonstrated that over 12 weeks of weekly injections, subjects experienced improved skin hydration, smoother texture, and histologically increased elastic filaments. Nevertheless, it is important to interpret these findings with caution, as the literature remains limited and many methodological details (e.g., concentration of extracts, injection depth, molecular weight spectrum of peptides) remain proprietary or unpublished.

From a mechanistic viewpoint, the improvement in collagen and elastin content results from the convergence of several processes: up-regulated gene expression of collagen I and III, increased tropoelastin synthesis, reduced degradation of matrix via down-regulation of MMPs, improved matrix organization and linkage, and augmented hydration which itself supports fibroblast viability and matrix deposition. For example, fibroblast cultures treated with collagen peptides showed reduced MMP release and increased elastin synthesis [270]. The skin-placenta-mesenchyme cocktails add to this by delivering a complex mixture of peptides, amino acids, growth factors and ECM fragments which in concert enhance fibroblast activity, reduce oxidative damage, improve cellular hydration and accelerate remodeling of the dermis from the inside out.

Hydration improvement is a fundamental component of the therapeutic effect. Many of the amino acids and peptides in placental and mesenchymal extracts act as osmolytes and water-binding molecules, while increased matrix glycosaminoglycan and proteoglycan production enhances the dermal capacity for water retention. Improved hydration leads to increased skin turgor, more uniform light scattering in the dermis and a reduction of visible roughness and fine lines. The histochemical analyses in the cohort study of skin-placenta-mesenchyme-collagen-elastin injections showed improved dermal hydration and a reduction in senile lentigo and uneven pigmentation, hence suggesting that the cocktail's effects extend beyond matrix restoration to pigmentary improvement and overall skin revitalization [271].

In terms of wrinkle reduction, the improved matrix firmness and elastic recoil reduce the depth of superficial rhytides, while increased hydration and smoother surface texture reduce tactile and visual cues of ageing. The alignment of newly synthesized collagen and elastin fibres, in a more organized fashion, results in improved mechanical properties of the skin. While large randomized clinical trials are still lacking, the mechanistic framework and existing pilot data make a compelling case that xenogeneic organ-specific cocktails such as skin-placenta-mesenchyme-collagen-elastin have a credible place in the armamentarium of aesthetic dermatology.

I want to conclude this chapter with the following statements that I come to realize that the formulation of xenogeneic organ-specific peptides and cell-derived extracts combining skin, placenta, mesenchyme and the key matrix proteins collagen and elastin represents an innovative approach to mesotherapy and facial rejuvenation. By harnessing the inherent signaling capacity of peptides, growth factors and ECM fragments, and by delivering them intradermally, one may stimulate fibroblast activation, enhanced matrix synthesis, improved hydration, and ultimately reduction of visible ageing changes. While further controlled research is necessary to define optimal delivery protocols, molecular weight spectra, dosing regimens and long-term durability, this cocktail-based paradigm represents a promising bridge between molecular regenerative biology and practical aesthetic therapy.

While the current peer-reviewed literature on injectable peptide mesotherapy is growing, it remains relatively limited in both scope and methodological rigor. Most available studies are small-scale, lack robust controls, and often involve heterogeneous peptide formulations, making direct comparisons and standardized recommendations difficult. Nevertheless, this emerging field presents multiple promising avenues for future research, each of which could significantly refine the clinical application of peptide-based therapies and elevate the standard of care in aesthetic dermatology.

One of the most pressing needs is for larger, multicenter randomized controlled trials (RCTs) that rigorously compare the efficacy and safety profiles of various peptide formulations. These studies should be designed to include placebo or sham injection arms to control for the mechanical and psychological effects of needling itself, which may independently contribute to collagen remodeling via microtrauma-induced fibroblast activation. Stratification by peptide type, molecular weight, and formulation vehicle will be essential to determine the specific contributions of individual components. Such trials would also allow for the generation of higher-level evidence and facilitate the development of standardized treatment guidelines.

In addition to study design, the temporal dimension of treatment efficacy remains inadequately characterized. Longer-term follow-up is critically needed to assess the durability of clinical improvements, such as skin tightening, wrinkle reduction, and dermal remodeling. Determining optimal maintenance intervals is equally important, as current protocols often vary widely, ranging from monthly to quarterly treatments, with little evidence to guide frequency or duration.

From a mechanistic standpoint, future studies should aim to delineate how peptides of different molecular weights and structures modulate fibroblast activity, extracellular matrix remodeling, and the biosynthesis of key proteins such as collagen types I, III, and VII, elastin, and tropoelastin. It is particularly important to elucidate whether low molecular weight peptides primarily serve as signaling molecules, while higher molecular weight peptides offer structural or scaffold-like functions when injected intradermally. These insights would enhance our understanding of how-to tailor peptide combinations to target specific aspects of cutaneous aging.

There is also a clear rationale for evaluating the synergistic effects of combining peptide mesotherapy with other established rejuvenation modalities, such as fractional lasers, microneedling, radiofrequency devices, and platelet-rich plasma (PRP). But in my 40 over years all over the world I come to realize that NOP and MOs are better than PRP. These energy-based or regenerative therapies already stimulate dermal remodeling through controlled injury or growth factor release. Introducing peptides into the post-treatment window may amplify the fibroblastic response and lead to enhanced collagen deposition and elastogenesis. Comparative studies assessing monotherapy versus combination protocols would help define the additive or synergistic value of peptides in integrated aesthetic regimens.

Beyond peptide composition, the mode of delivery is another key variable. Optimizing the delivery system, including the viscosity and pH of the carrier solution, particle size, and peptide stability could enhance bioavailability and tissue integration. Furthermore, refining injection parameters such as depth (superficial dermis vs deep dermis), spacing, volume per injection point, and total treatment area will be essential to standardize procedures and improve reproducibility. Detailed safety profiling, particularly over long-term use and repeated courses is also necessary to establish peptides as a low-risk option in aesthetic dermatology.

The differential clinical outcomes observed in the comparative case study of NOP and MO peptide formulations underscore a fundamental principle: more is not necessarily better. Rather, the therapeutic efficacy appears to depend on the strategic selection of peptides with complementary molecular weights, optimized delivery kinetics, and synergistic biological activities. MO, which combined low and mid-high molecular weight peptides, consistently outperformed NOP in measures of skin texture, wrinkle depth, collagen and elastin production, and overall patient satisfaction, hence suggesting that peptide diversity, rather than sheer concentration, may hold the key to efficacy.

Moreover, the application of advanced imaging techniques and molecular diagnostics, such as high-resolution ultrasound, optical coherence tomography, or non-invasive biomarker assays that may offer novel ways to evaluate treatment response objectively. Quantifying parameters such as dermal echogenicity, collagen density, elastin fiber architecture, and inflammatory markers could allow for personalized treatment protocols based on patient-specific dermal characteristics and biological responsiveness.

As the broader trend in cosmetic medicine continues to shift away from invasive surgical procedures toward minimally invasive, tissue-sparing interventions, peptide-based therapies are well positioned to meet the rising demand for subtle, natural-looking skin enhancement. They particularly cater to patients who seek improvements in overall cutaneous quality, such as enhanced smoothness, firmness, hydration, and glow rather than dramatic contouring or volumizing effects. For these individuals, injectable peptides represent a compelling option: biologically active, well-tolerated, and capable of engaging the skin's intrinsic regenerative pathways without overcorrection or loss of facial identity.

In this context, intradermally administered peptides may fill a unique therapeutic niche, bridging the gap between superficial skincare and more aggressive procedural interventions. With continued scientific validation, technological refinement, and clinical standardization, injectable peptides could become a cornerstone of personalized, regenerative dermatology thus offering patients not just aesthetic correction, but true skin revitalization grounded in molecular science.

Restoration of eyelashes and eyebrows in aesthetic dermatology

Dear Reader, at this point you may think that the topic of peptides in aesthetic dermatology is completed, however it is not, I assure you.

Aesthetic dermatology and facial rejuvenation are incomplete without restoration of eyelashes and eyebrows. Eyelashes and eyebrows hold an outsized influence in facial aesthetics, non-verbal communication, and ocular protection. The upper eyelid typically supports about 100 to 150 lashes arranged across two to three rows, while the lower eyelid has roughly half that number [272]. The eyebrows not only frame the eyes but also shepherd moisture and particulates away from the orbit and serve a pivotal role in facial expression, identity, and perception. Historically, efforts to enhance lash and brow appearance have ranged from cosmetic products such as mascara and eye-pencils to surgical implants, hair follicle transplants, skin-graft or laser-treatment procedures, and pharmacologic agents, among most notable prostaglandin analogues like bimatoprost. These interventions, however, often carry risks such as iris pigmentation change, conjunctival hyperemia, or anterior uveitis, or involve considerable invasiveness. In more recent years, interest has turned to *peptide-based therapies* for hair-follicle modulation (and by extension, for eyelash and eyebrow restoration). Peptides, being defined as short chains of amino acids, often less than 50 residues can act as signaling molecules in diverse tissue contexts and appear to play potential roles in hair-follicle proliferation, differentiation, and extracellular matrix modulation [272]. Notably, a study entitled "Peptides: A Novel Approach to Enhance Eyelash and Eyebrow Growth" by Alvin et al. (2020) evaluated nightly topical application of peptide-extract solutions combined with microneedling for eyelash and eyebrow enhancement over a 12-week interval. Our clinical study on Nanomized Hair Follicle Peptides: A Novel Aesthetic Therapy That Enhances Eyelash and Eyebrow Growth in Women, reports similar outcomes. In this chapter, we present a thorough review of the background, mechanism of action, clinical evidence, safety and tolerability considerations, and practical implementation of peptide-based therapies for eyelash and eyebrow restoration.

From an anatomical and physiological standpoint, eyelashes represent terminal hairs with a well-defined cycle of anagen (growth), catagen (transitional) and telogen (rest). Specifically, the upper-eyelid lashes exhibit a cycle duration of approximately five to eleven months [272]. The number of eyelash follicles is essentially fixed at birth, which implies that interventions must focus on stimulating or prolonging activity of existing follicles rather than generating entirely new ones [273]. Eyebrow follicles likewise follow hair-cycle dynamics and are influenced by hormonal, genetic, and mechanical factors. The anatomical position of the brow, sitting atop the orbital rim, tends to shift or descend slightly with age due to periorbital fat and bony resorption, contributing to brow thinning or a "tired" facial appearance. Traditional therapies have included prostaglandin F2α analogues (for example, bimatoprost) which are approved for eyelash growth but are associated with side-effects such as iris pigmentation changes, conjunctival hyperemia, and anterior uveitis. Scalp-hair follicle transplantation to the lash or brow margin is technically challenging, donor-site limited and invasive. Similarly, topical oils or herbal preparations, such as castor oil, argan oil or oat-protein, vitamin E blends are increasingly popular for lash/brow enhancement but lack robust clinical evidence.

Peptide therapeutics have been employed in medicine since the introduction of insulin therapy in the 1920s and garner appeal due to their high specificity, favourable safety profile and tunable structure. In cutaneous and hair-follicle biology, peptides such as copper-peptides (e.g., GHK-Cu), transforming growth factor-β (TGF-β) peptides and other biomimetic sequences have been shown to regulate hair-follicle growth, differentiation and extracellular-matrix remodeling. Because the dermal papilla and surrounding follicular stroma are recognized as critical regulators of hair-follicle activity, the hypothesis arises that peptides targeting these structures might improve follicle function. Additionally, microneedling has been shown to enhance topical delivery by creating micro-channels in the epidermis, thereby increasing skin permeability and facilitating uptake of peptides. Thus, the rationale is coherent: deliver low-molecular-weight peptide extracts (in one study ≤10 kDa) to eyelash and eyebrow follicular regions, via nightly topical application combined with periodic microneedling, with the goal of stimulating follicle activity (lengthening, thickening, even new follicle activation) while maintaining a favourable safety profile.

Although the precise molecular cascades remain incompletely defined, several plausible mechanisms support the use of peptides for lash and brow enhancement. One mechanism is the extension of the anagen (growth) phase: by modulating signaling pathways such as TGF-β, IGF or VEGF around the follicle, peptides may elongate the active growth phase of hair, thereby increasing both hair length and thickness. Another mechanism involves direct stimulation of the dermal papilla and matrix cells within the follicle. The dermal papilla acts as a key regulatory centre for hair growth; peptides may enhance fibroblast proliferation, cytokine release, and matrix remodeling within that compartment. A further mechanism is improved follicle anchorage and structural support: cosmetic/dermal formulations have employed peptides (for instance, acetyl tetrapeptide-3 or myristoyl tetrapeptide-6) shown to support ECM integrity and dermal thickness around follicles, thereby improving anchorage and reducing shedding. Peptide therapies may also promote activation of new or dormant follicles, our clinical study of eyebrow follicle scans reported new follicle presence at week 12, suggesting peptides may stimulate latent follicular units [272]. In addition, peptides may enhance the follicle micro-environment and micro-circulation via nitric-oxide signaling, reduce local inflammation, and improve nutrient supply and waste removal in the follicle niche. Finally, microneedling preludes the peptide delivery and represents a mechanism of enhanced uptake: pre-treatment with microneedles breaches the epidermal barrier and augments bioavailability of topically applied peptides. In aggregate, the therapeutic goal is to establish an enriched and stimulated follicular micro-environment in which the growth phase is prolonged, structural support is improved, and follicles are effectively reactivated, thereby producing longer, thicker lashes and brows.

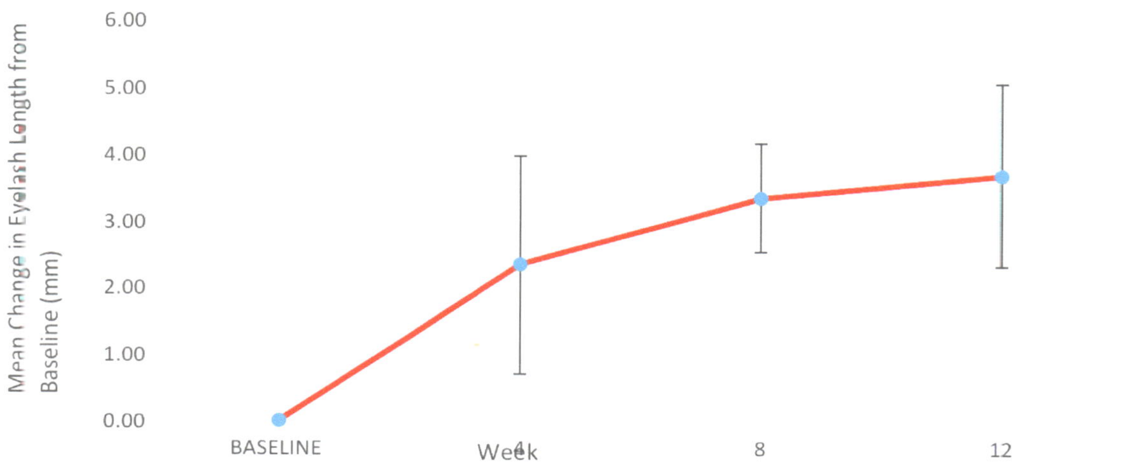

Fig 11.8. *Mean change in eyelash length from baseline, with standard deviation bars, throughout the 12 weeks treatment period (source: Alvin G. et al., 2022).*

An open-label cohort study was conducted over twelve weeks (November 2019 to January 2020) involving six healthy adult female subjects aged 21 to 46 years (mean 32 years) [272]. Subjects daily applied a peptide-extract solution to the upper eyelid margin and eyebrows and underwent microneedling sessions every two weeks (34-gauge hypodermic needle after topical 10 % lidocaine cream). Measurements included eyelash length (using an eyelash ruler with 0.01 mm resolution), the Global Eyelash Assessment (GEA) scale (1 = minimal to 4 = very marked) assessed by dermatologists, digital photographic evaluation of eyebrow thickness/density, and high-magnification (×200) micro-skin/hair diagnostics for eyebrow follicle thickness and new follicle presence. Baseline mean eyelash length was approximately 4 mm (range 3–5 mm). At twelve weeks, all six subjects experienced at least a ≥1-grade improvement in GEA score; five of six (83 %) improved by one grade and one subject (17 %) improved by two grades. Mean eyelash length gain was +2.3 ± 1.6 mm at week 4 ($p = 0.021$), +3.3 ± 0.82 mm at week 8 ($p = 0.013$), and +3.7 ± 1.4 mm at week 12 ($p = 0.014$). Eyebrow scans revealed increased individual follicle thickness and the presence of newly formed eyebrow follicles by week 12. No serious adverse events were recorded; one subject reported minor eyelid-margin discomfort at week 12 that was attributed to applicator trauma rather than the peptide product. These data suggest that topical peptide therapy, when combined with microneedling, can produce clinically meaningful improvements in eyelash length and prominence and eyebrow follicle density in a relatively short period with a favourable short-term safety profile.

However, several limitations merit emphasis. The small sample size ($n = 6$), open-label non-controlled design, the possible contribution of the microneedling intervention itself, the limited duration (12 weeks), and the study population restricted to healthy adult females with normal lash and brow density all limit generalizability. Details of the peptide formulation (specific sequence, stability, excipients) are sparsely reported, and the magnitude of effect may not apply to pathological lash/brow loss or male subjects. Hence, while the results are promising, they must be interpreted with caution.

Beyond the study conducted by my colleague Dr. Glen Alvin et al., further investigations of peptide- and glycosaminoglycan-based lash serums provide supplementary evidence. For example, a 2024 open-label trial of thirty female subjects aged 25–65 years assessed an enhancer serum containing peptides and glycosaminoglycans. At twelve weeks, statistically significant improvements from baseline were reported in eyelash length (+8.3 %), eyelash number (+5 %), eyelash width (+10.1 %), volume (+14.1 %), arc (+13.4 %) and angle (+28.3 %) of lash curvature, with Global Eyelash Assessment (GEA) scores significantly improved and patient satisfaction rising to 84.3 % [274]. Cosmetic-dermal literature describes common peptides employed in these contexts, such as GHK-Cu (copper peptide), acetyl tetrapeptide-3, biotinoyl tripeptide-1, and other biomimetic growth-factor peptides that support follicle health via extracellular matrix reinforcement, enhanced microvascular supply, signaling modulation and growth-phase extension. Delivery technology enhancements also play a role: nano- or micro-sized peptide carriers (including "nanomized" hair follicle peptides) have been suggested to improve penetration kinetics and bioavailability in follicular regions. Taken together, the evidence supports the concept of peptide-based lash/brow therapy as biologically plausible, technically feasible and commercially desirable; nevertheless, the clinical evidence remains limited and largely preliminary.

In terms of translation into practice, the protocol evidenced in the Australian study entailed nightly topical application of low-molecular-weight peptide extract to the upper eyelid margin (at the base of the eyelashes) and to the eyebrows, using a sterile applicator and allowing overnight contact without rinsing. Every two weeks the subjects underwent microneedling (34-gauge hypodermic needle) with prior topical anesthesia (10% lidocaine cream). Subjects were instructed to avoid additional eyelash or eyebrow treatments, tanning or sun exposure, and eye-drop use (including artificial tears) during the study period. Follow-up assessment occurred every two weeks for questionnaires and measurements and monthly for photographs; the total initial duration was twelve weeks. Candidate selection in the study comprised healthy adult females aged approximately 20–50 years, with normal eyelash and eyebrow density, no recent modification (e.g., lash extensions) and no medications influencing hair growth (such as steroids, immunosuppressants, topical eye medications). In practice, selection criteria should include absence of ocular surface disease, stable lash/brow baseline, and realistic expectation setting. Clinically relevant endpoints to monitor include lash length (e.g., ruler measurement in mm), GEA score for lash prominence, photographic assessment of brow density/thickness, and if available, high-magnification follicle scanning for brow follicle thickness and new-follicle count. Safety considerations must not be neglected: even though the trial reported no serious adverse events, the eyelid margin is a delicate region, and risks of ocular surface irritation, infection (especially with microneedling near the orbit), pigment changes or allergic reaction exist. Further, product migration into the eye is a potential concern, so formulations should be ophthalmic-safe or specifically approved for peri-ocular use; microneedling should be conducted by trained personnel under aseptic conditions.

From the available evidence, patients should be counseled that initial effect may appear after approximately four weeks, with the full effect typically observed between eight and twelve weeks (for example, mean lash-length gain of about 3.7 mm over twelve weeks in the cited study). Maintenance beyond twelve weeks remains empirical and may require ongoing nightly application and periodic professional treatment. Real-world compliance, cost (product + microneedling sessions) and incident lash/brow follicle status (e.g., severely depleted follicles) may attenuate outcomes compared with controlled-trial settings.

Peptide-based therapies represent an emerging and promising modality for eyelash and eyebrow restoration. Their biological rationale recruiting the pathway via enhancement of follicle growth, extracellular-matrix support, prolongation of anagen phase, improved anchorage and potential activation of latent follicles is compelling. The twelve-week open-label trial by Alvin et al. documented mean lash-length gains of ~3.7 mm, 100 % GEA improvement and favourable brow-follicle findings in a small cohort, without serious adverse events. Technological adjuncts (microneedling and nano-peptides) may enhance delivery and accelerate effect.

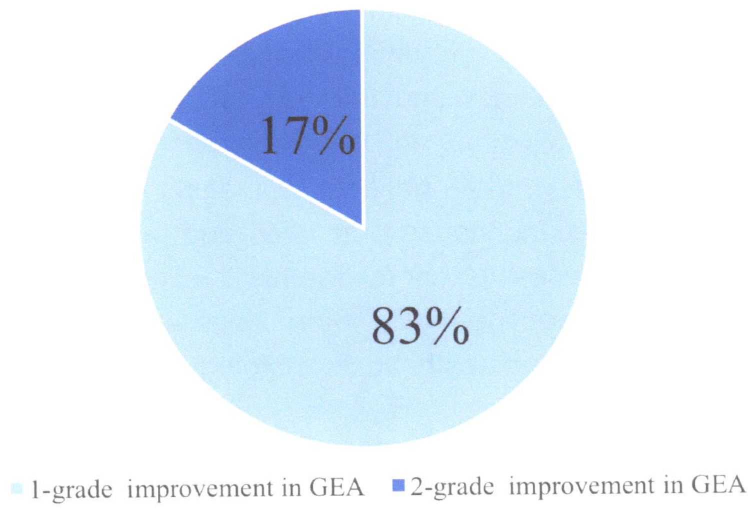

Fig 11.9. *Percentage of subjects according to grade enhancement in GEA score from baseline (source: Alvin G. et al., 2022).*

Nonetheless, the current evidence remains preliminary, with small sample sizes, open-label designs and restricted populations; hence, generalization to broader or clinical (e.g., alopecia-related) populations should be approached cautiously. For aesthetic practitioners and clinicians, nightly topical application plus periodic microneedling appears feasible, but requires adequate patient counseling—on evidence level, expectation setting, cost/commitment and monitoring for safety. For researchers, the field is ripe for further development: larger randomized controlled trials, mechanistic studies, formulation optimization and long-term durability data are needed. In sum, peptide therapy occupies an intermediate position between non-invasive cosmetic serums and more invasive prostaglandin or transplant approaches and may offer a biologically targeted and safety-favourable option for lash and brow enhancement.

In summary, peptides represent a biologically rational and increasingly clinically applied tool in the aesthetic dermatology armamentarium. Their ability to signal matrix synthesis, enhance fibroblast activity, support barrier integrity and improve skin texture provides a mechanistic foundation for their use. Injectable peptide therapies, especially within mesotherapy frameworks that offer further promise by bypassing topical delivery limitations. The referenced case study comparing two peptide formulations (NOP and MO) demonstrates that formulation design and molecular weight spectrum matter: MO (1–10 kDa + 45–65 kDa peptides) out-performed NOP (1–10 kDa only) in tightening, texture improvement, wrinkle reduction, collagen and elastin metrics and durability of effect. Nevertheless, robust controlled evidence remains limited, and clinicians must apply these interventions judiciously by selecting appropriate patients, managing expectations, integrating with adjunctive treatments, monitoring outcomes and providing maintenance as required. As the field advances, further research will refine best practice protocols, deepen understanding of peptide-matrix interactions and position peptide injections as part of evidence-based aesthetic dermatology care.

CHAPTER 12

Human Growth Hormone: Discovery, Synthesis, Physiology, and Clinical Applications in Regenerative Medicine

(With Dr. Dmytro Klokol, MD, PhD)

Historical Discovery and Biotechnological Synthesis

The concept that the anterior pituitary ("hypophysis") secretes factors which influence body growth dates to the late 19th and early 20th centuries. Clinically recognized disturbances of growth in children and of overgrowth (gigantism, acromegaly) in adults were observed in association with pituitary tumors. Autopsy studies demonstrated pituitary adenomas in many acromegaly cases, and animal experiments (e.g., injection of pituitary extracts or removal of the pituitary) established that extracts from pituitary glands could accelerate growth or retard it when the gland was removed [275][276][277].

Purification of human GH (hGH) from cadaveric pituitaries began in the 1950s. Early preparations (native hGH) provided proof that human pituitary-derived GH could stimulate growth in GH-deficient children. However, supply was strictly limited; millions of pituitaries were required to meet the needs of even a few patients. In the USA, the National Pituitary Agency (established in 1961) coordinated collection and distribution of human pituitaries for GH extraction [278][279].

The native GH supply route was interrupted by the discovery, in the mid-1980s, that some recipients of cadaveric pituitary GH developed Creutzfeldt-Jakob disease (CJD), presumably due to prion contamination. This led to the halt of use of pituitary-derived GH and to the regulatory acceptance and uptake of recombinant human GH (rhGH; also called biosynthetic GH) [277][280][279].

Recombinant synthesis of hGH was developed via expression of the human GH gene in *Escherichia coli*. The first recombinant GH preparation (initially with an extra methionine residue at the N-terminus, so called "Met-hGH") was approved by the US FDA in 1985 for treatment of GH deficiency in children. Production scale and methods rapidly improved, and many of the recombinant GH products became bioidentical to the 22 kDa form of pituitary GH. Comparative pharmacologic studies showed similar metabolic, growth-promoting activity, low antigenicity, and predictable pharmacokinetics compared to native preparations [279][231][280].

Physiology: Regulation, Receptor, and Mechanism of Action

Endogenous GH is produced by somatotrophs in the anterior pituitary under regulation by hypothalamic factors (growth hormone releasing hormone, GHRH) and somatostatin, as well as by various feedback signals (notably IGF-1 and metabolic states). Secretion is pulsatile, with higher peaks during sleep (especially slow-wave sleep), exercise, fasting, and other stressors. GH levels decline with age [282].

GH exerts its physiologic effects by binding to its cell surface receptor (GHR), which belongs to the class I cytokine receptor family. The receptor does not itself have intrinsic tyrosine kinase activity but is associated with intracellular non-receptor tyrosine kinase JAK2. Upon GH binding to GHR (which is thought to induce conformational changes and receptor dimerization), JAK2 is activated, leading to phosphorylation of both GHR and JAK2 on critical tyrosine residues. These phosphotyrosines serve as docking sites for signaling molecules including signal transducers and activators of transcription (STATs), especially STAT5b, as well as Shc, insulin receptor substrates (IRS1, IRS2), and adaptors leading to activation of the MAPK/ERK and PI3K/Akt pathways [282][276][283].

Many actions of GH are mediated indirectly via production of insulin-like growth factor 1 (IGF-1), principally by hepatocytes, but also locally in bone, muscle and other tissues. IGF-1 via its receptor (IGF-1R, a receptor tyrosine kinase) promotes cell proliferation, inhibits apoptosis, stimulates differentiation, and contributes to anabolic processes. The GH–IGF-1 axis is regulated by IGF binding proteins (IGF-BPs), which modulate IGF-1 bioavailability. Some GH effects are direct (lipolysis, modulation of carbohydrate metabolism, effects on immune cells) and these can be IGF-1 independent [282].

Negative regulation exists via multiple mechanisms: suppressor of cytokine signaling (SOCS) proteins, protein tyrosine phosphatases (e.g., SHP1, SHP2), receptor internalization and degradation, feedback by IGF-1, and interactions with nutritional, inflammatory, and metabolic status. With aging, there is often a decline in GH secretion (somatopause), reduced pulse amplitude, and increased somatostatin tone, among other regulatory shifts [280][282].

Mechanisms Relevant to Regenerative Medicine and Anti-Aging

Regenerative medicine seeks to restore structure and function, often by promoting tissue repair, stem/progenitor cell activity, reducing senescence, improving metabolic function, and preserving extracellular matrix. GH / IGF-1 axis intersects many of these processes.

GH promotes:

- Increased lean body mass, by stimulating protein synthesis in muscle, increasing amino acid uptake, reducing proteolysis; also, by enhancing myoblast fusion (in experimental models) via the IGF-1 pathway [284][282].
- Enhanced bone metabolism: increasing bone formation by stimulating osteoblast activity and increasing IGF-1 locally in bone, and systemic

IGF-1, with downstream effects in promoting skeletal growth in children and maintaining bone mass, reducing risk of osteoporosis [282].

- Lipid metabolism: GH increases lipolysis (mobilization of fat) and decreases adiposity in both experimental animals and humans; however, GH also has anti-insulin effects in carbohydrate metabolism which must be balanced [276].
- Effects on skin, connective tissue, and possibly extracellular matrix GH/IGF-1 have effects on collagen synthesis, skin thickness, wound healing in experimental settings. There are some human data (though limited) of improved skin quality.
- Possibly modulation of immune function and repair: GH may stimulate certain immune cell functions, improve protein anabolism post-injury or in catabolic states, and ameliorate muscle wasting. HIV/AIDS wasting syndrome is a well-characterized approved indication [285].

Evidence and Clinical Applications

From its approved uses to its off label / investigational applications in anti-aging and regenerative therapy, GH has been studied in various populations.

Approved indications in many countries include children with GH deficiency, children with growth disorders (Turner syndrome, small for gestational age, Prader-Willi syndrome, chronic renal insufficiency, etc.), adults with documented GH deficiency (often due to pituitary disease, surgery, or tumor), HIV/AIDS–associated cachexia or wasting, short bowel syndrome [285].

In terms of anti-aging or "age-related decline" settings in otherwise healthy older adults, some randomized controlled trials and observational studies have been conducted. A seminal study by Rudman et al. (1990) administered GH to older men and found increases in lean body mass, decreases in adipose tissue, and improved skin thickness but no significant improvement in muscle strength, and a constellation of side effects.

Additional studies have examined GH therapy in frail elderly, individuals with sarcopenia, or individuals recovering from injury or surgery. These show that GH can increase lean mass, modestly reduce fat mass, improve exercise capacity or quality of life in some circumstances, but the magnitude of benefit is variable, often modest, and often with trade-offs (side effects, cost, monitoring). Long-term data about lifespan extension or true reversal of aging processes in humans are lacking [285].

In regenerative medicine contexts (e.g., wound healing, coronary disease, organ regeneration), preclinical animal studies show promising results: GH / IGF-1 supplementation enhance healing, angiogenesis, cell survival, reduce apoptosis. Human data are more limited and often involve adjunctive roles, e.g., after surgical procedures, or in burn healing, or as part of combined regenerative / cell-based therapies. The evidence for GH alone achieving regeneration in complex organs is not yet robust.

Risks, Adverse Effects, and Limitations

Administration of exogenous GH, particularly in non-deficient individuals or in doses above physiologic replacement, carries significant risks. Known adverse effects include edema (fluid retention), arthralgias and myalgias, carpal tunnel syndrome (nerve compression), insulin resistance, hyperglycemia, possible worsening or induction of diabetes, and potential promotion of growth of neoplastic tissue (especially if there is risk of pre-existing cancer) because GH / IGF-1 signals are mitogenic [286].

In long term, excessive GH elevation leads to acromegaly, with characteristic tissue overgrowth, bone thickening, organomegaly, joint problems, cardiomyopathy, hypertension, and metabolic derangement. Even therapeutic GH must be carefully dosed, monitored, and adjusted. In anti-aging settings, often the risk/benefit ratio is less favorable compared to genuine deficiency. Regulatory bodies generally do *not* approve GH for anti-aging purposes, and off-label or illicit use is common (and potentially dangerous) [287].

Other limitations include variable response: age, gender, nutrition, co-morbidities, baseline GH/IGF-1 axis status, GH receptor sensitivity, IGF binding protein profile, presence of inflammation, all influence outcomes. There are also practical limitations: cost, need for injections, side effects, and ethical / legal regulation in many jurisdictions.

Evidence-Based Medical Data: What Is Well Established, What Is Tentative

What is well-established includes that GH replacement in patients with documented GH deficiency restores many of the features lost: improved bone mineral density, reduction in fat mass, increase in protein synthesis and muscle mass, improvement in exercise capacity and quality of life. Many studies in children show predictable increases in growth velocity and final height (when treatment is started early enough) with safety profiles that are acceptable in experienced hands. Recombinant hGH products are bioequivalent to native GH in many biochemical and physiologic endpoints (Human Growth Hormone. Drug Enforcement Administration. Diversion Control Division. Drug & Chemical Evaluation Section.).

What remains tentative or under-investigated includes whether GH therapy in otherwise healthy older adults (without proven deficiency) meaningfully slows aging, improves lifespan, or reduces incidence of age-related diseases in a safe manner. Some improvements (body composition, skin thickness, possibly bone density) are seen, but functional improvements (strength, endurance), and long-term safety (especially cancer risk, diabetes risk) are much less well-characterized. The optimal dosing regimens for regenerative purposes, or how to combine GH with other peptides or therapies (stem cells, growth factors, etc.), are still largely experimental.

Clinical trials are often small in sample size, of short duration, with heterogeneous endpoints. There is also risk of bias, and difficultly in blinding in some studies. Regulatory oversight restricts many uses.

Practical & Ethical Considerations and Future Directions

In considering GH for anti-aging or regenerative medicine, key practical elements include establishing whether there is true GH deficiency, monitoring IGF-1 levels, glucose tolerance, and screening for cancers. Dosing ideally mimics physiologic secretion (pulsatile where possible, lower doses rather than supraphysiologic). The circle of risks is greater in older patients, especially those with other co-morbidities (e.g., metabolic syndrome). Cost, access, and legal status differ by country;

in many places use of GH for anti-aging or athletic enhancement is off-label or outright regulated against. Ethical concerns include fairness, the border between treatment and enhancement, and long-term unknowns.

Key areas for further research include better understanding of GH / IGF-1 axis in aging, mechanisms of GH resistance (e.g., through inflammation, oxidative stress, epigenetic modifications), development of GH analogues or modified-release GH formulations that optimize beneficial vs deleterious effects, combination therapies (e.g. GH + peptides, nutraceuticals, lifestyle) to support regeneration, and large randomized controlled trials of GH in aging populations focusing on functional outcomes, safety over many years (including cancer incidence, metabolic disease).

Also, there is interest in using GH in tissue engineering, wound healing, possibly in neuroregeneration, and understanding its roles in stem/progenitor activation. But translation into routine clinical practice in regenerative medicine remains limited by safety concerns and the need for more robust evidence.

Human Growth Hormone in Anti-Aging & Regenerative Medicine: Clinical Trials & Peptide-Therapy Protocols

Several randomized controlled trials (RCTs) and long-term observational studies have characterized effects of recombinant human GH (rhGH, somatropin) in adult populations with GH deficiency (AGHD), elderly persons, or non-deficient but aging individuals. These provide the strongest basis for protocols, as well as known risks and magnitude of effect.

In a 5-year prospective study of 118 adult-onset GH deficient subjects (mean age ~49 years), GH replacement resulted in sustained increases in lean body mass, reductions in total adipose fat, and increments in bone mineral content (particularly lumbar spine L2-L4 and femur neck) over the course of therapy. The mean starting dose was approximately 0.98 mg/day, gradually decreased to ~0.48 mg/day by year 5. Improvements in lipid profile (reduced total cholesterol, LDL; increased HDL) were observed [288].

A dose-response trial in Japanese AGHD patients (96 subjects) randomized into low-dose (0.006 mg/kg/day) vs high-dose (0.012 mg/kg/day) rhGH vs placebo over 24 weeks, with a subsequent long-term open label extension, showed that both GH doses increased IGF-I SDS, increased lean body mass, decreased total fat mass and cholesterol; the high dose produced more marked reduction in trunk fat mass than the low dose [289].

In elderly populations without diagnosed GH deficiency, a systematic review of 18 unique study populations (508 subjects total) found GH treatment over ~27 weeks (mean) with dosage around 14 µg/kg/day (varied) led to significant decreases in fat mass (≈2.1-2.8 kg) and increases in lean body mass (~2.1 kg), without significant weight change. Other observed effects included modest reductions in cholesterol. Adverse effects included edema, joint pain / stiffness [290][291].

Another RCT involving healthy elderly men (age 65-80), examined GH alone, testosterone (Te) alone, and GH + Te together. GH doses were adjusted over ~8 weeks to reach IGF-I in upper half of age-specific reference range; Te was via transdermal patch. The GH + Te arm (and GH alone) increased lean mass; GH+Te uniquely produced improvements in aerobic capacity, mid-thigh muscle cross-section, and reductions in fat mass. Muscle strength improvements were inconsistent. Quality of life showed modest improvements [292].

There are also data in malnourished or catabolic elderly patients. A double-blind RCT of low-dose rhGH (0.09 IU/kg, ~0.03 mg/kg depending on conversion, 3×/week) for 4 weeks in malnourished elderly showed some improvements in nutritional status but limited evidence of functional gains in that short period [293].

More recently, therapies with once-weekly GH analogs (e.g., lonapegsomatropin / TransCon hGH) in adult GH deficiency have shown in phase 3 trials similar or superior gains in body composition compared to daily dosing: increases in total lean mass, reductions in trunk fat, improved trunk fat percent, over 38 weeks. This provides evidence that less frequent dosing (long-acting formulations) may be effective in the deficient population [294].

Meta-analyses, including a systematic review of more than 50 RCTs (3,400+ AGHD patients) indicate that GH therapy reliably reduces body fat by ~2-3 kg, increases lean body mass by ~1-2 kg, improves quality of life metrics in many but not all studies. Adverse effect rates (edema, joint stiffness, carpal tunnel) are significantly increased. Bone mineral density effects are more modest and require longer duration [295].

Clinical / Peptide Therapy Protocols: GH, GH Secretagogues, Combination Approaches

In regenerative medicine and anti-aging practice, beyond treating GH deficiency, there are protocols involving GH secretagogues, peptides, and combinations to optimize GH/IGF-1 signaling while attempting to minimize risks. Much of this is not formally validated in large clinical trials; many protocols derive from smaller studies or from research / 'off-label' contexts. These protocols can be grouped broadly as: direct rhGH replacement, secretagogue/analog peptides (GHRH analogs, GHRP/GHSR peptides), long-acting GH analogs, and combined hormone therapy (e.g., GH + sex steroids). Key factors: dose, frequency, monitoring, cycle length, patient selection.

For adult GH deficiency, typical starting doses are titrated based on age, risk factors, and IGF-1 levels. Younger or lower body weight patients often require higher per-kg doses; older or particularly sensitive patients (co-morbidities: insulin resistance, risk of malignancy) start lower. A frequently used scheme is starting in the range of ~0.2-0.5 mg/day, with adjustment every few weeks so that IGF-1 levels reach mid-normal to high-normal for age. Over longer therapy (years), total doses may be reduced once body composition stabilizes. Long-acting formulations are emerging, enabling once-weekly dosing (as in the lonapegsomatropin trial) which may improve compliance and reduce peak-side-effect amplitude [296].

These aim to stimulate endogenous GH release rather than providing exogenous GH, potentially reducing risk of overshoot, preserving pulsatility, and allowing more physiological control. Several peptides / analogs are used. Below are commonly used agents and how they are deployed in protocols, though emphasizing that many of these are not approved and are investigational:

> *GHRH analogs*: Sermorelin, Tesamorelin, CJC-1295 (with or without Drug Affinity Complex "DAC"). These mimic the hypothalamic GHRH, stimulating GH release from somatotrophs. With DAC modification, half-life is extended (albumin binding), enabling less frequent dosing (e.g., 1-2×/week vs daily).

GHRP / ghrelin secretagogues: Peptides like GHRP-2, GHRP-6, Ipamorelin. They act via growth hormone secretagogue receptor (GHSR), often producing more potent pulses, though can have other downstream effects (e.g., ghrelin receptor mediated appetite, possible cortisol/prolactin influences depending on peptide).

Many anti-aging protocols combine GHRH analogs (e.g., CJC-1295) with a secretagogue (e.g. Ipamorelin) to mimic both longer baseline elevation and pulsatile peaks. Some protocols use "nighttime dosing" to synchronize with sleep, given physiological GH surge during slow-wave sleep.

The table below provides examples of Peptide Therapy Protocols derived from clinical practice and research [293][292].

Table 12.1. Human Growth Hormone protocols

Protocol Context	Agents / Peptides Used	Dose / Frequency & Cycle	Purposes / Expected Outcomes
Aging healthy adults for body composition / anti-aging	CJC-1295 (no DAC) + Ipamorelin	~100-200 µg each, nightly before bed; cycle 8-12 weeks, followed by 4-week off period to prevent receptor desensitization	Aims: improved lean body mass, reduced fat, improved sleep / recovery; seeking moderate IGF-1 increase while limiting side effects. (Derived from research / practice reports)

Protocol Context	Agents / Peptides Used	Dose / Frequency & Cycle	Purposes / Expected Outcomes
Malnourished elderly / catabolic patients	Low-dose rhGH (~0.09 IU/kg BW, 3×/week) + nutritional support	Short duration (~4 weeks), with intensive dietary intervention; followed by monitoring functional outcomes	Aimed at nutritional repletion, reduced morbidity, improved functional status; caution for insulin resistance
AGHD patients using long-acting GH analog	Lonapegsomatropin once weekly, or daily somatropin comparator	38-week randomized trial; dose adjusted for age/oral estrogen status; IGF-1 target ≤ specified SD score; regular monitoring of body composition, trunk fat, lean mass	Outcome: significant increase in lean mass, reduced trunk fat with once-weekly drug, similar or better than daily therapy; potential improvement in convenience/compliance.
Combination GH + Testosterone in healthy elderly men	Low dose rhGH titrated + transdermal testosterone	6 months duration, GH adjusted over 8 weeks; Te given continuously; placebo-controlled design	Expected enhancements in lean mass, fat reduction, some gains in aerobic capacity; improves quality of life; mixed results for strength.

Any protocol (direct GH or peptide-secretagogue) must include rigorous monitoring: baseline and periodic measurement of IGF-1, glucose (fasting, possibly OGTT), lipid profile, body composition (via DXA or other reliable method), assessment for edema, joint pain, carpal tunnel symptoms, and screening / surveillance for neoplasia (personal/family history). Especially in older patients or those with co-morbidities (insulin resistance, cardiovascular risk, prior cancer) start with conservative doses.

Common side effects observed in GH trials include edema, arthralgia, carpal tunnel syndrome, insulin resistance or hyperglycemia. Higher GH doses correlate with greater side effect burden. In the Japanese dose-response study, adverse event rates were acceptable but dose-related increases in IGF-I were more marked (and therefore theoretical risk of over-growth, possible tumor promotion) at higher doses [289].

In healthy elderly meta-analyses, while lean and fat mass changes are consistent, bone mineral density improvements are less pronounced over short to medium term. Long duration (years) may be required to see appreciable changes. Risk of adverse metabolic effects (e.g., impaired glucose tolerance) remains [290][295].

Based on the clinical trial evidence plus current practice with peptides / secretagogues, one can outline illustrative protocols that balance benefit vs risk. These are *hypothetical guidelines* grounded in what data exists; actual clinical use should be individualized.

Protocol A: Direct GH Replacement in Diagnosed AGHD

- Confirm diagnosis: GH stimulation tests (where available), IGF-1 measurement, clinical features.
- Initiate rhGH at a low dose, e.g., for adults ~0.2-0.5 mg/day, or weight-based (for example 0.006–0.012 mg/kg/day as in the Japanese trial) depending on age and comorbidity. Titrate upward over 4-8 weeks to achieve IGF-1 within mid-range of age-appropriate normal.
- Monitor body composition (lean mass, fat mass), bone mineral density (baseline and yearly), metabolic parameters (glucose, lipids), and adverse symptoms every 1-3 months initially, then every 6-12 months.

- Duration: long term; many benefits accrue over 1-5 years. In some studies, dose is reduced after stabilization of body composition, but not discontinued, to maintain gains.

Protocol B: GH Secretagogue / Peptide Adjunct for Anti-Aging / Regenerative Maintenance (Non-Deficient Individuals)

- Patient selection: aging adult with modest decline in GH/IGF-1 (e.g., based on IGF-1 measurement), with body composition concerns (increased fat, reduced muscle mass), good metabolic baseline, no active neoplasia.
- Agents: combination of GHRH analog (e.g., CJC-1295; with or without DAC), plus a secretagogue (e.g., Ipamorelin, GHRP-2) to mimic physiological pulses. Possibly also lifestyle supports (sleep, diet, resistance exercise).
- Sample dose schedule: GHRH analog e.g., CJC-1295 (no DAC) 100-200 µg subcutaneously nightly before sleep + Ipamorelin 100-300 µg 30-60 minutes before bed; cycle length ~8-12 weeks; followed by 4 weeks off to reduce receptor desensitization. Some clinicians might employ DAC-modified GHRH (e.g., CJC-1295 with DAC) at lower frequency (e.g., 1-2×/week) to provide baseline stimulation, combined with nightly pulses.
- Monitoring: IGF-1 (to avoid supra-physiologic), glucose tolerance, signs of water retention / joint discomfort, periodic lipid panel, body composition (lean/fat mass) every 3 months. Potentially imaging or screening relevant to cancer risk if indicated.
- Expected effects: modest increase in lean body mass (1-3 kg over several months), reduction in fat mass (2-4 kg depending on baseline), improvements in skin quality, sleep, possibly quality of life metrics. Less robust evidence for permanent regenerative changes (bone density, organ regeneration) unless combined with other interventions (e.g., resistance training, nutritional optimization, possibly stem/progenitor cell therapies).

Protocol C: Use of Long-Acting GH Analogs

- For diagnosed deficiency or in settings where compliance with daily injections is problematic, consider weekly GH analogs (e.g., lonapegsomatropin) as per recent phase 3 trial. Use doses adjusted for age/oral estrogen status. Target IGF-1 levels similarly.
- Monitor similarly but be aware that long-acting formulations may have different pharmacokinetics, possibly different side effect dynamics (peaks/troughs may differ). Their impact in non-deficient aging populations has been less studied.

Protocol D: Combination Hormone Therapy

In older men with low testosterone and GH/IGF-1 decline, combining GH replacement or secretagogue use with testosterone may enhance effects on lean mass, aerobic capacity, fat reduction, and quality of life more than either alone. This should only be done under endocrine supervision, with testosterone monitored (serum levels, lipids, prostate health, hematocrit).

Example: In the RCT discussed, GH + Te over 6 months vs GH alone vs Te alone vs placebo. GH dose titrated for upper half of age specific IGF-1 reference; Te delivered via transdermal patches; follow-ups every several weeks. Outcomes included lean mass, midthigh muscle cross-section, aerobic capacity [292].

Despite promising data, several key questions remain inadequately answered in human studies:

- Long-term safety: particularly in non-deficient aging individuals, with respect to cancer risk, cardiovascular disease, glucose intolerance / diabetes. Existing trials are often short- to medium-duration (<1 year in many anti-aging studies).
- Functional outcomes vs surrogate markers: many studies show improvements in body composition (lean mass, fat reduction), but less consistent data on strength, endurance, mobility, bone fracture risk, organ function.

- Optimal dosing regimens: daily vs weekly vs secretagogue combinations; timing relative to sleep, meals, exercise; personalization by age, sex, baseline GH/IGF-1 status.
- Interaction with other regenerative therapies: how GH or secretagogues integrate with stem cell therapies, tissue engineering, peptide cocktails, nutritional and lifestyle interventions.
- Biomarkers to guide therapy: better normative data for IGF-1 across ages; markers of GH resistance; effect of IGF-binding proteins (IGF-BPs), of low-grade inflammation; genetic / epigenetic modulators.
- Regulatory / ethical oversight: defining acceptable risk, delineating treatment vs enhancement, ensuring evidence-based practice.

In sum, GH and its secretagogues offer measurable improvements in body composition, metabolic parameters, and some quality-of-life metrics in GH deficient and some aging populations; their use in regenerative medicine holds promise, especially when combined with other therapies. Protocols combining GHRH analogs + secretagogues are attractive because they aim to restore more natural GH rhythms and potentially lower risk.

However, clinical use should be conservative: starting with low doses, frequent monitoring, ensuring patient individualization, being alert for adverse metabolic or proliferative signals. Use in non-deficient anti-aging settings remains off-label in many jurisdictions and should be considered experimental. Long follow-up, rigorous endpoints (strength, functional capacity, long term safety) should be prioritized.

Human Growth Hormone has a well-elucidated biology, with deep historical roots in endocrinology and growth disorders. With the advent of recombinant synthesis, supply and safety improved substantially. Many physiologic and anabolic effects of GH make it an attractive candidate in regenerative medicine and anti-aging therapy. However, evidence in non-deficient / aging populations remains incomplete. Clinical use must be guided by stringent diagnostic criteria, careful dosing, long-term monitoring, and an honest appraisal of risk vs benefit. As of now GH functions best where there is deficiency or in specific wasting/regenerative contexts as a panacea for aging it remains hypothetical rather than established.

THE LAST CHAPTER OF THIS BOOK

Peptides in Bodybuilding and Athletic Body Recomposition

(By Dr. Dmytro Klokol, MD, PhD)

Body composition is a constant tension in the life of competitive and recreational athletes alike. Building muscle (hypertrophy), reducing fat (lipolysis), enhancing recovery, improving performance and delaying injury accumulate into a complex interplay of training, diet, rest, and increasingly, biologic adjuncts. Bodybuilding, once the exclusive realm of training, nutrition, and discipline, has evolved into a sophisticated fusion of exercise physiology, molecular science, and targeted biological optimization. As a medical doctor, biomedical researcher, and bodybuilder with over 33 years in the gym, I have observed firsthand how the integration of therapeutic peptides into the athlete's toolkit has reshaped the landscape of physique development, performance enhancement, and injury resilience.

Peptides are the short chains of amino acids that mimic or modulate endogenous signaling represent a frontier of performance enhancement and body recomposition. Their utility in bodybuilding lies in their ability to fine-tune physiological processes: accelerating fat loss, enhancing muscle hypertrophy, improving recovery, protecting joints and tendons, and optimizing metabolic balance. They act not as blunt force agents, but as biological amplifiers of internal systems already active in well-trained individuals. Having been a bodybuilder, coach and medical advisor for bodybuilders, and a clinician for over three decades, I have witnessed how training and nutrition push human limits, but also how biologic adjuncts, when used responsibly, can help shift the margin. This chapter explores the science and practice of anabolic and regenerative peptides in bodybuilding: their mechanisms, dosing protocols, phases (bulking vs cutting), stacking, risks, and ethical-clinical considerations.

Mechanisms of Action: Understanding What Peptides Do

Peptides used in bodybuilding and recomposition work via several modes. Understanding how peptides work requires examining the signaling pathways and cellular targets they influence. Unlike synthetic hormones that override natural feedback systems, most peptides function by stimulating endogenous pathways, mimicking natural ligands, or stabilizing physiological processes under stress. First are growth hormone secretagogues (GHS) or GH-releasing hormone (GHRH) analogues (e.g., CJC-1295, Ipamorelin, GHRP-6), which increase GH and downstream IGF-1 signaling, thereby stimulating protein synthesis, satellite cell activation, recovery, and general anabolic environment. Secondly, some peptides act more locally or via regeneration by promoting tissue repair, angiogenesis, collagen formation, tendon and ligament healing (e.g., BPC-157). Third, certain peptides are lipolytic: that is, they help mobilize fat or enhance metabolic rate during cutting or recomposition phases (e.g., HGH Fragment 176-191). Fourth, mitochondrial peptides or peptides that support mitochondrial function aid energy metabolism, reduce oxidative stress, reduce fatigue, and may support lean mass preservation during caloric deficits.

From over three decades of experience, I see that the athletes who respond best are those whose metabolic systems are reasonably healthy, who have trained the training fundamentals (volume, progressive overload, nutrition) first and peptides amplify but cannot replace those.

Dear Reader, for us to grasp how peptides exert their effects, it is essential to explore the cellular signaling pathways and molecular receptors they engage. Being a naturally occurring molecules or close to it, Peptides typically enhance the body's own biochemical functions. I propose to explore the internal signaling cascades through which peptides work by either imitating naturally occurring messenger molecules or reinforcing physiological balance during periods of stress or injury.

1. Anabolic Signaling via GH/IGF-1 Axis

Peptides like CJC-1295, Ipamorelin, GHRP-6, and Tesamorelin work by stimulating the anterior pituitary gland to release growth hormone (GH), which in turn activates hepatic production of insulin-like growth factor-1 (IGF-1). IGF-1 is a potent mitogen, driving myofiber hypertrophy, muscle protein synthesis, and satellite cell activation. The beauty of these secretagogues is that they preserve the body's pulsatile GH rhythm, reducing the risk of suppression associated with exogenous hGH injections.

CJC-1295 (especially with DAC) has a long half-life, sustaining elevated GH over days, while Ipamorelin acts with a shorter half-life and minimal prolactin or cortisol elevation, making it ideal for daily anabolic support with fewer side effects.

2. Lipolysis and Fat Mobilization

Peptides like HGH Fragment 176–191 act selectively on adipose tissue metabolism. This fragment of the GH molecule retains its lipolytic properties without stimulating IGF-1, minimizing systemic anabolic effects and thus reducing the risk of acromegaly or insulin resistance.

By increasing lipase activity and promoting adipocyte apoptosis, HGH Fragment 176–191 enhances the oxidation of fatty acids during caloric deficit phases. Its role becomes critical during cutting or recomposition cycles, when the goal is maximal fat loss with minimal muscle catabolism.

3. Tissue Regeneration and Injury Recovery

One of the most transformative categories in peptide therapy is regenerative peptides such as BPC-157 (Body Protection Compound) and TB-500 (Thymosin

Beta-4). These peptides do not directly increase muscle size but support the structural and vascular infrastructure essential for high-performance training.

BPC-157 enhances angiogenesis, collagen remodeling, tenocyte migration, and suppresses inflammatory cytokines like TNF-α and IL-6. Athletes often use BPC-157 during injury recovery, joint instability, or tendonitis, with reported accelerated healing and pain reduction.

4. Mitochondrial Optimization and Energy Metabolism

A newer but rapidly expanding area involves mitochondrial peptides. These peptides promote mitochondrial biogenesis, electron transport chain efficiency, and anti-oxidative capacity through signaling pathways like SIRT1/PGC-1α/AMPK. Insulin can be mentioned here as well as it can enhance muscle growth, nutrient uptake, and recovery, especially when used with steroids and growth hormone.

In practice, these peptides enhance training endurance, reduce central fatigue, and support muscle preservation during intense caloric restriction or overtraining. Their neuroprotective and anti-inflammatory effects also make them valuable in aging athletes or those prone to CNS fatigue.

Key Peptides: Anabolic, Regenerative, and Lipolytic Agents

Some of the most prominent peptides that are currently widely used in athletic body recomposition include [297]:

- BPC-157: healing, anti-inflammatory, regeneration of connective tissue often used in recovery from injury.
- HGH-Fragment 176-191 (AOD-9604 fragment): lipolytic, helps with fat reduction, less effect on IGF-1, potentially fewer GH-associated side effects.
- CJC-1295 (with or without DAC) & Ipamorelin: GH axis modulators, increased GH/IGF-1, used for hypertrophy, improved recovery, sleep, and lean gains.

- Mitochondrial peptides: mitochondrial support, improved energy, reduced oxidative stress.
- Myostatin inhibitors (e.g., FS-344 / Follistatin 344 or variants): release the "brake" on muscle growth. Animal studies and some anecdotal human experience exist.
- GLP-1 agonists: more known for fat loss, appetite control, metabolic health; may help in recomposition by reducing fat while preserving lean mass under correct diet/training.

Phased Use of Peptides in Bodybuilding

Peptides are best deployed strategically, depending on the goal of the training phase. The approach differs significantly between bulking, cutting, and recovery periods.

Bulking Phase

During the bulking phase the main objective is to maximize lean mass accrual while maintaining joint and connective tissue integrity.

Recommended Peptides:

- CJC-1295 (w/DAC): 100–200 mcg 2× per week
- Ipamorelin: 200–300 mcg 2–3× daily (morning, post-workout, pre-bed)
- Follistatin or Myostatin Inhibitors: short-term cycles (2–4 weeks) for aggressive hypertrophy
- BPC-157: 500 mcg/day for joint/tendon support

Expected Outcomes:

- Enhanced muscle protein synthesis and recovery
- Increased IGF-1 levels and improved sleep quality
- Joint stability and reduced overuse injuries
- Elevated training volume and better muscular fullness

Cutting/Recomposition Phase

The prime objectives of the cutting phase is to reduce body fat while preserving or slightly increasing lean muscle mass.

Recommended Peptides:

- HGH-Fragment 176–191: 250–500 mcg/day split dosing (AM + PM)
- CJC-1295 / Ipamorelin (lower dose)
- GLP-1 agonists (where legal and indicated): for appetite control
- BPC-157 or TB-500: reduce inflammation from increased cardio

Expected Outcomes:

- Fat mobilization, especially abdominal and visceral fat
- Muscle sparing during calorie deficits
- Improved vascularity and muscle definition
- Stable mood, cognitive function, and endurance under dietary stress

Recovery Phase

This phase, albeit often disregarded by many athletes, is nevertheless very important. The main objective of this phase is to heal connective tissue, reduce inflammation, and restore hormonal homeostasis. For seasoned athletes this phase can be considered as a maintenance phase as well.

Recommended Peptides:

- BPC-157: 500–1000 mcg/day split dosing
- TB-500: 2–5 mg weekly in severe injuries
- Low-dose GH secretagogues: 2–3×/week to maintain baseline IGF-1

Table 1. Practical Protocols of peptides in bodybuilding: dosing, cycles, stacking Strategies

Phase	Peptide(s)	Dosing Strategy	Cycle Duration	Possible Stacking
Bulking	CJC-1295 (with DAC) + Ipamorelin	CJC-1295: ~100-200 µg, 2× per week; Ipamorelin: ~200-300 µg 2-3× daily (e.g., morning + post-workout + before sleep)	8-12 weeks	Add Myostatin inhibitor (FS-344) in 4-6-week sub cycles; mitochondrial peptides; recovery peptides (BPC-157) for joint support
Cutting / Recomposition	HGH-Fragment 176-191 + GH Secretagogues + Mitochondrial Peptides	Fragment 176-191: ~250-500 µg/day (split doses); CJC-1295 or Ipamorelin at lowered doses (e.g., 100-150 µg/d or fewer injections); mitochondrial peptides daily or on training days	6-10 weeks	GLP-1 agonists (if metabolic strain), plus lots of anti-inflammatory & joint support (BPC etc.)

Phase	Peptide(s)	Dosing Strategy	Cycle Duration	Possible Stacking
Recovery / Maintenance	BPC-157 + mitochondrial peptides + lower dose GH secretagogues	BPC-157: 250-500 µg/day or 500-1000 µg split; mitochondrial peptides several times per week; GH secretagogues ≈ 2×/week	4-8 weeks	Focus less on hypertrophy, more on mobility, recovery, sleep, nutrition

Stacking and proper cycle planning is a cornerstone of peptide therapy. It means selecting complementary peptides to target multiple pathways while minimizing overlapping risks.

Classic GH Stack:

- CJC-1295 + Ipamorelin (synergistic GH release)
- Add Mito Organelles for energy and performance support

Recomp Stack:

- CJC-1295 + HGH Fragment 176–191
- Add mitochondrial peptides + GLP-1 for fat loss synergy

Recovery Stack:

- BPC-157 + TB-500 + Mito peptides
- Supports post-surgical or chronic joint injury recovery

Cycle Duration:

- Typical peptide cycles range 6–12 weeks, followed by 2–4 weeks off.
- Repeated cycles over a year show cumulative benefits in muscle quality, body composition, and injury resilience.

Side Effects and Risk Management

Despite their targeted nature, peptides are not free from adverse effects. Common concerns include:

- GH Secretagogues: Edema, water retention, insulin resistance, carpal tunnel syndrome, elevated IGF-1
- Lipolytic Peptides: Possible muscle loss if diet/training are not managed
- Regenerative Peptides: Minimal, but rare reactions at injection sites
- Mitochondrial Peptides: Usually well tolerated; monitor fatigue, metabolic markers

Safety Best Practices:

- Bloodwork: IGF-1, fasting glucose, HbA1c, lipids, liver and kidney function
- Medical supervision: source pharmaceutical-grade products
- Cycling: always include rest periods to prevent desensitization

Insulin Use in Bodybuilding—Mechanisms, Applications, and Scientific Basis

This conversation will not be complete if I skip the insulin topic.

Insulin, traditionally viewed through the lens of glucose metabolism, holds a central place in the hormonal arsenal of performance-enhancing protocols used in bodybuilding. Far beyond its role in blood sugar regulation, insulin is a potent anabolic hormone that influences amino acid uptake, glycogen synthesis, and inhibition of protein catabolism. These properties, combined with its ability to shuttle nutrients into muscle cells, have made it a subject of interest, as well as controversy, in physique sports.

In bodybuilding, insulin is not used therapeutically but rather strategically, aiming to enhance muscle growth, increase recovery speed, and improve nutrient partitioning. However, its use requires deep biochemical understanding and meticulous planning due to the inherent risks of hypoglycemia and metabolic disruption.

Insulin exerts several anabolic and anti-catabolic effects that are exploited by bodybuilders. These include:

- Enhanced Muscle Protein Synthesis: Insulin increases amino acid uptake into skeletal muscle and stimulates the mTOR pathway, synergizing with IGF-1 and resistance training to promote hypertrophy.
- Inhibition of Protein Breakdown: It suppresses proteolysis (muscle protein breakdown), thus preserving lean mass during calorie-restricted or high-intensity training phases.
- Glycogen Storage and Volumization: Insulin facilitates rapid glucose uptake by muscle cells, promoting muscle glycogen supercompensation and cell volumization, which enhances the "full" look bodybuilders seek especially during carb-loading protocols.
- Nutrient Shuttling: Insulin increases cellular permeability, driving not just glucose but creatine, amino acids, electrolytes, and IGF-1 into the muscle cell. This improves both anabolism and muscle recovery post-training.
- Synergy with IGF-1 and GH: When used alongside exogenous IGF-1 or growth hormone, insulin amplifies their anabolic effects by creating a nutrient-rich, growth-promoting environment at the cellular level.

So what are the scientific rationale for Insulin use in bodybuilding, if such even exist? While insulin is not FDA-approved for enhancement purposes, its anabolic properties are well-documented in scientific literature:

- Protein Metabolism: Studies have shown that insulin infusion reduces leucine oxidation and nitrogen loss, effectively reducing muscle catabolism during both fasting and exercise-induced stress [298].

- Post-Exercise Recovery: Insulin administration post-resistance training enhances glycogen resynthesis and improves net muscle protein balance, particularly when combined with carbohydrates and amino acids [299][300].
- Synergy with GH/IGF-1 Axis: Research supports the concept that insulin is permissive to IGF-1 expression and activity, and that insulin deficiency impairs GH's anabolic signaling [301].

These findings validate the theoretical and practical rationale for bodybuilders using insulin to potentiate post-training recovery, increase muscle cell volume, and prevent muscle degradation during intense dieting phases.

Insulin Protocols and Application in Bodybuilding

Insulin protocols in bodybuilding vary, depending on training phase, goals, and insulin type (rapid-acting vs. intermediate-acting). Below are common applications:

1. Post-Workout Protocol (Rapid-Acting Insulin, e.g., Humalog, Novolog)
    - Timing: Administered immediately post-workout
    - Dosage: 4–10 IU (individualized), followed by rapid-absorbing carbohydrates (~10g per 1 IU insulin), protein (e.g., 30–50g whey), and creatine
    - Objective: Maximize anabolic window by increasing glucose and amino acid uptake
2. Intra-Workout Protocol
    - Timing: Microdoses (2–4 IU) 10–15 minutes pre-training
    - Nutrition: Consumed with intra-workout shake containing 20–30g essential amino acids + 30–50g dextrose/maltodextrin
    - Objective: Increase training endurance and prevent muscle breakdown

3. Carb-Loading and "Fullness" for Contest Prep

    - Timing: In final 3–5 days before competition
    - Dosage: Very low-dose insulin paired with controlled carb intake
    - Objective: Achieve extreme muscle fullness via glycogen supercompensation while monitoring sodium and fluid balance

Caution: All insulin protocols must be matched with precise nutrient timing and blood glucose monitoring. Misuse can lead to severe hypoglycemia, unconsciousness, or even death.

While insulin offers significant anabolic potential, it also carries high physiological and ethical risks:

- Hypoglycemia: The most immediate danger, manifesting as dizziness, confusion, tremors, seizures, and potentially coma if unaddressed.
- Fat Gain: Insulin promotes lipogenesis if caloric intake exceeds energy expenditure or is mistimed.
- Insulin Resistance: Chronic or high-dose use can impair beta-cell sensitivity, increasing the risk of metabolic syndrome.
- Dependency and downregulation: Athletes may lose the ability to optimize glucose metabolism naturally if endogenous insulin pathways are neglected.

In competitive settings, insulin is banned by WADA (World Anti-Doping Agency) unless a therapeutic use exemption (TUE) is granted for diabetic athletes.

Wrapping up the topic of Insulin use in athletic body recomposition I must emphasize that it is a *tool for experts, not amateurs*.

Insulin, when used in bodybuilding, is not a shortcut but a high-risk tool for experienced athletes under medical guidance. Its mechanisms are grounded in real science, and its anabolic synergy with GH, IGF-1, and amino acids is well-supported by experimental evidence. But it remains a double-edged sword, demanding an intimate understanding of human metabolism, timing, and nutrient kinetics.

For athletes and coaches interested in its application, the emphasis must be on education, safety, and clinical supervision. In the right hands, insulin can help sculpt a world-class physique. In the wrong hands, it can endanger lives.

Personal Perspective: Peptides at the Frontlines of Performance, Recovery, and Reinvention

Peptides didn't just change my approach to medicine and sports science, instead they changed my life as a competitive bodybuilder, athlete, coach, and physician. This isn't a theoretical exploration for me. It's the lived reality of more than three decades inside gyms, laboratories, and clinics, where iron meets biology and theory meets physiology.

I began experimenting with recombinant human growth hormone (rhGH) even before I started my competitive career (which also came quite late in my life), not for vanity or shortcuts, but as a response to the chronic wear-and-tear that decades of heavy lifting inevitably brought. Shoulder strains, lower back tightness, neck pain, medial epicondylitis and early signs of cartilage degradation . . . they were all constant companions. GH changed that trajectory. Administered consistently at physiologic doses, it gave me the recovery edge I needed. My sleep deepened, my joints ached less, soft tissue healed faster, and my muscle bellies became fuller, denser, that is what competitors call "3D." But more than size, it gave me durability and enabled the long-term game in a sport that often burns people out before they reach their true potential.

Over the years, I refined my protocols. During cutting phases and contest prep, I began stacking GHRP-6—a growth hormone-releasing peptide, which I administered early in the morning followed by fasted cardio and at least 2 hours of fasting before first meal of the day. I'd take it first thing in the morning, subcutaneously, then hit the treadmill or stairmaster while fasted. The synergy between GH pulse stimulation and elevated lipolysis during fasted cardio was incredible. My body fat melted off more efficiently, especially in the stubborn zones like lower back and glutes. Then, I'd administer a dose of GH later in the evening, thus capitalizing on the body's natural circadian GH rhythm and promoting overnight recovery.

On particularly intense hypertrophy cycles, I experimented with IGF-1 LR3, combined with low doses of insulin during and post-workout. The intra-workout protocol would involve sipping a carb-rich solution infused with electrolytes and essential amino acids, timed precisely with the IGF/insulin stack. The result was dramatic cell volumization, enhanced nutrient shuttling, and faster post-training recovery. Of course, this protocol requires meticulous glycemic control and should never be used without a solid medical understanding, but under correct conditions, the results were phenomenal. Pumps were massive, recovery was rapid, and lean mass accretion was tangible over a span of weeks.

Then came CJC-1295, which became a cornerstone of my post-workout recovery stack. Its longer half-life and DAC (drug affinity complex) modification allowed for sustained GH release, complementing the acute effects of peptides like Ipamorelin or GHRP-6. Post-leg day or after heavy compound lifting, I'd use CJC-1295 to amplify the repair and remodeling phase that follows intense training. Subjectively, it improved sleep quality, skin texture, and most importantly the muscle density and retention during aggressive training blocks.

But the real revelation came with BPC-157 ("body protection compound"). Years of lifting had left me with chronic rotator cuff inflammation and partial bilateral biceps tendon tears. At one point, I was told that I'd even may need surgery or completely forget about the sport. Saddest part was when my left distal biceps tendon tear happened just 2 weeks out of one of the shows. But I wasn't ready to quit training. I began a dual protocol: oral BPC-157, twice daily, combined with localized injectable BPC-157 directly into the affected region. The pain subsided within days. Range of motion returned. And over the course of several weeks, I was training through what would've sidelined me for months. That was when I learned one of the most critical lessons of my clinical experience: dose matters. In my own case, 500 to 600 mcg per shot allowed substantially more than typical starting protocols, it became the threshold for real, tangible results. Lower doses simply didn't yield the same regenerative effect.

Since then, BPC-157 has become a staple in my injury recovery toolkit, not just for myself, but for athletes I coached and consulted and patients I treat. It doesn't just mask pain; it heals at the cellular level, reducing cytokine-driven inflammation and stimulating angiogenesis where tissues are starved of oxygen and blood flow.

Yet even BPC-157 has its limits and that's where exosomes enter the picture.

In cases of chronic joint degeneration, post-surgical recovery, or severe muscle tears, I've found that localized injection of nano-purified exosomes, derived from MSC cultures, outperforms peptides in terms of speed, precision, and depth of healing. These extracellular vesicles carry hundreds of growth factors, RNA species, and signaling proteins, modulating gene expression and orchestrating repair in a way that even the best-designed peptide can't always match. They don't stimulate; they reprogram.

When I tore my right long head biceps, I used both BPC-157 and exosomes injected via self-administration with a non-dominant left hand. The recovery, which would have typically taken 12–16 weeks, was functionally complete in just over 4 weeks. When I had to go for the umbilical hernia repair, peptides allowed me to start cardio on day 4 after surgery, return to gym after 1-week post-surgery and do the leg day after 2 weeks. In all my years as both physician and athlete, nothing has come close to the synergy of exosomes and peptides in accelerating deep tissue regeneration.

And still, years of personal experience and numerous observations taught me one thing—Peptides are not magic bullets. They are tools, yes—powerful, nuanced, and often misunderstood. When used responsibly, they can restore the body's regenerative intelligence, rekindling the processes that time, overtraining, and inflammation try to shut down. For me, they have extended not only my physical performance but my understanding of what modern medicine can offer.

The next generation of athletes and physicians won't be asking whether peptides work. They'll be asking how best to personalize them, how to optimize their use by training phase, injury profile, metabolic phenotype, and recovery response.

That is the frontier. And we are already living it.

References

Chapter 1

1. Fosgerau K, Hoffmann T. Peptide therapeutics: current status and future directions. Drug Discov Today. 2015 Jan;20(1):122-8. doi: 10.1016/j.drudis.2014.10.003. Epub 2014 Oct 17. PMID: 25450771.

2. Angell Y, Holford M, Moos WH. Building on Success: A Bright Future for Peptide Therapeutics. Protein Pept Lett. 2018;25(12):1044-1050. doi: 10.2174/0929866525666181114155542. PMID: 30430932.

3. Henninot A, Collins JC, Nuss JM. The Current State of Peptide Drug Discovery: Back to the Future? J Med Chem. 2018 Feb 22;61(4):1382-1414. doi: 10.1021/acs.jmedchem.7b00318. Epub 2017 Aug 11. PMID: 28737935.

4. Wang L, Wang N, Zhang W, Cheng X, Yan Z, Shao G, Wang X, Wang R, Fu C. Therapeutic peptides: current applications and future directions. Signal Transduct Target Ther. 2022 Feb 14;7(1):48. doi: 10.1038/s41392-022-00904-4. PMID: 35165272; PMCID: PMC8844085.

5. Kim J, Kim J, Choi C, Bae J, Choi HJ. Structural insights into GPCR signaling activated by peptide ligands: from molecular mechanism to therapeutic application. Exp Mol Med. 2025 Jul;57(7):1467-1481. doi: 10.1038/s12276-025-01497-y. Epub 2025 Jul 8. PMID: 40629042; PMCID: PMC12322139.

6. Otvos L Jr and Wade JD (2014) Current challenges in peptide-based drug discovery. Front. Chem. 2:62. doi: 10.3389/fchem.2014.0006.

7. Khazanov, N. A., and Carlson, H. A. (2013). Exploring the composition of protein-ligand binding sites on a large scale. PLoS Comput. Biol. 9: e1003321. doi: 10.1371/journal.pcbi.1003321.

8. Md Fadilah NI, Shahabudin NA, Mohd Razif RA, Sanyal A, Ghosh A, Baharin KI, Ahmad H, Maarof M, Motta A, Fauzi MB. Discovery of bioactive peptides as therapeutic agents for skin wound repair. J Tissue Eng. 2024 Sep 29; 15:20417314241280359. doi: 10.1177/20417314241280359. PMID: 39398382; PMCID: PMC11468004.

9. Muttenthaler M., King G.F., D.J. Adams, P.F. Alewood, Trends in peptide drug discovery, Nat. Rev. Dr.

10. Hosio M, Jaks V, Lagus H, Vuola J, Ogawa R, Kankuri E. Primary Ciliary Signaling in the Skin-Contribution to Wound Healing and Scarring. Front Cell Dev Biol. 2020 Nov 13; 8:578384. doi: 10.3389/fcell.2020.578384. PMID: 33282860; PMCID: PMC7691485.

11. Zhao X, Guan JL. Focal adhesion kinase and its signaling pathways in cell migration and angiogenesis. Adv Drug Deliv Rev. 2011 Jul 18;63(8):610-5. doi: 10.1016/j.addr.2010.11.001. Epub 2010 Nov 29. PMID: 21118706; PMCID: PMC3132829.

12. Guo, Y., Pan, W., Liu, S., Shen, Z., Xu, Y., & Hu, L. (2020). ERK/MAPK signalling pathway and tumorigenesis (Review). Experimental and Therapeutic Medicine, 19, 1997-2007.

13. Jin P, Duan X, Huang Z, Dong Y, Zhu J, Guo H, Tian H, Zou CG, Xie K. Nuclear receptors in health and disease: signaling pathways, biological functions and pharmaceutical interventions. Signal Transduct Target Ther. 2025 Jul 28;10(1):228. doi: 10.1038/s41392-025-02270-3. PMID: 40717128; PMCID: PMC12301492.

14. Lee, Changhan & Zeng, Jennifer & Drew, Brian & Sallam, Tamer & Martin-Montalvo, Alejandro & Wan, Junxiang & Kim, Su-Jeong & Mehta, Hemal & Hevener, Andrea & Cabo, Rafael. (2015). The Mitochondrial-Derived Peptide MOTS-c Promotes Metabolic Homeostasis and Reduces Obesity and Insulin Resistance. Cell metabolism. 21. 443-454. 10.1016/j.cmet.2015.02.009.

15. Wan W, Zhang L, Lin Y, Rao X, Wang X, Hua F, Ying J. Mitochondria-derived peptide MOTS-c: effects and mechanisms related to stress, metabolism and aging. J Transl Med. 2023 Jan 20;21(1):36. doi: 10.1186/s12967-023-03885-2. PMID: 36670507; PMCID: PMC9854231.

16. Chatterjee D, Sivashanmugam K. Immunomodulatory peptides: new therapeutic horizons for emerging and re-emerging infectious diseases. Front Microbiol. 2024

Dec 20; 15:1505571. doi: 10.3389/fmicb.2024.1505571. PMID: 39760081; PMCID: PMC11695410.

17. Arun M, Rajasingh S, Madasamy P, Rajasingh J. Immunomodulatory and Regenerative Functions of MSC-Derived Exosomes in Bone Repair. Bioengineering. 2025; 12(8):844.

18. Lee C, Kim MJ, Kumar A, Lee HW, Yang Y, Kim Y. Vascular endothelial growth factor signaling in health and disease: from molecular mechanisms to therapeutic perspectives. Signal Transduct Target Ther. 2025 May 19;10(1):170 doi: 10.1038/s41392-025-02249-0. PMID: 40383803; PMCID: PMC12086256.

19. Lv S, Cai H, Xu Y, Dai J, Rong X, Zheng L. Thymosin-β 4 induces angiogenesis in critical limb ischemia mice via regulating Notch/NF-κB pathway. Int J Mol Med. 2020 Oct;46(4):1347-1358. doi: 10.3892/ijmm.2020.4701. Epub 2020 Aug 11. PMID: 32945357; PMCID: PMC7447324.

20. Krymchenko R, Avila-Martinez N, Gansevoort M, Bakker GJ, Gomes MLNP, Vlig M, Versteeg EMM, Boekema BKHL, van Kuppevelt TH, Daamen WF. Collagen-elastin dermal scaffolds enhance tissue regeneration and reduce scarring in preclinical models. Mater Today Bio. 2025 Aug 25; 34:102239. doi: 10.1016/j.mtbio 2025.102239. PMID: 40917518; PMCID: PMC12408406.

21. Lee JE, Lee Y-J, Yoon J-K. Advanced 3D In Vitro Liver Fibrosis Models: Spheroids, Organoids, and Liver-on-Chips. Biomimetics. 2025; 10(10):639.

22. Sahoo S, Losordo DW. Exosomes and cardiac repair after myocardial infarction. Circ Res. 2014 Jan 17;114(2):333-44. doi: 10.1161/CIRCRESAHA.114.300639. PMID: 24436429.

23. Pearman NA, Ronander E, Smith AM, Morris GA. The identification and characterisation of novel bioactive peptides derived from porcine liver. Curr Res Food Sci. 2020 Nov 25; 3:314-321. doi: 10.1016/j.crfs.2020.11.002. PMID: 33336193; PMCID: PMC7733001.

24. Banga A.K. CRC press; 2015. Therapeutic Peptides and Proteins: Formulation, Processing, and Delivery Systems.

25. Jukniené I, Zaborskiené G, Stankevičiené J. Identification for Antioxidant Peptides in Porcine Liver and Heart Hydrolysates Using SWATH-MS Analysis. Processes. 2024; 12(12):2944.

26. Slivka JP, Bauer C, Younsi A, Wong MBF, Chan MKS, Skutella T. Exploring the Molecular Tapestry: Organ-Specific Peptide and Protein Ultrafiltrates and Their Role

in Therapeutics. Int J Mol Sci. 2024 Mar 1;25(5):2863. doi: 10.3390/ijms25052863. PMID: 38474110; PMCID: PMC10931619.

27. Barman, P., Joshi, S., Sharma, S. et al. Strategic Approaches to Improvise Peptide Drugs as Next Generation Therapeutics. Int J Pept Res Ther 29, 61 (2023).

28. Mukherjee AB, Wanjari UR, Gopalakrishnan et al., Evolving strategies and application of proteins and peptide therapeutics in cancer treatment, Biomedicine & Pharmacotherapy, 2023, 163, 114832.

29. Chan MKS, Wong MBF, Klokol D, et al. Exploring the toxicity and carcinogenic potential of 300 KDA "Mito Organelles"™ cellular extracts through MTT and BALB/C-3T3 cell transformation assays: a vital component of peptide and protein biomedical research and safety study. J Stem Cell Res Ther. 2024;9(1):9-15. DOI: 10.15406/jsrt.2024.09.00166.

30. Wang L, Zhou X, Lu T. Role of mitochondria in physiological activities, diseases, and therapy. Mol Biomed. 2025 Jun 19;6(1):42. doi: 10.1186/s43556-025-00284-5. PMID: 40536597; PMCID: PMC12179052.

31. Tung C, Varzideh F, Farroni E, Mone P, Kansakar U, Jankauskas SS, Santulli G. Elamipretide: A Review of Its Structure, Mechanism of Action, and Therapeutic Potential. Int J Mol Sci. 2025 Jan 23;26(3):944. doi: 10.3390/ijms26030944. PMID: 39940712; PMCID: PMC11816484.

32. Lee C, Zeng J, Drew BG, Sallam T, Martin-Montalvo A, Wan J, Kim SJ, Mehta H, Hevener AL, de Cabo R, Cohen P. The mitochondrial-derived peptide MOTS-c promotes metabolic homeostasis and reduces obesity and insulin resistance. Cell Metab. 2015 Mar 3;21(3):443-54. doi: 10.1016/j.cmet.2015.02.009. PMID: 25738459; PMCID: PMC4350682.

33. Coppé JP, Desprez PY, Krtolica A, Campisi J. The senescence-associated secretory phenotype: the dark side of tumor suppression. Annu Rev Pathol. 2010; 5:99-118. doi: 10.1146/annurev-pathol-121808-102144. PMID: 20078217; PMCID: PMC4166495.

34. Martini H, Passos JF. Cellular senescence: all roads lead to mitochondria. FEBS J. 2023 Mar;290(5):1186-1202. doi: 10.1111/febs.16361. Epub 2022 Jan 30. PMID: 35048548; PMCID: PMC9296701.

35. Stojanovic B, Jovanovic I, Dimitrijevic Stojanovic M, Stojanovic BS, Kovacevic V, Radosavljevic I, Jovanovic D, Miletic Kovacevic M, Zornic N, Arsic AA, Eric S, Mirkovic

N, Nesic J, Jakovljevic S, Lazarevic S, Milivojcevic Bevc I, Milosevic B. Oxidative Stress-Driven Cellular Senescence: Mechanistic Crosstalk and Therapeutic Horizons. Antioxidants (Basel). 2025 Aug 12;14(8):987. doi: 10.3390/antiox14080987. PMID: 40867884; PMCID: PMC12383077.

36. Wang S, Long H, Hou L, Feng B, Ma Z, Wu Y, Zeng Y, Cai J, Zhang DW, Zhao G. The mitophagy pathway and its implications in human diseases. Signal Transduct Target Ther. 2023 Aug 16;8(1):304. doi: 10.1038/s41392-023-01503-7. PMID: 37582956; PMCID: PMC10427715.

37. Shires SE, Gustafsson ÅB. Regulating Renewable Energy: Connecting AMPKα2 to PINK1/Parkin-Mediated Mitophagy in the Heart. Circ Res. 2018 Mar 2;122(5):649-651. doi: 10.1161/CIRCRESAHA.118.312655. PMID: 29496793; PMCID: PMC5836749.

38. Zhao B, Qiang L, Joseph J, Kalyanaraman B, Viollet B, He YY. Mitochondrial dysfunction activates the AMPK signaling and autophagy to promote cell survival. Genes Dis. 2016 Mar;3(1):82-87. doi: 10.1016/j.gendis.2015.12.002. Epub 2016 Jan 4. PMID: 28066797; PMCID: PMC5215801.

39. Covarrubias AJ, Perrone R, Grozio A, Verdin E. NAD+ metabolism and its roles in cellular processes during ageing. Nat Rev Mol Cell Biol. 2021 Feb;22(2):119-141. doi: 10.1038/s41580-020-00313-x. Epub 2020 Dec 22. PMID: 33353981; PMCID: PMC7963035.

40. Ye X., Li M., Hou T., Gao T., Zhu W., Yang Y. Sirtuins in glucose and lipid metabolism. Oncotarget. 2017; 8: 1845-1859.

41. Tripathi U, Chaib S, Gerdes EOW, Hogan KA, Zhu Y. Development of a novel senolytic by precise disruption of FOXO4-p53 complex. EBioMedicine. 2021 Dec; 74:103693. doi: 10.1016/j.ebiom.2021.103693. Epub 2021 Nov 9. PMID: 34768086; PMCID: PMC8601985.

42. Lafontaine J, Cardin GB, Malaquin N, Boisvert JS, Rodier F, Wong P. Senolytic Targeting of Bcl-2 Anti-Apoptotic Family Increases Cell Death in Irradiated Sarcoma Cells. Cancers (Basel). 2021 Jan 21;13(3):386. doi: 10.3390/cancers13030386. PMID: 33494434; PMCID: PMC7866159.

43. Chan MKS, Wong MBF, Chernykh V, Iemeliyanova M, Alvin G, Nishkumai O, Shyshkina N, Lakey JRT, Skutella T. Mitochondrial Peptides and Cell Extracts in Regenerative Medicine and Anti-Aging Therapies: Therapeutic Potential of Mito Organelles. J Stem Cell Res. 6(2):1-11.

44 Rui, C., Chan, M.K.S., Skutella, T. (2024). Stem Cell Therapies and Ageing: Unlocking the Potential of Regenerative Medicine. In: Korolchuk, V.I., Harris, J.R. (eds) Biochemistry and Cell Biology of Ageing: Part V, Anti-Ageing Interventions. Subcellular Biochemistry, vol 107. Springer, Cham.

45 Mike KS Chan, Michelle BF Wong, Krista Casazza, Dmytro Klokol, Ian Jenkins and Jonathan RT Lakey. Next-Generation Regenerative Therapies in Companion Animals: Integrating Stem Cells, Mitochondrial Peptides, and Nanomized Peptides for Targeted Tissue Repair. Am J Biomed Sci & Res. 2025 28(4) AJBSR.MS.ID.003697, DOI: 10.34297/AJBSR.2025.28.003697.

46 Mike KS Chan, Michelle BF Wong, Krista Casazza, Dmytro Klokol, Olha Nishkumai, et al. Peptide-Based Precision Therapeutics for Cardiac Disease: Targeting Mitochondrial Dysfunction, Fibrosis, and Inflammation. Am J Biomed Sci & Res. 2025 27(3) AJBSR. MS.ID.003560, DOI: 10.34297/AJBSR.2025.27.003560.

47 Abu Shelbayeh O, Arroum T, Morris S, Busch KB. PGC-1α Is a Master Regulator of Mitochondrial Lifecycle and ROS Stress Response. Antioxidants (Basel). 2023 May 10;12(5):1075. doi: 10.3390/antiox12051075. PMID: 37237941; PMCID: PMC10215733.

48 Mike KS Chan, Michelle BF Wong, Krista Casazza, Waldemar Lerhardt, Eric Mathur, et al. Adekunle Oluwatoyin M, Oladipupo Dotun O, et al. Organo-Specific Nano Peptides and Mitochondrial Modulators for Therapeutic Rejuvenation and Disease Modification: A Translational Perspective. Am J Biomed Sci & Res. 2025 28(2) AJBSR. MS.ID.003664, DOI: 10.34297/AJBSR.2025.28.003664.

49 Mirhaji, S.S., Pirhaghi, M., Soleimanpour, M., Saboury, A.A. (2025). Peptide-Based Systems for Regenerative Medicine. In: Ghorbani, F., Ghalandari, B., Liu, C. (eds) Principles of Bioinspired and Biomimetic Regenerative Medicine. Biomaterials, Bioengineering and Sustainability, vol 3. Springer, Cham.

Chapter 2

50 Vecchio I, Tornali C, Bragazzi NL, Martini M. The Discovery of Insulin: An Important Milestone in the History of Medicine. Front Endocrinol (Lausanne). 2018 Oct 23; 9:613. doi: 10.3389/fendo.2018.00613. PMID: 30405529; PMCID: PMC6205949.

51 Camerino C. The Long Way of Oxytocin from the Uterus to the Heart in 70 Years from Its Discovery. Int J Mol Sci. 2023 Jan 29;24(3):2556. doi: 10.3390/ijms24032556. PMID: 36768879; PMCID: PMC9916674.

52. du Vigneaud et al. Britannica: "Oxytocin | Definition, Discovery, Effects, & Facts," 2025https://www.britannica.com/science/oxytocin.

53. Carter CS, Kenkel WM, MacLean EL, Wilson SR, Perkeybile AM, Yee JR, Ferris CF, Nazarloo HP, Porges SW, Davis JM, Connelly JJ, Kingsbury MA. Is Oxytocin "Nature's Medicine"? Pharmacol Rev. 2020 Oct;72(4):829-861. doi: 10.1124/pr.120.019398. PMID: 32912963; PMCID: PMC7495339.

54. Angelousi A, Margioris AN, Tsatsanis C. ACTH Action on the Adrenals. [Updated 2020 Jun 13]. In: Feingold KR, Ahmed SF, Anawalt B, et al., editors. Endotext [Internet]. South Dartmouth (MA): MDText.com, Inc.; 2000-. Available from: https://www.ncbi.nlm.nih.gov/books/NBK279118/.

55. Cawley NX, Li Z, Loh YP. 60 YEARS OF POMC: Biosynthesis, trafficking, and secretion of pro-opiomelanocortin-derived peptides. J Mol Endocrinol. 2016 May;56(4):T77-97. doi: 10.1530/JME-15-0323. Epub 2016 Feb 15. PMID: 26880796; PMCID: PMC4899099.

56. Allen MJ, Sharma S. Physiology, Adrenocorticotropic Hormone (ACTH) [Updated 2023 Aug 8]. In: StatPearls [Internet]. Treasure Island (FL): StatPearls Publishing; 2025 Jan-. Available from: https://www.ncbi.nlm.nih.gov/books/NBK500031/.

57. Manning M, Misicka A, Olma A, Bankowski K, Stoev S, Chini B, Durroux T, Mouillac B, Corbani M, Guillon G. Oxytocin and vasopressin agonists and antagonists as research tools and potential therapeutics. J Neuroendocrinol. 2012 Apr;24(4):609-28. doi: 10.1111/j.1365-2826.2012.02303.x. PMID: 22375852; PMCID: PMC3490377.

58. A.-M.J. Lengyel. Novel mechanisms of growth hormone regulation: growth hormone-releasing peptides and ghrelin. Braz J Med Biol Res 39 (8) • Aug 2006https://doi.org/10.1590/S0100-879X2006000800002.

59. Bowers CY. History to the discovery of ghrelin. Methods Enzymol. 2012; 514:3-32. doi: 10.1016/B978-0-12-381272-8.00001-5. PMID: 22975043.

60. Lefrère JJ, Berche P. La thérapeutique du docteur Brown-Séquard [Doctor Brown-Sequard's therapy]. Ann Endocrinol (Paris). 2010 Mar;71(2):69-75. French. doi: 10.1016/j.ando.2010.01.003. Epub 2010 Feb 18. PMID: 20167305.

61. Cussons AJ, Bhagat CI, Fletcher SJ, Walsh JP. Brown-Séquard revisited: a lesson from history on the placebo effect of androgen treatment. Med J Aust. 2002 Dec 2-16;177(11-12):678-9. doi: 10.5694/j.1326-5377. 2002.tb05014.x. PMID: 12463999.

62 Nair CG, Babu MJ, Menon R, Jacob P. Hypocalcaemia following total thyroidectomy: An analysis of 806 patients. Indian J Endocrinol Metab. 2013 Mar;17(2):298-303. doi: 10.4103/2230-8210.109718. PMID: 23776907; PMCID: PMC3683209.

63 Sarkar S, Banerjee S, Sarkar R, Sikder B. A Review on the History of 'Thyroid Surgery'. Indian J Surg. 2016 Feb;78(1):32-6. doi: 10.1007/s12262-015-1317-5. Epub 2015 Dec 18. PMID: 27186037; PMCID: PMC4848216.

64 https://time.com/archive/6802534/medicine-the-healing-lamb/ The Youth Doctors narrative, Time Magazine. Time, 1955.

65 Cordero OJ, Piñeiro A, Nogueira M. Thymic peptides and preparations: an update. Arch Immunol Ther Exp (Warsz). 1999;47(2):77-82. PMID: 10202559.

66 Avolio F, Martinotti S, Khavinson VK, Esposito JE, Giambuzzi G, Marino A, Mironova E, Pulcini R, Robuffo I, Bologna G, Simeone P, Lanuti P, Guarnieri S, Trofimova S, Procopio AD, Toniato E. Peptides Regulating Proliferative Activity and Inflammatory Pathways in the Monocyte/Macrophage THP-1 Cell Line. Int J Mol Sci. 2022 Mar 25;23(7):3607. doi: 10.3390/ijms23073607. PMID: 35408963; PMCID: PMC8999041.

67 Hannappel E, Davoust S, Horecker BL. Thymosins beta 8 and beta 9: two new peptides isolated from calf thymus homologous to thymosin beta 4. Proc Natl Acad Sci U S A. 1982 Mar;79(6):1708-11. doi: 10.1073/pnas.79.6.1708. PMID: 6952223; PMCID: PMC346049.

68 Review of Thymic Peptides and Hormones: From Their Properties to Clinical Application." (2024). *International Journal of Peptide Research and Therapeutics*, 31, Article 10.

69. Besman, M., Zambrowicz, A. & Matwiejczyk, M. Review of Thymic Peptides and Hormones: From Their Properties to Clinical Application. Int J Pept Res Ther 31, 10 (2025).

70. Naylor PH, Mutchnick MG. Thymus-derived peptides in the treatment of viral chronic hepatitis. Dig Dis. 1996 Nov-Dec;14(6):362-70. doi: 10.1159/000171570. PMID: 9030468.

71. Mike RK Chan & Michelle BF Wong. Thymus Therapy: the past, present and future. ISBN 9791220150583, 332 pp.

72. Almeida JR. The Century-Long Journey of Peptide-Based Drugs. Antibiotics (Basel). 2024 Feb 20;13(3):196. doi: 10.3390/antibiotics13030196. PMID: 38534631; PMCID: PMC10967573.

73. Lau JL, Dunn MK. Therapeutic peptides: Historical perspectives, current development trends, and future directions. Bioorg Med Chem. 2018 Jun 1;26(10):2700-2707. doi: 10.1016/j.bmc.2017.06.052. Epub 2017 Jul 1. PMID: 28720325.

74. Lau, Jolene & Dunn, Michael. (2017). Therapeutic Peptides: Historical Perspectives, Current Development Trends, and Future Directions. Bioorganic & Medicinal Chemistry. 26. 10.1016/j.bmc.2017.06.052.

75. Merry TL, Chan A, Woodhead JST, Reynolds JC, Kumagai H, Kim SJ, Lee C. Mitochondrial-derived peptides in energy metabolism. Am J Physiol Endocrinol Metab. 2020 Oct 1;319(4): E659-E666. doi: 10.1152/ajpendo.00249.2020. Epub 2020 Aug 10. PMID: 32776825; PMCID: PMC7750512.

76. 303. Chan MKS, Jambo SA, Jumat MI, Landa F, Saili NS, et al. Human Cytology: Classification and Quantitative Cell Landscape with Numbers, Types and Functional Diversity. J Stem Cell Res. 6(1):1-42.

Chapter 3

77. Mascolo MG, Perdichizzi S, Rotondo F, et al. BALB/c 3T3 cell transformation assay for the prediction of carcinogenic potential of chemicals and environmental mixtures. Toxicol In Vitro. 2010;24(4):1292–1300.

78. Kakunaga T. A quantitative system for assay of malignant transformation by chemical carcinogens using a clone derived from BALB-3T3. Int J Cancer. 1973;12(2):463–473.

79. Chan, M. K., Wong, M. B., Pan, S. Y., Chernykh, V., Shyshkina, N., Yemeliyanova, M., Klokol, D., Nishkumai, O., Alvin, G., Kobzev, O., Dubynska, S. & Lakey, J. (2025). Carcinogenicity And Oncogenicity of Precursor/Progenitor Stem Cells of the Xenogeneic Origin: The Balb/C-3t3 Cell Transformation Assay. SSP Modern Pharmacy and Medicine, 5(3), 20-37.

80. Mike K S Chan, Michelle B F Wong, Krista Casazza, Jonathan R T Lakey, et al. Short-Peptides May be the Key to Long Life. Am J Biomed Sci & Res. 2025 26(2) AJBSR.MS.ID.003423, DOI: 10.34297/AJBSR.2025.26.003423.

81. Lakey J, Wells A, Good A, Damyar K, Tucker TR, et al (2022) Protective Effects of Stem Cell-Derived Peptides in Preventing Autoimmune Diabetes in the Non-Diabetic Mouse Model. American Journal of Biomedical Science & Research.

82. Merry TL, Chan A, Woodhead JST, Reynolds JC, Kumagai H, et al (2020) Mitochondrial-derived peptides in energy metabolism. Am J Physiol Endocrinol Metab 319(4): E659-E666.

83 Chan MK, Wong MB, Klokol D, Nishkumai O, Lakey JRT, et al (2024) Peptides in Cardiology: Preventing Cardiac Aging and Reversing Heart Disease. Adv Clin Med Res 5(4): 1-16.

84 Wells A, Good A., Damyar K, Michael Alexander, Jonathan RT Lakey, et al., Mass Spectrometry Analysis of Novel Stem Cell-Derived Peptides. Am J Biomed Sci & Res. 2022—16(2). AJBSR.MS.ID.002215. DOI: 10.34297/AJBSR.2022.16.002215.

85 Slivka JP, Bauer C, Younsi A, Wong MBF, Chan MKS, Skutella T. Exploring the Molecular Tapestry: Organ-Specific Peptide and Protein Ultrafiltrates and Their Role in Therapeutics. Int J Mol Sci. 2024 Mar 1;25(5):2863. doi: 10.3390/ijms25052863. PMID: 38474110; PMCID: PMC10931619.

86 Steinberg R., Koch H.G. The Largely Unexplored Biology of Small Proteins in Pro- and Eukaryotes. FEBS J. 2021; 288:7002–7024. doi: 10.1111/febs.15845.

87 Elsayed YY, Kühl T, Imhof D. Regulatory Guidelines for the Analysis of Therapeutic Peptides and Proteins. J Pept Sci. 2025 Mar;31(3): e70001. doi: 10.1002/psc.70001. PMID: 39921384; PMCID: PMC11806371.

88 Choules MP, Bisson J, Gao W, Lankin DC, McAlpine JB, Niemitz M, Jaki BU, Franzblau SG, Pauli GF. Quality Control of Therapeutic Peptides by 1H NMR HiFSA Sequencing. J Org Chem. 2019 Mar 15;84(6):3055-3073. doi: 10.1021/acs.joc.8b02704. Epub 2019 Feb 22. PMID: 30793905; PMCID: PMC6452441.

89 Swietlow A; Lax R Quality control in peptide manufacturing: specifications for GMP peptides. Pept. Chem 2004, 7, 22–24.

90 Kabsch W; Sander C Dictionary of protein secondary structure: Pattern recognition of hydrogen-bonded and geometrical features. Biopolymers 1983, 22 (12), 2577–2637.

91 Masgras I, Carrera S, de Verdier PJ, Brennan P, Majid A, Makhtar W, Tulchinsky E, Jones GDD, Roninson IB, Macip S. Reactive oxygen species and mitochondrial sensitivity to oxidative stress determine induction of cancer cell death by p21. J Biol Chem. 2012 Mar 23;287(13):9845-9854. doi: 10.1074/jbc.M111.250357. Epub 2012 Feb 6. PMID: 22311974; PMCID: PMC3322987.

92 Szeto, Hazel. (2008). Cell-Permeable, Mitochondrial-Targeted, Peptide Antioxidants. 10.1007/978-0-387-76678-2_31.

93 Wang Q, Zhang M., Tomita T., et al., Selected reaction monitoring approach for validating peptide biomarkers, Proc. Natl. Acad. Sci. U.S.A. 114 (51) 13519-13524, https://doi.org/10.1073/pnas.1712731114 (2017).

94. Sakai A, Sasaki K, Muramatsu D, et al. A Bhas 42 cell transformation assay on 98 chemicals: the characteristics and performance for the prediction of chemical carcinogenicity. Mutat Res. 2010;702(1):100–122.

95. Puig M, Shubow S. Immunogenicity of therapeutic peptide products: bridging the gaps regarding the role of product-related risk factors. Front Immunol. 2025 Jun 18; 16:1608401. doi: 10.3389/fimmu.2025.1608401. PMID: 40607385; PMCID: PMC12213570.

96. Achilleos K, Petrou C, Nicolaidou V, Sarigiannis Y. Beyond Efficacy: Ensuring Safety in Peptide Therapeutics through Immunogenicity Assessment. J Pept Sci. 2025 Jun;31(6):e70016. doi: 10.1002/psc.70016. PMID: 40256940; PMCID: PMC12010466.

97. Reddy GN, Laltanpuii C, Sonti R. Review on in vivo profiling of drug metabolites with LC-MS/MS in the past decade. Bioanalysis. 2021 Nov;13(22):1697-1722. doi: 10.4155/bio-2021-0144. Epub 2021 Oct 26. PMID: 34696599.

98. Shankar G, Arkin S, Cocea L, Devanarayan V, Kirshner S, Kromminga A, Quarmby V, Richards S, Schneider CK, Subramanyam M, Swanson S, Verthelyi D, Yim S; American Association of Pharmaceutical Scientists. Assessment and reporting of the clinical immunogenicity of therapeutic proteins and peptides-harmonized terminology and tactical recommendations. AAPS J. 2014 Jul;16(4):658-73. doi: 10.1208/s12248-014-9599-2. Epub 2014 Apr 24. PMID: 24764037; PMCID: PMC4070270.

99. Koren E, Zuckerman LA, Mire-Sluis AR. Immune responses to therapeutic proteins in humans—clinical significance, assessment and prediction. Curr Pharm Biotechnol. 2002;3(4):349–360. doi: 10.2174/1389201023378175.

Chapter 4

100. Casanova A, Wevers A, Navarro-Ledesma S, Pruimboom L. Mitochondria: It is all about energy. Front Physiol. 2023 Apr 25; 14:1114231. doi: 10.3389/fphys.2023.1114231. PMID: 37179826; PMCID: PMC10167337.

101. Pliouta, L., Lampsas, S., Kountouri, A., Korakas, E., Thymis, J., Kassi, E., Oikonomou, E., Ikonomidis, I., & Lambadiari, V. (2025). Mitochondrial Dysfunction in the Development and Progression of Cardiometabolic Diseases: A Narrative Review. Journal of Clinical Medicine, 14(11), 3706.

102. Miller B, Kim SJ, Kumagai H, Mehta HH, Xiang W, Liu J, Yen K, Cohen P. Peptides derived from small mitochondrial open reading frames: Genomic, biological, and therapeutic implications. Exp Cell Res. 2020 Aug 15;393(2):112056. doi: 10.1016/j.yexcr.2020.112056. Epub 2020 May 6. PMID: 32387288; PMCID: PMC7778388.

103. Lee C, Kim KH, Cohen P. MOTS-c: A novel mitochondrial-derived peptide regulating muscle and fat metabolism. Free Radic Biol Med. 2016 Nov; 100:182-187. doi: 10.1016/j.freeradbiomed.2016.05.015. Epub 2016 May 20. PMID: 27216708; PMCID: PMC5116416.

104. Ma ZW, Liu DX. Humanin decreases mitochondrial membrane permeability by inhibiting the membrane association and oligomerization of Bax and Bid proteins. Acta Pharmacol Sin. 2018 Jun;39(6):1012-1021. doi: 10.1038/aps.2017.169. Epub 2017 Dec 21. PMID: 29265109; PMCID: PMC6256269.

105. Mohtashami Z, Singh MK, Salimiaghdam N, Ozgul M, Kenney MC. MOTS-c, the Most Recent Mitochondrial Derived Peptide in Human Aging and Age-Related Diseases. Int J Mol Sci. 2022 Oct 9;23(19):11991. doi: 10.3390/ijms231911991. PMID: 36233287; PMCID: PMC9570330.

106. Kim S, Kim NY, Park JY, Park HM, Lim CM, Kim J, Lee HP, Hong JT, Yoon DY. MMPP Exerts Anti-Inflammatory Effects by Suppressing MD2-Dependent NF-κB and JNK/AP-1 Pathways in THP-1 Monocytes. Pharmaceuticals (Basel). 2023 Mar 23;16(4):480. doi: 10.3390/ph16040480. PMID: 37111237; PMCID: PMC10146917.

107. Yang B, Yu Q, Chang B, Guo Q, Xu S, Yi X, Cao S. MOTS-c interacts synergistically with exercise intervention to regulate PGC-1α expression, attenuate insulin resistance and enhance glucose metabolism in mice via AMPK signaling pathway. Biochim Biophys Acta Mol Basis Dis. 2021 Jun 1;1867(6):166126. doi: 10.1016/j.bbadis.2021.166126. Epub 2021 Mar 13. PMID: 33722744.

108. Daiber A, Xia N, Steven S, Oelze M, Hanf A, Kröller-Schön S, Münzel T, Li H. New Therapeutic Implications of Endothelial Nitric Oxide Synthase (eNOS) Function/Dysfunction in Cardiovascular Disease. Int J Mol Sci. 2019 Jan 7;20(1):187. doi: 10.3390/ijms20010187. PMID: 30621010; PMCID: PMC6337296.

109. Gong Z, Goetzman E, Muzumdar RH. Cardio-protective role of Humanin in myocardial ischemia-reperfusion. Biochim Biophys Acta Gen Subj. 2022 Feb;1866(2):130066. doi: 10.1016/j.bbagen.2021.130066. Epub 2021 Dec 9. PMID: 34896254.

110. Kwiecinski, Jacek & Lennen, Ross & Gray, Gillian & Borthwick, Gary & Boswell, Lyndsey & Baker, Andrew & Newby, David & Dweck, Marc & Jansen, Maurits.

(2020). Progression and regression of left ventricular hypertrophy and myocardial fibrosis in a mouse model of hypertension and concomitant cardiomyopathy. Journal of Cardiovascular Magnetic Resonance. 22. 10.1186/s12968-020-00655-7.

111. Wei, Ming & Gan, Lu & Liu, Zheng & Liu, Li & Chang, Jin-Rui & Yin, Da-Chuan & Cao, Hui-Ling & Su, Xing-Li & Smith, Wanli W. (2019). Mitochondrial-Derived Peptide MOTS-c Attenuates Vascular Calcification and Secondary Myocardial Remodeling via Adenosine Monophosphate-Activated Protein Kinase Signaling Pathway. Cardiorenal Medicine. 10. 1-9. 10.1159/000503224.

112. Luo YH, Xie L, Li JY, Xie Y, Li MQ, Zhou L. Serum MOTS-C Levels are Decreased in Obese Children and Associated with Vascular Endothelial Function. Diabetes Metab Syndr Obes. 2023 Apr 12; 16:1013-1020. doi: 10.2147/DMSO.S403934. PMID: 37077579; PMCID: PMC10106799.

113. Dhingra R, Vasan RS. Biomarkers in cardiovascular disease: Statistical assessment and section on key novel heart failure biomarkers. Trends Cardiovasc Med. 2017 Feb;27(2):123-133. doi: 10.1016/j.tcm.2016.07.005. Epub 2016 Jul 28. PMID: 27576060; PMCID: PMC5253084.

114. Szeto HH, Liu S. Cardiolipin-targeted peptides rejuvenate mitochondrial function, remodel mitochondria, and promote tissue regeneration during aging. Arch Biochem Biophys. 2018 Dec 15; 660:137-148. doi: 10.1016/j.abb.2018.10.013. Epub 2018 Oct 23. PMID: 30359579.

115. Rochette L, Rigal E, Dogon G, Malka G, Zeller M, Vergely C, Cottin Y. Mitochondrial-derived peptides: New markers for cardiometabolic dysfunction. Arch Cardiovasc Dis. 2022 Jan;115(1):48-56. doi: 10.1016/j.acvd.2021.10.013. Epub 2021 Dec 28. PMID: 34972639.

116. Hashimoto Y., Niikura T., Ito Y., Sudo H., Hata M., Arakawa E., Abe Y., Kita Y., Nishimoto I. Detailed Characterization of Neuroprotection by a Rescue Factor Humanin against Various Alzheimer's Disease-Relevant Insults. J. Neurosci. 2001; 21:9235–9245. doi: 10.1523/JNEUROSCI.21-23-09235.2001.

117. Oh YK, Bachar AR, Zacharias DG, Kim SG, Wan J, Cobb LJ, Lerman LO, Cohen P, Lerman A. Humanin preserves endothelial function and prevents atherosclerotic plaque progression in hypercholesterolemic ApoE deficient mice. Atherosclerosis. 2011 Nov;219(1):65-73. doi: 10.1016/j.atherosclerosis.2011.06.038. Epub 2011 Jun 25. PMID: 21763658; PMCID: PMC3885346.

118. Wang X, Wu Z, He Y, Zhang H, Tian L, Zheng C, Shang T, Zhu Q, Li D, He Y. Humanin prevents high glucose-induced monocyte adhesion to endothelial cells by targeting KLF2. Mol Immunol. 2018 Sep; 101:245-250. doi: 10.1016/j.molimm.2018.07.008. Epub 2018 Jul 18. PMID: 30029058.

119. Meyrelles, S.S., Peotta, V.A., Pereira, T.M. et al. Endothelial Dysfunction in the Apolipoprotein E-deficient Mouse: insights into the influence of diet, gender and aging. Lipids Health Dis 10, 211 (2011).

120. Widmer RJ, Flammer AJ, Herrmann J, Rodriguez-Porcel M, Wan J, Cohen P, Lerman LO, Lerman A. Circulating humanin levels are associated with preserved coronary endothelial function. Am J Physiol Heart Circ Physiol. 2013 Feb 1;304(3):H393-7. doi: 10.1152/ajpheart.00765.2012. Epub 2012 Dec 7. PMID: 23220334; PMCID: PMC3774506.

121. Sivandzade F, Prasad S, Bhalerao A, Cucullo L. NRF2 and NF-κB interplay in cerebrovascular and neurodegenerative disorders: Molecular mechanisms and possible therapeutic approaches, Redox Biology, 2019, 21,101059, 2213-2317.

122. Li M, Liu Z, Cao X, Xiao W, Wang S, Zhao C, Zhao Y, Xie Y. [Gly14]-Humanin ameliorates high glucose-induced endothelial senescence via SIRT6. Sci Rep. 2024 Dec 28;14(1):30924. doi: 10.1038/s41598-024-81878-x. PMID: 39730568; PMCID: PMC11681169.

123. Zheng, M., Li, H., Zhao, J., Li, J., Yang, W., & Zhang, X. (2021). The mitochondrial-derived peptide MOTS-c attenuates oxidative stress injury and the inflammatory response of H9c2 cells through the Nrf2/ARE and NF-κB pathways. Journal of Cellular Biochemistry, 122(6), 634-645.

124. Birk A, Arain S, Musumeci D, Garcia-Marin V, MacNeil MA. Targeting High-Density Aromatic Peptides to Cardiolipin Optimizes the Mitochondrial Membrane Potential and Inhibits Oxidative Stress. FASEB Bioadv. 2025 Sep 29;7(10):e70052. doi: 10.1096/fba.2024-00061. PMID: 41035613; PMCID: PMC12479369.

125. 303.Gibson CM, Duffy D, Korjian S, Bahit MC, Chi G, Alexander JH, Lincoff AM, Heise M, Tricoci P, Deckelbaum LI, Mears SJ, Nicolau JC, Lopes RD, Merkely B, Lewis BS, Cornel JH, Trebacz J, Parkhomenko A, Libby P, Sacks FM, Povsic TJ, Bonaca M, Goodman SG, Bhatt DL, Tendera M, Steg PG, Ridker PM, Aylward P, Kastelein JJP, Bode C, Mahaffey KW, Nicholls SJ, Pocock SJ, Mehran R, Harrington RA; AEGIS-II Committees and Investigators. Apolipoprotein A1 Infusions and Cardiovascular Outcomes after Acute Myocardial Infarction. N Engl J Med. 2024

May 2;390(17):1560-1571. doi: 10.1056/NEJMoa2400969. Epub 2024 Apr 6. PMID: 38587254.

Chapter 5

126. Green C, Zaman V, Blumenstock K, Banik NL, Haque A. Dysregulation of Metabolic Peptides in the Gut-Brain Axis Promotes Hyperinsulinemia, Obesity, and Neurodegeneration. Biomedicines. 2025 Jan 8;13(1):132. doi: 10.3390/biomedicines13010132. PMID: 39857716; PMCID: PMC11763097.

127. Al-Suhaimi EA, Shehzad A. Leptin, resistin and visfatin: the missing link between endocrine metabolic disorders and immunity. Eur J Med Res. 2013 May 1;18(1):12. doi: 10.1186/2047-783X-18-12. PMID: 23634778; PMCID: PMC3655867.

128. Makki, Kassem, Froguel, Philippe, Wolowczuk, Isabelle, Adipose Tissue in Obesity-Related Inflammation and Insulin Resistance: Cells, Cytokines, and Chemokines, International Scholarly Research Notices, 2013, 139239, 12 pages, 2013.

129. Khan M, Joseph F. Adipose tissue and adipokines: the association with and application of adipokines in obesity. Scientifica (Cairo). 2014; 2014:328592. doi: 10.1155/2014/328592. Epub 2014 Sep 17. PMID: 25309775; PMCID: PMC4182896.

130. Burgos-Morón E, Abad-Jiménez Z, Marañón AM, Iannantuoni F, Escribano-López I, López-Domènech S, Salom C, Jover A, Mora V, Roldan I, Solá E, Rocha M, Víctor VM. Relationship Between Oxidative Stress, ER Stress, and Inflammation in Type 2 Diabetes: The Battle Continues. J Clin Med. 2019 Sep 4;8(9):1385. doi: 10.3390/jcm8091385.

131. Besse-Patin A, Estall JL. An Intimate Relationship between ROS and Insulin Signalling: Implications for Antioxidant Treatment of Fatty Liver Disease. Int J Cell Biol. 2014; 2014:519153. doi: 10.1155/2014/519153. Epub 2014 Feb 12. PMID: 24672550; PMCID: PMC3944655.

132. Kim SJ, Xiao J, Wan J, Cohen P, Yen K. Mitochondrially derived peptides as novel regulators of metabolism. J Physiol. 2017 Nov 1;595(21):6613-6621. doi: 10.1113/JP274472. Epub 2017 Jul 18. PMID: 28574175; PMCID: PMC5663826.

133. Kal S, Mahata S, Jati S, Mahata SK. Mitochondrial-derived peptides: Antidiabetic functions and evolutionary perspectives. Peptides. 2024 Feb; 172:171147. doi: 10.1016/j.peptides.2023.171147. Epub 2023 Dec 29. PMID: 38160808; PMCID: PMC10838678.

134. Kim S, Mehta HH, Wan J, Kuehnemann C, Chen J, Hu J, Hoffman AR, Cohen P. Mitochondrial peptides modulate mitochondrial function during cellular senescence. Aging (Albany NY). 2018 Jun 10; 10:1239-1256.

135. Kong BS, Lee C, Cho YM. Mitochondrial-Encoded Peptide MOTS-c, Diabetes, and Aging-Related Diseases. Diabetes Metab J. 2023 May;47(3):315-324. doi: 10.4093/dmj.2022.0333. Epub 2023 Feb 24. PMID: 36824008; PMCID: PMC10244198.

136. Zhou, Q., Yin, S., Lei, X. et al. The correlation between mitochondrial derived peptide (MDP) and metabolic states: a systematic review and meta-analysis. Diabetol Metab Syndr 16, 200 (2024).

137. Nambidi, S., Pallatt, S., Banerjee, A. et al. Klotho protein: a multifaceted regulator in aging and cancer dynamics. Mol Biol Rep 52, 507 (2025).

138. Chan MKS, Wong MBF, Casazza K, Klokol D, et al. Klotho, Obesity, and Inflammation: A Triad of Metabolic Regulation. Am J Biomed Sci & Res. 2025 25(6) AJBSR. MS.ID.003376, DOI: 10.34297/AJBSR.2025.25.003376.

139. Chan MKS, Sardar SN, Rahim MSA, Wang MBW et al. Neuromuscular and Muscular-Skeletal Modulations as The Antiaging Strategy of Physical Adaptation in Non-Communicable Diseases. J Neurol Sci Res. 5(1):1-24.

140. Castillo-Díaz, L. A., Ruiz-Pacheco, J. A., Elsawy, M. A., Reyes-Martínez, J. E., & Enríquez-Rodríguez, A. I. (2020). Self-Assembling Peptides as an Emerging Platform for the Treatment of Metabolic Syndrome. International Journal of Nanomedicine, 15, 10349–10370.

141. Müller TD, Finan B, Bloom SR, D'Alessio D, Drucker DJ, Flatt PR, Fritsche A, Gribble F, Grill HJ, Habener JF, Holst JJ, Langhans W, Meier JJ, Nauck MA, Perez-Tilve D, Pocai A, Reimann F, Sandoval DA, Schwartz TW, Seeley RJ, Stemmer K, Tang-Christensen M, Woods SC, DiMarchi RD, Tschöp MH. Glucagon-like peptide 1 (GLP-1). Mol Metab. 2019 Dec;30:72-130. doi: 10.1016/j.molmet.2019.09.010. Epub 2019 Sep 30. PMID: 31767182; PMCID: PMC6812410.

142. Durak A, Akkus E, Canpolat AG, Tuncay E, Corapcioglu D, Turan B. Glucagon-like peptide-1 receptor agonist treatment of high carbohydrate intake-induced metabolic syndrome provides pleiotropic effects on cardiac dysfunction through alleviations in electrical and intracellular Ca2+ abnormalities and mitochondrial dysfunction. Clin Exp Pharmacol Physiol. 2022 Jan;49(1):46-59. doi: 10.1111/1440-1681.13590. Epub 2021 Oct 27. PMID: 34519087.

143. Luna-Marco C, de Marañon AM, Hermo-Argibay A, Rodriguez-Hernandez Y, Hermenejildo J, Fernandez-Reyes M, Apostolova N, Vila J, Sola E, Morillas C, Rovira-Llopis S, Rocha M, Victor VM. Effects of GLP-1 receptor agonists on mitochondrial function, inflammatory markers and leukocyte-endothelium interactions in type 2 diabetes. Redox Biol. 2023 Oct; 66:102849. doi: 10.1016/j.redox.2023.102849. Epub 2023 Aug 14. PMID: 37591012; PMCID: PMC10457591

144. Granata A, Maccarrone R, Anzaldi M, Leonardi G, Pesce F, Amico F, Gesualdo L, Corrao S. GLP-1 receptor agonists and renal outcomes in patients with diabetes mellitus type 2 and diabetic kidney disease: state of the art. Clin Kidney J. 2022 Mar 12;15(9):1657-1665. doi: 10.1093/ckj/sfac069. PMID: 36003669; PMCID: PMC9394722.

145. Rizvi AA, Rizzo M. The Emerging Role of Dual GLP-1 and GIP Receptor Agonists in Glycemic Management and Cardiovascular Risk Reduction. Diabetes Metab Syndr Obes. 2022 Apr 5; 15:1023-1030. doi: 10.2147/DMSO.S351982. PMID: 35411165; PMCID: PMC8994606.

146. Zheng Y, Wei Z, Wang T. MOTS-c: A promising mitochondrial-derived peptide for therapeutic exploitation. Front Endocrinol (Lausanne). 2023 Jan 25; 14:1120533. doi: 10.3389/fendo.2023.1120533. PMID: 36761202; PMCID: PMC9905433.

147. Pacini, Lorenzo & Muthyala, Manoj Kumar & Zitterbart, Robert & Rovero, Paolo & Papini, Anna. (2024). Sustainable Scale-Up of GLP-1 Agonist Peptides through Green Solid Phase Peptide Synthesis. 2050-2050. 10.17952/37EPS. 2024.P2050.

148. Mike K S Chan, Michelle B F Wong, Krista Casazza, Dmytro Klokol, et al. Beyond the Powerhouse: Mitochondrial Organelles as Master Regulators of Wellness. Am J Biomed Sci & Res. 2025 27(3) AJBSR.MS.ID.00352, DOI: 10.34297/AJBSR.2025.27.003552.

149. Nambidi, S., Pallatt, S., Banerjee, A. et al. Klotho protein: a multifaceted regulator in aging and cancer dynamics. Mol Biol Rep 52, 507 (2025).

150. Knights AJ, Funnell AP, Pearson RC, Crossley M, Bell-Anderson KS. Adipokines and insulin action: A sensitive issue. Adipocyte. 2014 Apr 1;3(2):88-96. doi: 10.4161/adip.27552. Epub 2014 Jan 8. PMID: 24719781; PMCID: PMC3979885.

151. Iwaniak A, Darewicz M, Minkiewicz P. Peptides Derived from Foods as Supportive Diet Components in the Prevention of Metabolic Syndrome. Compr Rev Food Sci Food Saf. 2018 Jan;17(1):63-81. doi: 10.1111/1541-4337.12321. Epub 2017 Nov 27. PMID: 33350059.

152. Iwaniak, A., & Mogut, D. (2020). Metabolic Syndrome-Preventive Peptides Derived from Milk Proteins and Their Presence in Cheeses: A Review. Applied Sciences, 10(8), 2772.

153. Axel Kattar, Angel Concheiro & Carmen Alvarez-Lorenzo. (2021) Diabetic eye: associated diseases, drugs in clinic, and role of self-assembled carriers in topical treatment. Expert Opinion on Drug Delivery 18:11, pages 1589-1607.

154. Yuan Q, Zeng ZL, Yang S, Li A, Zu X, Liu J. Mitochondrial Stress in Metabolic Inflammation: Modest Benefits and Full Losses. Oxid Med Cell Longev. 2022 Nov 22; 2022:8803404. doi: 10.1155/2022/8803404. PMID: 36457729; PMCID: PMC9708372.

155. Lakey JRT, Wells A., Good A., Klokol D., Chan MKS, Song MBF. et al. Protective Effects of Stem Cell-Derived Peptides in Preventing Autoimmune Diabetes in the Non-Diabetic Mouse Model. Am J Biomed Sci & Res. 2022—16(5). AJBSR. MS.ID.002264. DOI:10.34297/AJBSR.2022.16.002264.

156. Sandsdal, R.M., Juhl, C.R., Jensen, S.B.K. et al. Combination of exercise and GLP-1 receptor agonist treatment reduces severity of metabolic syndrome, abdominal obesity, and inflammation: a randomized controlled trial. Cardiovasc Diabetol 22, 41 (2023).

157. Sandsdal RM, Juhl CR, Jensen SBK, Lundgren JR, Janus C, Blond MB, Rosenkilde M, Bogh AF, Gliemann L, Jensen JB, Antoniades C, Stallknecht BM, Holst JJ, Madsbad S, Torekov SS. Combination of exercise and GLP-1 receptor agonist treatment reduces severity of metabolic syndrome, abdominal obesity, and inflammation: a randomized controlled trial. Cardiovasc Diabetol. 2023 Feb 25;22(1):41. doi: 10.1186/s12933-023-01765-z. PMID: 36841762; PMCID: PMC9960425.

158. Zakaria H, Jabri H, Alshehhi S, Caccelli M, Debs J, Said Y, Kattan J, Almarzooqi N, Hashemi A, Almarzooqi I. Glucagon-Like Peptide-1 Receptor Agonists Combined With Personalized Digital Health Care for the Treatment of Metabolic Syndrome in Adults With Obesity: Retrospective Observational Study. Interact J Med Res. 2025 Mar 27;14: e63079. doi: 10.2196/63079. PMID: 40146920; PMCID: PMC11967752.

Chapter 6

159. Mike KS Chan, Michelle BF Wong, Krista Casazza, Waldemar Lernhardt, Dmytro Klokol, et al. Recalibrating Retinal Immunity: Peptide-Based Strategies for Durable

Vision Preservation in Retinitis Pigmentosa. Am J Biomed Sci & Res. 2025 28(1) AJBSR. MS.ID.003638, DOI: 10.34297/AJBSR.2025.28.003638.

160. Chan MKS, Wong MBF, Nishkumari O., Alvin G., Lemeliyanova M. and Klokol D. Treatment of Glaucoma with Progenitor/Precursor Stem Cells: Current Approaches and Future Prospects. J Stem Cell Res. 6(1):1-6.

161. Luger TA, Brzoska T. alpha-MSH related peptides: a new class of anti-inflammatory and immunomodulating drugs. Ann Rheum Dis. 2007 Nov;66 Suppl 3(Suppl 3): iii52-5. doi: 10.1136/ard.2007.079780. PMID: 17934097; PMCID: PMC2095288.

162. Zhu Y, Luo M, Bai X, Li J, Nie P, Li B, Luo P. SS-31, a Mitochondria-Targeting Peptide, Ameliorates Kidney Disease. Oxid Med Cell Longev. 2022 Jun 6; 2022:1295509. doi: 10.1155/2022/1295509. PMID: 35707274; PMCID: PMC9192202.

163. Goldstein AL, Hannappel E, Sosne G, Kleinman HK. Thymosin β4: a multi-functional regenerative peptide. Basic properties and clinical applications. Expert Opin Biol Ther. 2012 Jan;12(1):37-51. doi: 10.1517/14712598.2012.634793. Epub 2011 Nov 10. PMID: 22074294.

164. Rao RV, Bredesen DE. Misfolded proteins, endoplasmic reticulum stress and neurodegeneration. Curr Opin Cell Biol. 2004 Dec;16(6):653-62. doi: 10.1016/j.ceb.2004.09.012. PMID: 15530777; PMCID: PMC3970707.

165. Rajeswaren V, Wong JO, Yabroudi D, Nahomi RB, Rankenberg J, Nam MH, Nagaraj RH. Small Heat Shock Proteins in Retinal Diseases. Front Mol Biosci. 2022 Apr 11; 9:860375. doi: 10.3389/fmolb.2022.860375. PMID: 35480891; PMCID: PMC9035800.

166. Laliotou B, Liversidge J, Forrester JV, Dick AD. Interphotoreceptor retinoid binding protein is a potent tolerogen in Lewis rat: suppression of experimental autoimmune uveoretinitis is retinal antigen specific. Br J Ophthalmol. 1997 Jan;81(1):61-7. doi: 10.1136/bjo.81.1.61. PMID: 9135411; PMCID: PMC1722010.

167. Wang S, Li W, Chen M, Cao Y, Lu W, Li X. The retinal pigment epithelium: Functions and roles in ocular diseases. Fundam Res. 2023 Nov 28;4(6):1710-1718. doi: 10.1016/j.fmre.2023.08.011. PMID: 39734536; PMCID: PMC11670733.

168. Karamali, F., Behtaj, S., Babaei-Abraki, S. et al. Potential therapeutic strategies for photoreceptor degeneration: the path to restore vision. J Transl Med 20, 572 (2022).

169. Somaa FA, Wang TY, Niclis JC, Bruggeman KF, Kauhausen JA, Guo H, McDougall S, Williams RJ, Nisbet DR, Thompson LH, Parish CL. Peptide-Based Scaffolds

Support Human Cortical Progenitor Graft Integration to Reduce Atrophy and Promote Functional Repair in a Model of Stroke. Cell Rep. 2017 Aug 22;20(8):1964-1977. doi: 10.1016/j.celrep.2017.07.069. PMID: 28834757.

170. Akhter MH, Ahmad I, Alshahrani MY, Al-Harbi AI, Khalilullah H, Afzal O, Altamimi ASA, Najib Ullah SNM, Ojha A, Karim S. Drug Delivery Challenges and Current Progress in Nanocarrier-Based Ocular Therapeutic System. Gels. 2022 Jan 28;8(2):82. doi: 10.3390/gels8020082. PMID: 35200463; PMCID: PMC8871777.

171. Suk JS, Xu Q, Kim N, Hanes J, Ensign LM. PEGylation as a strategy for improving nanoparticle-based drug and gene delivery. Adv Drug Deliv Rev. 2016 Apr 1;99(Pt A):28-51. doi: 10.1016/j.addr.2015.09.012. Epub 2015 Oct 9. PMID: 26456916; PMCID: PMC4798869.

172. Thorp EB, Boada C, Jarbath C, Luo X. Nanoparticle Platforms for Antigen-Specific Immune Tolerance. Front Immunol. 2020 May 20; 11:945. doi: 10.3389/fimmu.2020.00945. PMID: 32508829; PMCID: PMC7251028.

Chapter 7

173. Bloomingdale P, Karelina T, Ramakrishnan V, Bakshi S, Véronneau-Veilleux F, Moye M, Sekiguchi K, Meno-Tetang G, Mohan A, Maithreye R, Thomas VA, Gibbons F, Cabal A, Bouteiller JM, Geerts H. Hallmarks of neurodegenerative disease: A systems pharmacology perspective. CPT Pharmacometrics Syst Pharmacol. 2022 Nov;11(11):1399-1429. doi: 10.1002/psp4.12852. Epub 2022 Aug 17. PMID: 35894182; PMCID: PMC9662204.

174. Spires-Jones TL, Attems J, Thal DR. Interactions of pathological proteins in neurodegenerative diseases. Acta Neuropathol. 2017 Aug;134(2):187-205. doi: 10.1007/s00401-017-1709-7. Epub 2017 Apr 11. PMID: 28401333; PMCID: PMC5508034.

175. Singh K, Gupta JK, Kumar S, Soni U. A Review of the Common Neurodegenerative Disorders: Current Therapeutic Approaches and the Potential Role of Bioactive Peptides. Curr Protein Pept Sci. 2024;25(7):507-526. doi: 10.2174/011389203727522124 0327042353. PMID: 38561605.

176. Mesias A, Borges S, Pintado M, Baptista-Silva S. Bioactive peptides as multipotent molecules bespoke and designed for Alzheimer's disease. Neuropeptides. 2025 Jun; 111:102515. doi: 10.1016/j.npep.2025.102515. Epub 2025 Mar 4. PMID: 40056763.

177. Gulisano W, Maugeri D, Baltrons MA, Fà M, Amato A, Palmeri A, D'Adamio L, Grassi C, Devanand DP, Honig LS, Puzzo D, Arancio O. Role of Amyloid-β and Tau Proteins in Alzheimer's Disease: Confuting the Amyloid Cascade. J Alzheimers Dis. 2018;64(s1): S611-S631. doi: 10.3233/JAD-179935. Erratum in: J Alzheimers Dis. 2019;68(1):415. doi: 10.3233/JAD-189015. PMID: 29865055; PMCID: PMC8371153.

178. Mojarad-Jabali S, Roh KH. Peptide-based inhibitors and nanoparticles: Emerging therapeutics for Alzheimer's disease. Int J Pharm. 2025 Jan 25; 669:125055. doi: 10.1016/j.ijpharm.2024.125055. Epub 2024 Dec 7. PMID: 39653296.

179. Kazim, S.F., Iqbal, K. Neurotrophic factor small-molecule mimetics mediated neuroregeneration and synaptic repair: emerging therapeutic modality for Alzheimer's disease. Mol Neurodegeneration 11, 50 (2016). https://doi.org/10.1186/s13024-016-0119-y.

180. Kazim SF, Iqbal K. Neurotrophic factor small-molecule mimetics mediated neuroregeneration and synaptic repair: emerging therapeutic modality for Alzheimer's disease. Mol Neurodegener. 2016 Jul 11;11(1):50. doi: 10.1186/s13024-016-0119-y. PMID: 27400746; PMCID: PMC4940708.

181. Zou Z, Wu F, Chen L, Yao H, Wang Z, Chen Y, Qi M, Jiang Y, Tang L, Gan X, Kong L, Yang Z, Huang X, Shu W, Li B, Tan X, Huang L, Bai S, Wu L, Mo J, Hu H, Liu H, Zou R, Wei Y. The J bs-5YP peptide can alleviate dementia in senile mice by restoring the transcription of Slc40a1 to secrete the excessive iron from brain. J Adv Res. 2025 Mar; 69:51-59. doi: 10.1016/j.jare.2024.03.014. Epub 2024 Mar 23. PMID: 38527587; PMCID: PMC11954793.

182. Yang H, Wang F, Zhao P, Ullah S, Ma Y, Zhao G, Cheng Y, Li Q, Li T, Qiao M, Song L, Zhang L, Galaverna G, Huang X, Li N. Black soybean peptide mediates the AMPK/SIRT1/NF-κB signaling pathway to alleviate Alzheimer's-related neuroinflammation in lead-exposed HT22 cells. Int J Biol Macromol. 2025 Jan; 286:138404. doi: 10.1016/j.ijbiomac.2024.138404. Epub 2024 Dec 4. PMID: 39643189.

183. Sun MK, Alkon DL. Alzheimer's therapeutic development: shifting neurodegeneration to neuroregeneration. Trends Pharmacol Sci. 2024 Mar;45(3):197-209. doi: 10.1016/j.tips.2024.01.012. Epub 2024 Feb 14. PMID: 38360510; PMCID: PMC10939773.

184. Preethy H A, Rajendran K, Sukumar AJ, Krishnan UM. Emerging paradigms in Alzheimer's therapy. Eur J Pharmacol. 2024 Oct 15; 981:176872. doi: 10.1016/j.ejphar.2024.176872. Epub 2024 Aug 6. PMID: 39117266.

185. Pintado-Grima C, Bárcenas O, Iglesias V, Santos J, ManglCarlos Pintado-Grima, Oriol Bárcenas, Valentín Iglesias, Jaime Santos, Zoe Manglano-Artuñedo, Irantzu Pallarès, Michał Burdukiewicz, Salvador Ventura, aSynPEP-DB: a database of biogenic peptides for inhibiting α-synuclein aggregation, Database, Volume 2023, 2023, baad084.

186. Artuñedo Z, Pallarès I, Burdukiewicz M, Ventura S. aSynPEP-DB: a database of biogenic peptides for inhibiting α-synuclein aggregation. Database (Oxford). 2023 Nov 27;2023: baad084. doi: 10.1093/database/baad084. PMID: 38011719; PMCID: PMC10681447.

187. Sorrentino, Vincenzo & Auwerx, Johan. (2018). Repairing Mitochondrial Dysfunction in Disease. Annual Review of Pharmacology and Toxicology. 58. 10.1146/annurev-pharmtox-010716-104908.

188. Tsekrekou M, Giannakou M, Papanikolopoulou K, Skretas G. Protein aggregation and therapeutic strategies in SOD1- and TDP-43- linked ALS. Front Mol Biosci. 2024 May 24; 11:1383453. doi: 10.3389/fmolb.2024.1383453. PMID: 38855322; PMCID: PMC11157337.

189. Blokhuis AM, Groen EJ, Koppers M, van den Berg LH, Pasterkamp RJ. Protein aggregation in amyotrophic lateral sclerosis. Acta Neuropathol. 2013 Jun;125(6):777-94. doi: 10.1007/s00401-013-1125-6. Epub 2013 May 15. PMID: 23673820; PMCID: PMC3661910.

190. Mike KS Chan, Michelle BF Wong, Wenyi Guo, Michael Alexander, and Jonathan RT Lakey. Peptides Therapy for Neurodegenerative Disorders. Am J Biomed Sci & Res. 2024—22(6). AJBSR.MS.ID.003027. DOI:10.34297/AJBSR.2024.22.003027.

191. Zhang Q, Liu J, Chen L, Zhang M. Promoting Endogenous Neurogenesis as a Treatment for Alzheimer's Disease. Mol Neurobiol. 2023 Mar;60(3):1353-1368. doi: 10.1007/s12035-022-03145-2. Epub 2022 Nov 29. PMID: 36445633.

192. Wei M, Wu T, Chen N. Bridging neurotrophic factors and bioactive peptides to Alzheimer's disease. Ageing Res Rev. 2024 Feb; 94:102177. doi: 10.1016/j.arr.2023.102177. Epub 2023 Dec 22. PMID: 38142891.

193. Mike K S Chan, Michelle B F Wong, Krista Casazza, Ian Jenkins and Jonathan R T Lakey*. Peptide Neuromodulation inAutism Spectrum Disorder: Targeting Neuroinflammation, Mitochondrial Dysfunction, and Synaptic Plasticity. Am J Biomed Sci & Res. 202527(2) AJBSR.MS.ID.003532, DOI: 10.34297/AJBSR.2025.27.003532.

194. Yang HM. Overcoming the Blood-Brain Barrier: Advanced Strategies in Targeted Drug Delivery for Neurodegenerative Diseases. Pharmaceutics. 2025 Aug 11;17(8):1041. doi: 10.3390/pharmaceutics17081041. PMID: 40871062; PMCID: PMC12388969.

195. Salloway SP, Sevingy J, Budur K, Pederson JT, DeMattos RB, Von Rosenstiel P, Paez A, Evans R, Weber CJ, Hendrix JA, Worley S, Bain LJ, Carrillo MC. Advancing combination therapy for Alzheimer's disease. Alzheimers Dement (N Y). 2020 Oct 7;6(1): e12073. doi: 10.1002/trc2.12073. PMID: 33043108; PMCID: PMC7539671.

196. Sharma D, Dhiman I, Das S, Das DK, Pramanik DD, Dash SK, Pramanik A. Recent Advances in Therapeutic Peptides: Innovations and Applications in Treating Infections and Diseases. ACS Omega. 2025 Apr 23;10(17):17087-17107. doi: 10.1021/acsomega.5c02077. PMID: 40352490; PMCID: PMC12059905.

197. Hlávka JP, Kinoshita AT, Jeyasingh D, Huang C, Mirsafian L, Jacobson M. Emerging Alzheimer's disease treatment paradigms: A late-stage clinical trial review. Alzheimers Dement (N Y). 2024 Dec 27;10(4):e70022. doi: 10.1002/trc2.70022. PMID: 39748848; PMCID: PMC11694526.

198. Preethy H A, Rajendran K, Sukumar AJ, Krishnan UM. Emerging paradigms in Alzheimer's therapy. Eur J Pharmacol. 2024 Oct 15; 981:176872. doi: 10.1016/j.ejphar.2024.176872. Epub 2024 Aug 6. PMID: 39117266.

199. Xu X, Pang Y, Fan X. Mitochondria in oxidative stress, inflammation and aging: from mechanisms to therapeutic advances. Signal Transduct Target Ther. 2025 Jun 11;10(1):190. doi: 10.1038/s41392-025-02253-4. PMID: 40500258; PMCID: PMC12159213.

200. Kim A, Joseph S, Khan A, Epstein CJ, Sobel R, Huang TT. Enhanced expression of mitochondrial superoxide dismutase leads to prolonged in vivo cell cycle progression and up-regulation of mitochondrial thioredoxin. Free Radic Biol Med. 2010 Jun 1;48(11):1501-12. doi: 10.1016/j.freeradbiomed.2010.02.028. Epub 2010 Feb 25. PMID: 20188820; PMCID: PMC2945707.

201. Adamu A, Li S, Gao F, Xue G. The role of neuroinflammation in neurodegenerative diseases: current understanding and future therapeutic targets. Front Aging Neurosci. 2024 Apr 12; 16:1347987. doi: 10.3389/fnagi.2024.1347987. PMID: 38681666; PMCID: PMC11045904.

Chapter 8

202. Wehkamp J, Schmid M, Stange EF. Defensins and other antimicrobial peptides in inflammatory bowel disease. Curr Opin Gastroenterol. 2007 Jul;23(4):370-8. doi: 10.1097/MOG.0b013e328136c580. PMID: 17545771.

203. Zhang M, Sun K, Wu Y, Yang Y, Tso P and Wu Z (2017) Interactions between Intestinal Microbiota and Host Immune Response in Inflammatory Bowel Disease. Front. Immunol. 8:942. doi: 10.3389/fimmu.2017.00942.

204. Chengmei Gea, Zhen Wanga, Yu Wangb, Meihao Wei. Peptide-based therapeutic and delivery strategies for inflammatory bowel disease: challenges and future directions. RSC Adv., 2025, 15, 25560-25578.

205. Gopalakrishnan S, Tripathi A, Tamiz AP, Alkan SS, Pandey NB. Larazotide acetate promotes tight junction assembly in epithelial cells. Peptides. 2012 May;35(1):95-101. doi: 10.1016/j.peptides.2012.02.016. Epub 2012 Feb 28. PMID: 22401910.

206. Gopalakrishnan S, Durai M, Kitchens K, Tamiz AP, Somerville R, Ginski M., Paterson, B.M., Murray, J.A., Verdu E.F., Alkan S.S., Pandey N.B. Larazotide acetate regulates epithelial tight junctions in vitro and in vivo. Peptides. 2012 May;35(1):86-94. doi: 10.1016/j.peptides.2012.02.015. Epub 2012 Feb 27. PMID: 22401908.

207. Slifer ZM, Hernandez L, Pridgen TA, Carlson AR, Messenger KM, Madan J, Krishnan BR, Laumas S, Blikslager AT. Larazotide acetate induces recovery of ischemia-injured porcine jejunum via repair of tight junctions. PLoS One. 2021 Apr 22;16(4):e0250165. doi: 10.1371/journal.pone.0250165. PMID: 33886649; PMCID: PMC8061941.

208. Leffler DA, Kelly CP, Abdallah HZ, Colatrella AM, Harris LA, Leon F, Arterburn LA, Paterson BM, Lan ZH, Murray JA. A randomized, double-blind study of larazotide acetate to prevent the activation of celiac disease during gluten challenge. Am J Gastroenterol. 2012 Oct;107(10):1554-62. doi: 10.1038/ajg.2012.211. Epub 2012 Jul 24. PMID: 22825365; PMCID: PMC3463856.

209. Ghazvini K, Taghiabadi Z, Karimi MA, Hosseini Bafghi M, Paryan M, Amirfakhrian R. Anti-Inflammatory Peptides as Promising Therapeutics Agent Against Inflammatory Bowel Diseases: A Systematic Review. JGH Open. 2025 Jun 29;9(7):e70212. doi: 10.1002/jgh3.70212. PMID: 40589771; PMCID: PMC12206851.

210. Deogil Kim, Dong Woo Lee, Eui Kyun Jeong, Hoo Cheol Lee, Yoon Shin Park, Jue Yeon Lee, Chong Pyung Chung, Yoon Jeong Park, NIPEP-IBD; A SYNTHETIC

PEPTIDE TARGETING NOVEL MOLECULE, INTEGRIN BETA 1, TO RESTITUTE INTESTINAL EPITHELIAL CELLS FOR INFLAMMATORY BOWEL DISEASE (IBD) TREATMENT, Inflammatory Bowel Diseases, Volume 28, Issue Supplement_1, February 2022, Page S64.

211. Zhang L, Wei X, Zhang R, Petitte JN, Si D, Li Z, Cheng J, Du M. Design and Development of a Novel Peptide for Treating Intestinal Inflammation. Front Immunol. 2019 Aug 6; 10:1841. doi: 10.3389/fimmu.2019.01841. PMID: 31447849; PMCID: PMC6691347.

212. Shan, W., Zhang, W., Xue, F. et al. Schistosoma japonicum peptide SJMHE1 inhibits acute and chronic colitis induced by dextran sulfate sodium in mice. Parasites Vectors 14, 455 (2021).

213. Xie WY, Ji ZH, Ren WZ, Zhao PS, Wei FH, Hu J, Yuan B, Gao W. Wheat peptide alleviates DSS-induced colitis by activating the Keap1-Nrf2 signaling pathway and maintaining the integrity of the gut barrier. Food Funct. 2024 May 20;15(10):5466-5484. doi: 10.1039/d3fo04413k. PMID: 38690672.

214. Grimstad T, Bjørndal B, Cacabelos D, et al. A salmon peptide diet alleviates experimental colitis as compared with fish oil. Journal of Nutritional Science. 2013;2:e2. doi:10.1017/jns.2012.23.

215. Ullah H, Deng T, Ali M, Farooqui NA, Alsholi DM, Siddiqui NZ, Rehman AU, Ali S, Ilyas M, Wang L, Xin Y. Sea Conch Peptides Hydrolysate Alleviates DSS-Induced Colitis in Mice through Immune Modulation and Gut Microbiota Restoration. Molecules. 2023 Sep 28;28(19):6849. doi: 10.3390/molecules28196849. PMID: 37836692; PMCID: PMC10574497.

216. Wei X, Zhang L, Zhang R, Wu R, Si D, Ahmad B, Petitte JN, Mozdziak PE, Li Z, Guo H, Zhang M. A highly efficient hybrid peptide ameliorates intestinal inflammation and mucosal barrier damage by neutralizing lipopolysaccharides and antagonizing the lipopolysaccharide-receptor interaction. FASEB J. 2020 Dec;34(12):16049-16072. doi: 10.1096/fj.201903263RRR. Epub 2020 Oct 15. PMID: 33058296.

217. Taherali F, Chouhan N, Wang F, Lavielle S, Baran M, McCoubrey LE, Basit AW, Yadav V. Impact of Peptide Structure on Colonic Stability and Tissue Permeability. Pharmaceutics. 2023 Jul 15;15(7):1956. doi: 10.3390/pharmaceutics15071956. PMID: 37514143; PMCID: PMC10384666.

218. Wei X, Zhang L, Zhang R, Koci M, Si D, Ahmad B, Cheng J, Wang J, Aihemaiti M, Zhang M. A Novel Cecropin-LL37 Hybrid Peptide Protects Mice Against EHEC

Infection-Mediated Changes in Gut Microbiota, Intestinal Inflammation, and Impairment of Mucosal Barrier Functions. Front Immunol. 2020 Jun 30; 11:1361. doi: 10.3389/fimmu.2020.01361. PMID: 32695115; PMCID: PMC7338479.

219. Mike KS Chan, Michelle BF Wong, Krista Casazza, Ian Jenkins and Jonathan RT Lakey. Rebuilding the Barrier: Peptide-Based Strategies for Intestinal Regeneration. Am J Biomed Sci & Res. 2025 26(6) AJBSR.MS.ID.003494, DOI: 10.34297/AJBSR.2025.26.003494.

220. Mike KS Chan, Ian Jenkins, Michelle BF Wong, Krista Casazza, Dmytro Klokol, et al. Restoring Immune Balance and Intestinal Integrity in Crohn's Disease: A Framework for Targeted Regenerative and Immunomodulatory Therapies. Am J Biomed Sci & Res. 2025 27(4) AJBSR.MS.ID.003587, DOI: 10.34297/AJBSR.2025.27 003587.

Chapter 9

221. Cross M, Smith E, Hoy D, et al. The global burden of osteoarthritis: estimates from the Global Burden of Disease 2010 study. Ann Rheum Dis. 2014;73(7):1323–1330. doi:10.1136/annrheumdis-2013-204763.

222. Hunter DJ, Bierma-Zeinstra S. Osteoarthritis. Lancet. 2019;393(10182):1745–1759. doi:10.1016/S0140-6736(19)30417-9.

223. Martel-Pelletier J, Barr AJ, Cicuttini FM, Conaghan PG, Cooper C, Goldring MB, Goldring SR, Jones G, Teichtahl AJ, Pelletier JP. Osteoarthritis. Nature Reviews Disease Primers. 2016; 1:16072. doi:10.1038/nrdp.2016.72 OUCI.

224. Hawker, Gillian. (2019). Osteoarthritis is a serious disease. Clinical and experimental rheumatology. 37 Suppl 120. 3-6.

225. Chan MTK, Klokol D, Jonathan R.T. Lakey, et al. Novel Bioregenerative Options for Chondrocyte Restoration in Osteoarthritis. Stem Cells Regen Med. 2022; 6(1): 1-8.

226. Sophia Fox AJ, Bedi A, Rodeo SA. The basic science of articular cartilage: structure, composition, and function. Sports Health. 2009 Nov;1(6):461-8. doi: 10.1177/1941738109350438. PMID: 23015907; PMCID: PMC3445147.

227. Kan S, Duan M, Liu Y, Wang C, Xie J. Role of Mitochondria in Physiology of Chondrocytes and Diseases of Osteoarthritis and Rheumatoid Arthritis. Cartilage. 2021 Dec;13(2_suppl):1102S-1121S. doi: 10.1177/19476035211063858. Epub 2021 Dec 11. PMID: 34894777; PMCID: PMC8804744.

228. Musumeci, G., Aiello, F. C., Szychlinska, M. A., Di Rosa, M., Castrogiovanni, P., & Mobasheri, A. (2015). Osteoarthritis in the XXIst century: risk factors and behaviours that influence disease onset and progression. International journal of molecular sciences, 16(3), 6093-6112.

229. Vaamonde-García, C., Riveiro-Naveira, R. R., Valcárcel-Ares, M. N., Hermida-Carballo, L., Blanco, F. J., & López-Armada, M. J. (2012). Mitochondrial dysfunction increases inflammatory responsiveness to cytokines in normal human chondrocytes. Arthritis & Rheumatism, 64(9), 2927-2936.

230. Kiełbowski, K., Herian, M., Bakinowska, E., Banach, B., Sroczyński, T., & Pawlik, A. (2023). The role of genetics and epigenetic regulation in the pathogenesis of osteoarthritis. International Journal of Molecular Sciences, 24(14), 11655.

231. Archibald, J. (2020). Molecular Mechanisms Leading to Interleukin-1β Release by Macrophages in Response to Wear and Corrosion Products from Metal Implants (Doctoral dissertation, Université d'Ottawa/University of Ottawa).

232. Tan, S., Sun, Y., Li, S., Wu, H., & Ding, Y. (2025). The impact of mitochondrial dysfunction on osteoarthritis cartilage: current insights and emerging mitochondria-targeted therapies. Bone Research, 13(1), 77.

233. Mike K S Chan, Michelle B F Wong, Krista Casazza, Dmytro Klokol, Olha Nishkumai, et.al. Novel Progression from Cell-Based Therapies to Increasingly Refined, Cell-Free Approaches. Am J Biomed Sci & Res. 2024 25(1) AJBSR.MS.ID.003279, DOI: 10.34297/AJBSR.2024.25.003279.

234. Liu Q, Jia Z, Duan L, Xiong J, Wang D, Ding Y. Functional peptides for cartilage repair and regeneration. Am J Transl Res. 2018 Feb 15;10(2):501-510. PM D: 29511444; PMCID: PMC5835815.

235. Liao HJ, Chen HT, Chang CH. Peptides for Targeting Chondrogenic Induction and Cartilage Regeneration in Osteoarthritis. Cartilage. 2024 Sep 18:19476035241276406. doi: 10.1177/19476035241276406. Epub ahead of print. PMID: 39291443; PMCID: PMC11556548.

236. Zhang M, Zhou Q, Liang QQ, Li CG, Holz JD, Tang D, Sheu TJ, Li TF, Shi Q, Wang YJ. IGF-1 regulation of type II collagen and MMP-13 expression in rat endplate chondrocytes via distinct signaling pathways. Osteoarthritis Cartilage. 2009 Jan;17(1):100-6. doi: 10.1016/j.joca.2008.05.007. Epub 2008 Jul 1. PMID: 18595745.

237. Chang CH, Tsai WC, Hsu YH, Pang JH. Pentadecapeptide BPC 157 enhances the growth hormone receptor expression in tendon fibroblasts. Molecules. 2014 Nov 19;19(11):19066-77. doi: 10.3390/molecules191119066. PMID: 25415472; PMCID: PMC6271067.

238. Lu YC, Ho TC, Huang CH, Yeh SI, Chen SL, Tsao YP. PEDF peptide plus hyaluronic acid stimulates cartilage regeneration in osteoarthritis via STAT3-mediated chondrogenesis. Bone Joint Res. 2024 Apr 1;13(4):137-148. doi: 10.1302/2046-3758.134. BJR-2023-0179.R2. PMID: 38555936; PMCID: PMC10981997.

239. Schultz, C. (2019) Targeting the extracellular matrix for delivery of bioactive molecules to sites of arthritis. British Journal of Pharmacology, 176: 26–37.

Chapter 10

240. Yan F, Mo X, Liu J, Ye S, Zeng X, Chen D. Thymic function in the regulation of T cells, and molecular mechanisms underlying the modulation of cytokines and stress signaling (Review). Mol Med Rep. 2017 Nov;16(5):7175-7184. doi: 10.3892/mmr.2017.7525. Epub 2017 Sep 19. PMID: 28944829; PMCID: PMC5865843.

241. Damsker JM, Hansen AM, Caspi RR. Th1 and Th17 cells: adversaries and collaborators. Ann N Y Acad Sci. 2010 Jan; 1183:211-21. doi: 10.1111/j.1749-6632.2009.05133. x. PMID: 20146717; PMCID: PMC2914500.

242. Xing Y, Ye Y, Zuo H, Li Y. Progress on the Function and Application of Thymosin β4. Front Endocrinol (Lausanne). 2021 Dec 21; 12:767785. doi: 10.3389/fendo.2021.767785. PMID: 34992578; PMCID: PMC8724243.

243. Anderson G, Cosway EJ, James KD, Ohigashi I, Takahama Y. Generation and repair of thymic epithelial cells. J Exp Med. 2024 Oct 7;221(10):e20230894. doi: 10.1084/jem.20230894. Epub 2024 Jul 9. Erratum in: J Exp Med. 2024 Oct 7;221(10):e2023089409042024c. doi: 10.1084/jem.2023089409042024c. PMID: 38980292; PMCID: PMC11232892.

244. Chan MKS, Wong MBF, Skutella T, Moya R, Klokol D (2023) Clinical Experience of Thymic Regeneration with Thymus Extracts, Thymic Peptides and Stem Cells in General Medicine, Oncology and Anti-Aging Medicine: A Review. J Stem Cell Res Dev Ther 9: 106.

245. Wolf E, Milazzo S, Boehm K, Zwahlen M, Horneber M. Thymic peptides for treatment of cancer patients. Cochrane Database Syst Rev. 2011 Feb 16;2011(2):CD003993. doi: 10.1002/14651858.CD003993.pub3. PMID: 21328265; PMCID: PMC6481824.

246. Qian L, Zhu Y, Deng C, Liang Z, Chen J, Chen Y, Wang X, Liu Y, Tian Y, Yang Y. Peroxisome proliferator-activated receptor gamma coactivator-1 (PGC-1) family in physiological and pathophysiological process and diseases. Signal Transduct Target Ther. 2024 Mar 1;9(1):50. doi: 10.1038/s41392-024-01756-w. PMID: 38424050; PMCID: PMC10904817.

247. Ngo V, Duennwald ML. Nrf2 and Oxidative Stress: A General Overview of Mechanisms and Implications in Human Disease. Antioxidants (Basel). 2022 Nov 27;11(12):2345. doi: 10.3390/antiox11122345. PMID: 36552553; PMCID: PMC9774434.

248. Terman A, Kurz T, Navratil M, Arriaga EA, Brunk UT. Mitochondrial turnover and aging of long-lived postmitotic cells: the mitochondrial-lysosomal axis theory of aging. Antioxid Redox Signal. 2010 Apr;12(4):503-35. doi: 10.1089/ars.2009.2598. PMID: 19650712; PMCID: PMC2861545.

249. Burtscher J, Soltany A, Visavadiya NP, Burtscher M, Millet GP, Khoramipour K, Khamoui AV. Mitochondrial stress and mitokines in aging. Aging Cell. 2023 Feb;22(2):e13770. doi: 10.1111/acel.13770. Epub 2023 Jan 15. PMID: 36642986; PMCID: PMC9924952.

250. Sha L, Zhang H, Zhang X. Thymosin α1 combined with XELOX improves immune function and reduces serum tumor markers in colorectal cancer patients after radical surgery. Open Life Sci. 2024 Apr 13;19(1):20220793. doi: 10.1515/biol-2022-0793. PMID: 38623586; PMCID: PMC11017181.

251. Garaci, Enrico & Pica, Francesca & Rasi, Guido & Favalli, Cartesio. (2001). Thymosin alpha 1 in the treatment of cancer: From basic research to clinical application. International journal of immunopharmacology. 22. 1067-76. 10.1016/S0192-0561(00)00075-8.

252. Huang C, Fei L, Xu W, Li W, Xie X, Li Q, Chen L. Efficacy Evaluation of Thymosin Alpha 1 in Non-severe Patients With COVID-19: A Retrospective Cohort Study Based on Propensity Score Matching. Front Med (Lausanne). 2021 Apr 23; 8:664776. doi: 10.3389/fmed.2021.664776. PMID: 33968969; PMCID: PMC8102900.

253. Sharma H, Moroni L. Recent Advancements in Regenerative Approaches for Thymus Rejuvenation. Adv Sci (Weinh). 2021 May 7;8(14):2100543. doi: 10.1002/advs.202100543. PMID: 34306981; PMCID: PMC8292900.

254. Ramos-Zaldívar H, Reyes-Perdomo K, Espinoza-Moreno N, Dox-Cruz E, Urbina T, Caballero A, Dominguez E, Calix S, Monterroso-Reyes J, Vásquez E, Ortiz T, Rodríguez-Machado H, Solis M, Silva I, Galeano M, Alvarado A, Medina A,

Guerrero-Díaz L, Jiménez-Faraj J, Santos C, Arita W, Montufar D, Sabillón J, Sorto M, Navarro X, Palomo-Bermúdez V, Andino H, Guzman S, Reyes M, Pazf E, Enamorado J, Sagastume Y, Rivera A, Sarmiento C, Pineda X, Puerto V, Landaverde J, Reyes S, Perdomo I, Rivera J, Girón W, Sabillón K, Leiva P, Toro K, Montes-Gambarelli J, Flores C, Salas-Huenuleo E, Andia M. SAFETY AND EFFICACY OF THYMIC PEPTIDES IN THE TREATMENT OF HOSPITALIZED COVID-19 PATIENTS IN HONDURAS. Georgian Med News. 2022 Sep;(330):99-105. PMID: 36427851.

255. Schulof RS. Thymic peptide hormones: basic properties and clinical applications in cancer. Crit Rev Oncol Hematol. 1985;3(4):309-76. doi: 10.1016/s1040-8428(85)80035-4. PMID: 3902261.

256. Dinetz E., Lee E. Comprehensive Review of the Safety and Efficacy of Thymosin Alpha 1 in Human Clinical Trials. Altern There, 2024, 30(1), 6-12.

257. Dardenne M. Role of thymic peptides as transmitters between the neuroendocrine and immune systems. Ann Med. 1999 Oct;31 Suppl 2:34-9. PMID: 10574153.

258. 302.Wu J, Pei F, Zhou L, Li W, Sun R, Li Y, Wang Z, He Z, Zhang X, Jin X, Long Y, Cui W, Wang C, Chen E, Zeng J, Yan J, Lin Q, Zhou F, Huang L, Shang Y, Duan M, Zheng W, Zhu D, Kou Q, Zhang S, Liu Y, Yao C, Shang M, Peng S, Zhou Q, Cheng KK, Guan X; TESTS study collaborator group. The efficacy and safety of thymosin α1 for sepsis (TESTS): multicentre, double blinded, randomised, placebo controlled, phase 3 trial. BMJ. 2025 Jan 15;388:e082583. doi: 10.1136/bmj-2024-082583. Erratum in: BMJ. 2025 May 30;389:r1098. doi: 10.1136/bmj.r1098. PMID: 39814420; PMCID: PMC11780596.

Chapter 11

259. Pond, D., McBride, A. T., Davids, L. M., Reddy, B. D., & Limbert, G. (2018). Microstructurally-based constitutive modelling of the skin–Linking intrinsic ageing to microstructural parameters. Journal of Theoretical Biology, 444, 108-123.

260. El-Domyati M, El-Ammawi TS, Moawad O, El-Fakahany H, Medhat W, Mahoney MG, Uitto J. Efficacy of mesotherapy in facial rejuvenation: a histological and immunohistochemical evaluation. Int J Dermatol. 2012 Aug;51(8):913-9. doi: 10.1111/j.1365-4632.2011.05184. x. PMID: 22788806; PMCID: PMC3513770.

261. Alvin G.et al., Cell Therapy: The New Approach to Dermatology and Dermatologic Surgery. Clin Surg. 2021; 5(8): 1-14.

262. Raikou V, Varvaresou A, Panderi I, Papageorgiou E. The efficacy study of the combination of tripeptide-10-citrulline and acetyl hexapeptide-3. a prospective, randomized controlled study. J Cosmet Dermatol. 2017;16(2):271-278. doi: 10.1111/jocd.12314.

263. Lim SH, Sun Y, Thiruvallur madanagopal T, Rosa V, Kang L. Enhanced skin permeation of anti-wrinkle peptides via molecular modification. Sci Rep. 2018;8(1):1596. doi:10.1038/s41598-017-18454-z.

264. An JH, Lee HJ, Yoon MS, Kim DH. Anti-wrinkle efficacy of cross-linked hyaluronic acid-based microneedle patch with Acetyl hexapeptide-8 and epidermal growth factor on Korean skin. Ann Dermatol. 2019;31(3):263-271. doi: 10.5021/ad.2019.31.3.263.

265. Blanes-Mira C, Clemente J, Jodas G, et al. A synthetic hexapeptide (Argireline) with antiwrinkle activity. Int J Cosmet Sci. 2002;24(5):303-310. doi: 10.1046/j.1467-2494.2002.00153. x.

266. Yaar M, Gilchrest BA. Photoaging: mechanism, prevention and therapy. Br J Dermatol. 2007; 157:874–887.

267. Farage MA, Miller KW, Berardesca E, et al. Clinical implications of aging skin: cutaneous disorders in the elderly. Am J Clin Dermatol. 2009; 10:73–86.

268. El-Domyati M, El-Ammawi TS, Medhat W, et al. Electro-optical synergy technique: a new and effective non-ablative approach to skin aging. J Clin Aesthet Dermatol. 2010; 3:22–30.

269. Alvin G.et al., Cell Therapy: The New Approach to Dermatology and Dermatologic Surgery. Clin Surg. 2021; 5(8): 1-14.

270. Klokol D. et al. Application of Cell Extracts from Skin, Placenta, Mesenchyme with Collagen and Elastin in Aesthetic Dermatology and Skin Revitalization: Evaluation of Outcomes in Cohort Study. American Journal of Advanced Drug Delivery. 2016, 4(5), 69-77.

271. Makrantonaki E, Zouboulis CC. Molecular mechanisms of skin aging: state of the art. Ann N Y Acad Sci. 2007;1119:40–50.

272. Chernykh V, Nallenthiran L, Yemeliyanova M. Efficacy and safety of a cosmeceutical regimen based on a combination of low molecular weight hyaluronic acid, placental peptides and extract of Malus domestica in improving signs of periorbital skin aging. J Stem Cell Res Ther. 2020;6(3):85–92. DOI: 10.15406/jsrt.2020.06.00147.

273. Edgar S, Hopley B, Genovese L, Sibilla S, Laight D, Shute J. Effects of collagen-derived bioactive peptides and natural antioxidant compounds on proliferation and matrix protein synthesis by cultured normal human dermal fibroblasts. Sci Rep. 2018 Jul 11;8(1):10474. doi: 10.1038/s41598-018-28492-w. PMID: 29992983; PMCID: PMC6041269.

274. Michalek IM, Lelen-Kaminska K, Caetano Dos Santos FL. Peptides stimulating synthesis of extracellular matrix used in anti-ageing cosmetics: Are they clinically tested? A systematic review of the literature. Australas J Dermatol. 2019 Nov;60(4):e267-e271. doi: 10.1111/ajd.13036. Epub 2019 Apr 2. PMID: 30941744.

275. Alvin G, Chernykh V, Chan M (2020) Peptides: A Novel Approach to Enhance Eyelash and Eyebrow Growth. J Dermatolog Clin Res 8(2): 1137.

276. Alvin, Glen. (2021). Peptides: A Comparison between Nanoparticles and Mito Organelles to Enhance Eyelash and Eyebrow Growth. Journal of Stem Cells. 16. 1.

277. Fernandez-Gonzalez P, Truchuelo-Díez MT, Gómez-Sánchez MJ. Open clinical trial evaluating the efficacy of a novel eyelash growth enhancer with peptides and glycosaminoglycans. J Cosmet Dermatol. 2024 Jun;23(6):2170-2180. doi: 10.1111/jocd.16265. Epub 2024 Apr 4. PMID: 38572527.

Chapter 12

278. Lindholm J. Growth hormone: historical notes. Pituitary. 2006;9(1):5-10. doi: 10.1007/s11102-006-7557-4. PMID: 16703403.

279. Dehkhoda F, Lee CMM, Medina J, Brooks AJ. The Growth Hormone Receptor: Mechanism of Receptor Activation, Cell Signaling, and Physiological Aspects. Front Endocrinol (Lausanne). 2018 Feb 13; 9:35. doi: 10.3389/fendo.2018.00035. PMID: 29487568; PMCID: PMC5816795.

280. Laron Z. The Era of Cadaveric Pituitary Extracted Human Growth Hormone (1958-1985): Biological and Clinical Aspects. Pediatr Endocrinol Rev. 2018 Sep;16(Suppl 1):11-16. doi: 10.17458/per.vol16.2018.la.hghcadavericpituitary. PMID: 30378778.

281. Blizzard RM. History of growth hormone therapy. Indian J Pediatr. 2012 Jan;79(1):87-91. doi: 10.1007/s12098-011-0609-4. Epub 2011 Nov 12. PMID: 22081428.

282. Jørgensen JT, Chirstensen T, Jørgensen M, Jakobsen G. Development, production and pharmacodynamics of human growth hormone. Indian J Pediatr. 1991 Sep-Oct;58 Suppl 1:23-32. doi: 10.1007/BF02750980. PMID: 1824371.

283. Alan D. Rogol, Edward O. Reiter; Growth and Growth Hormone through the Ages: Art and Science. Horm Res Paediatr 29 November 2022; 95 (6): 515–528.

284. Cronin MJ. Pioneering recombinant growth hormone manufacturing: pounds produced per mile of height. J Pediatr. 1997 Jul;131(1 Pt 2): S5-7. doi: 10.1016/s0022-3476(97)70002-7. PMID: 9255218.

285. Perrini, S., Laviola, L., Carreira, M. C., Cignarelli, A., Natalicchio, A., & Giorgino, F. (2010). The GH/IGF1 axis and signaling pathways in the muscle and bone: mechanisms underlying age-related skeletal muscle wasting and osteoporosis. Journal of Endocrinology, 205(3), 201-210. Retrieved Oct 13, 2025, from https://doi.org/10.1677/JOE-09-0431.

286. Carter-Su C, King AP, Argetsinger LS, Smit LS, Vanderkuur J, Campbell GS. Signalling pathway of GH. Endocr J. 1996 Oct;43 Suppl: S65-70. doi: 10.1507/endocrj.43.suppl_s65. PMID: 9076344.

287. Mahendra D. Mavalli, Marcas M. Bamman, Thomas L. Clemens. Distinct growth hormone receptor signaling modes regulate skeletal muscle development and insulin sensitivity in mice. J Clin Invest. 2010;120(11):4007-4020.

288. Nakatani S (2024) Potential of Human Growth Hormone: Benefits, Risks, and Therapeutic Applications. Advan Genet Eng. 13:253.

289. Marker PC, Unterberger CJ, Swanson SM. GH-dependent growth of experimentally induced carcinomas in vivo. Endocr Relat Cancer. 2023 Mar 29;30(5):e220403. doi: 10.1530/ERC-22-0403. PMID: 36826838; PMCID: PMC10140676.

290. Frederick Berro Rivera, Marianne Katharina Taliño, Marie Francesca Ansay, Gerard Francis Mangubat, Mer Lorraine Mahilum, Rajiv Hans Menghrajani, Siena Placino, Sung Whoy Cha, John Paul Aparece, Marc Gregory Yu, Michael Lawrenz Co, Edgar Lerma, Krishnaswami Vijayaraghavan, Peter A. McCullough. Cardiovascular Effects of Excess Growth Hormone: How Real is the Threat?. Rev. Cardiovasc. Med. 2023, 24(4), 95.

291. Götherström G, Svensson J, Koranyi J, Alpsten M, Bosaeus I, Bengtsson B, Johannsson G. A prospective study of 5 years of GH replacement therapy in GH-deficient adults: sustained effects on body composition, bone mass, and metabolic indices. J Clin Endocrinol Metab. 2001 Oct;86(10):4657-65. doi: 10.1210/jcem.86.10.7887. PMID: 11600522.

292. Chihara K, Fujieda K, Shimatsu A, Miki T, Tachibana K. Dose-dependent changes in body composition during growth hormone (GH) treatment in Japanese patients with adult GH deficiency: a randomized, placebo-controlled trial. Growth Horm IGF Res. 2010 Jun;20(3):205-11. doi: 10.1016/j.ghir.2010.01.003. Epub 2010 Feb 21. PMID: 20176498.

293. Liu H, Bravata DM, Olkin I, Nayak S, Roberts B, Garber AM, Hoffman AR. Systematic review: the safety and efficacy of growth hormone in the healthy elderly. Ann Intern Med. 2007 Jan 16;146(2):104-15. doi: 10.7326/0003-4819-146-2-200701160-00005. PMID: 17227934.

294. Liu H, Bravata DM, Olkin I, et al. Systematic review: the safety and efficacy of growth hormone in the healthy elderly. 2007. In: Database of Abstracts of Reviews of Effects (DARE): Quality-assessed Reviews [Internet]. York (UK): Centre for Reviews and Dissemination (UK); 1995-. Available from: https://www.ncbi.nlm.nih.gov/books/NBK74769/?utm_source=chatgpt.com].

295. Giannoulis MG, Sonksen PH, Umpleby M, Breen L, Pentecost C, Whyte M, McMillan CV, Bradley C, Martin FC. The effects of growth hormone and/or testosterone in healthy elderly men: a randomized controlled trial. J Clin Endocrinol Metab. 2006 Feb;91(2):477-84. doi: 10.1210/jc.2005-0957. Epub 2005 Dec 6. PMID: 16332938.

296. Chu LW, Lam KS, Tam SC, Hu WJ, Hui SL, Chiu A, Chiu KC, Ng P. A randomized controlled trial of low-dose recombinant human growth hormone in the treatment of malnourished elderly medical patients. J Clin Endocrinol Metab. 2001 May;86(5):1913-20. doi: 10.1210/jcem.86.5.7457. PMID: 11344184.

297. https://www.healio.com/news/endocrinology/20231227/onceweekly-human-gh-increases-total-body-lean-mass-for-adults-with-gh-deficiency?.

298. Hazem A, Elamin MB, Bancos I, Malaga G, Prutsky G, Domecq JP, Elraiyah TA, Abu Elnour NO, Prevost Y, Almandoz JP, Zeballos-Palacios C, Velasquez ER, Erwin PJ, Natt N, Montori VM, Murad MH. Body composition and quality of life in adults treated with GH therapy: a systematic review and meta-analysis. Eur J Endocrinol. 2012 Jan;166(1):13-20. doi: 10.1530/EJE-11-0558. Epub 2011 Aug 24. PMID: 21865409.

299. Juul Kildemoes R, Højby Rasmussen M, Agersø H, Overgaard RV. Optimal Monitoring of Weekly IGF-I Levels During Growth Hormone Therapy With Once-Weekly Somapacitan. J Clin Endocrinol Metab. 2021 Jan 23;106(2):567-576. doi: 10.1210/clinem/dgaa775. PMID: 33313798; PMCID: PMC7823237.

The Last Chapter

300. Chan MKS, Wong MBF, Chernykh V, Iemeliyanova M, Alvin G, and Klokol D. Emerging Anabolic and Regenerative Peptides in Athletic Body Re-composition and Bodybuilding: Mechanisms of Action, Dosing Strategies, and Evidence Review. J Stem Cell Res. 6(2):1-28.

301. Biolo G, Tipton KD, Klein S, Wolfe RR. An abundant supply of amino acids enhances the metabolic effect of exercise on muscle protein. Am J Physiol. 1997 Jul;273(1 Pt 1):E122-9. doi: 10.1152/ajpendo.1997.273.1.E122. PMID: 9252488.

302. Wolfe RR., The underappreciated role of muscle in health and disease. Am J Clin Nutr 2006; 84:475– 82.

303. Ivy JL, Katz AL, Cutler CL, Sherman WM, Coyle EF. Muscle glycogen synthesis after exercise: effect of time of carbohydrate ingestion. J Appl Physiol (1985). 1988 Apr;64(4):1480-5. doi: 10.1152/jappl.1988.64.4.1480. PMID: 3132449.

304. Clemmons DR. Metabolic actions of insulin-like growth factor-I in normal physiology and diabetes. Endocrinol Metab Clin North Am. 2012 Jun;41(2):425-43, vii-viii. doi: 10.1016/j.ecl.2012.04.017. PMID: 22682639; PMCID: PMC3374394.